TO PACE OR NOT TO PACE

New Developments in Biosciences: Their Implications for Laboratory Animal Science

Proceedings of the Third Symposium of
the Federation of European Laboratory Animal Science Associations,
held in Amsterdam, The Netherlands, 1–5 June 1987

edited by

Anton C. Beynen

Department of Laboratory Animal Science, Faculty of Veterinary Medicine, University of Utrecht, Utrecht, The Netherlands

and

Henk A. Solleveld

Preclinical Research and Development, Smith Kline & French Laboratories, Philadelphia, Pennsylvania, U.S.A.

1988

SPRINGER-SCIENCE+BUSINESS MEDIA, B.V.

Library of Congress Cataloging in Publication Data

Federation of European Laboratory Animal Science Associations.
Symposium (3rd : 1987 : Amsterdam, Netherlands)
New developments in biosciences : their implications for laboratory animal science : proceedings of the Third Symposium of the Federation of European Laboratory Animal Science Associations, held in Amsterdam, The Netherlands, 1-5 June 1987 / edited by Anton C. Beynen, Henk A. Solleveld.
p. cm.
ISBN 978-94-010-7973-0 ISBN 978-94-009-3281-4 (eBook)
DOI 10.1007/978-94-009-3281-4
1. Laboratory animals--Congresses. 2. Zoology, Experimental--Congresses. I. Beynen, Anton C., 1953- . II. Solleveld, H. A. III. Title.
QL55.F43 1987
591'.07'24--dc19 87-28193
CIP

Originally published by Martinus Nijhoff Publishers, Dordrecht in 1988
Softcover reprint of the hardcover 1st edition 1988

Preface

This volume includes chapters originally presented at the 3rd FELASA Symposium, held in Amsterdam, June 1-5, 1987. Special topics were "Immune Deficiency Syndromes in Man and Animals", "DNA Technology and Laboratory Animal Science", "Interactions of Behaviour, Housing and Welfare", and "Laboratory Animals as Models in Biomedical Research". In addition, there was a great number of presentations concerning other aspects of laboratory animal science.

We would like to thank the following persons for organizing the Symposium.
Mrs. M.A.G. Kuipers, M.Sc., President FELASA
Mrs. V. Baumans, D.V.M., Ph.D., Secretary FELASA
P. de Vrey, D.V.M., Treasurer
Mrs. I. Zaalmink, Organizing and Scientific Secretariat.

The editors would also like to express their gratitude to all the participants and authors for their contribution to this succesful symposium.

A.C. Beynen, Ph.D., Secretary Scientific Committee
H.A. Solleveld, Ph.D., Chairman Scientific Committee

<u>FELASA</u>

<u>Federation of European Laboratory Animal Science Associations</u>

Gesellschaft für Versuchstierkunde/Society for Laboratory Animal Science
Laboratory Animal Science Association
Nederlandse Vereniging voor Proefdierkunde
Scandinavian Federation for Laboratory Animal Science
Societé Française d'Expérimentation Animale

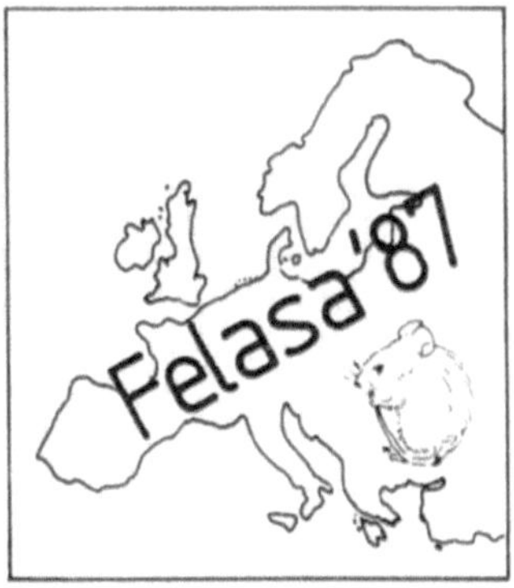

2ND EUROPEAN PACEMAKER COLLOQUIUM

Brussels – Belgium
April 21 and 22, 1977

TO PACE OR NOT TO PACE

CONTROVERSIAL SUBJECTS IN CARDIAC PACING

edited by

HILBERT J. TH. THALEN, M.D.
Department of Cardiology, University Hospital, Groningen, The Netherlands

and

J. WARREN HARTHORNE, M.D.
Cardiac Unit, Massachusetts General Hospital, Boston, U.S.A.

1978
MARTINUS NIJHOFF MEDICAL DIVISION
THE HAGUE/BOSTON/LONDON

ISBN-13: 978-94-009-9725-7 e-ISBN-13: 978-94-009-9723-3
DOI: 10.1007/978-94-009-9723-3

Printed in The Netherlands

This book is dedicated to

PAUL M. ZOLL,

who initiated the modern era of cardiac stimulation with his publication "Resuscitation of the heart in ventricular standstill by external electric stimulation" in the New England Journal of Medicine in 1952 and who continuously has played an active role in cardiac stimulation as he demonstrated with his participation in the final Round Table of this Colloquium – exactly 25 years after his first publication.

PREFACE

The increasing number of pacemaker patients correlates with the number of pacemaker meetings that attract physicians and medical engineers entering this expanding branch of medicine. The Pacemaker Colloquium organised in Brussels April 21st and 22nd 1977 was such a meeting. It was different from previous meetings as it had no surveys or summaries on patient series but instead it focused on controversial subjects that have emerged from pacing in the past and on new developments for the future.

Besides controversial papers on indications for temporary and long-term pacing, new technical developments were presented in Brussels, where for the first time the important lithium battery manufacturers demonstrated their data. The surveys on electrodes, especially the fixation mechanisms and the atrial electrodes, initiated an animated discussion. This all converged in a Round Table on the choice of the electrode-pacemaker combination. Pacemaker electrocardiography and the application of cardiac stimulation in various types of tachyarrhythmias formed two clinically oriented sessions.

After a survey of the various follow-up systems a series of presentations deals for the first time with the possibilities and difficulties of the application of computers in cardiac pacing. A Round Table on the organisation of the Pacemaker clinic closed this friendly and animated meeting.

It is our sincere hope that the publication of the presented papers and discussions in these Proceedings will help all those active in cardiac pacing to answer some of their problems and to improve the treatment of pacemaker patients.

HILBERT J. TH. THALEN

CONTENTS

SECTION II. TO PACE OR NOT TO PACE

SECTION III. ENERGY SOURCES AND ELECTRONIC CIRCUIT

SECTION IV. STIMULATION ELECTRODES

A. Atrial Electrodes

SECTION V. THE CHOICE OF THE PACEMAKER-ELECTRODE COMBINATION

ROUND TABLE

SECTION VI. PACEMAKER IMPLANTATION: SURGEON AND/OR CARDIOLOGIST

SECTION VII. PACEMAKER ELECTROCARDIOGRAPHY

SECTION VIII. TACHYCARDIA AND PACING

SECTION IX. PACEMAKER FOLLOW-UP METHODS

SECTION X. COMPUTER APPLICATION IN PACEMAKER REGISTRATION AND FOLLOW-UP

ROUND TABLE DISCUSSION

OFFICIAL CLOSURE

CONTRIBUTORS

E. Aliot, Clinique des Maladies Cardiovasculaires, Université de Nancy, Nancy, France.
S.S. Amram M.D., Dept. of Cardiology, Santa Maria Hospital, Lisbon, Portugal.
M. Ataii M.D., Queen Pahlavi Foundation, Cardiac Medical Center, Tehran, Iran.
A. Aubert Ph.D., Div. of Cardiology, Dept. of Internal Medicine, Univ. Clinic St. Raphael, Leuven, Belgium.
I. Babotai, Surgical Clinic A, Kantonsspital, Zürich, Switzerland.
S.S. Barold M.D., Div. of Cardiology, Dept. of Medicine, Genesee Hospital and University of Rochester, School of Medicine and Dentistry, Rochester, U.S.A.
P. Barrett, Dept. of Cardiology, Westminster Hospital, London, England.
J. Beyer, Chir. Klinik, University of Munich, Munich, F.R. Germany.
A. Bianchini, Cardiac Stimulation Center, Clinique d'Alleray, Paris, France.
M. Bilitch M.D., Los Angeles County/USC Medical Center, Los Angeles, U.S.A.
A.J. Blankestijn Ing, Marketing Dept. Vitatron Medical, Dieren, The Netherlands.
D.L. Bowers BSEE., Bellevue, Washington, U.S.A.
J. Bredikis M.D., Dept. of Cardiovascular Surgery, Kaunas Medical Institute, Kaunas, Lithuania, U.S.S.R.
G. Breithardt M.D., I. Med. Klinik B, University of Düsseldorf, Düsseldorf, F.R. Germany.
M. Broussely, Battery Department, SAFT, Poitiers, France.
Buchowiecki, Dept. of Cardiology, Medical Academy of Warsaw, Warsaw, Poland.
B.J.L. Candelon Ph.D., C.H.U. Rangueil, Toulouse, France.
M. Castellanet M.D., Div. of Clinical Physiology and Sect. of Cardiology, Memorial Hospital Medical Center, Long Beach, California, U.S.A.
J.K. Cywinski Ph.D. Dept. of Medical Engineering, Massachusetts General Hospital, Harvard Medical School, Boston, U.S.A.
J.H. Demoulin M.D., Div. of Cardiology, Institute of Medicine, University of Liège, Liège, Belgium.
H. Denolin M.D., Dept. of Cardiology, St. Pietershospital, Brussels, Belgium.
R. Dian M.D., Cardiac Stimulation Center, Clinique d'Alleray, Paris, France.
B. Dodinot M.D., Clinique des Maladies Cardiovasculaires, Université de Nancy, Nancy, France.
A. Dumcius M.D., Dept. of Cardiovascular Surgery, Kaunas Medical Institute, Kaunas, Lithuania, U.S.S.R.
J.P. van Durme M.D., Dept. of Cardiology, University Hospital, Ghent, Belgium.
A.J. Dziatkowiak M.D., Institute of Cardiology, Medical Academy, Lodz, Poland.
H. Ector M.D., Div. of Cardiology, Dept. of Internal Medicine, Univ. Clinic St. Raphael, Leuven, Belgium.
O. Elert M.D., Dept. of Thoracic Surgery, University Hospital, Frankfurt on Main, F.R. Germany.
M.H. Ellestad M.D., Div. of Clinical Physiology and Sect. of Cardiology, Memorial Hospital Medical Center, Long Beach, California, U.S.A.
R. Emanuel, Dept. of Cardiology, Westminster Hospital, London, England.
M. Falkoff M.D.,Div. of Cardiology, Dept. of Medicine, Genesee Hospital and University of Rochester, School of Medicine and Dentistry, Rochester, U.S.A.
G.A. Feruglio M.D., Institute of Cardiology, Ospedale Generale, Udine, Italy.
G. Fontaine M.D., Service de Cardiologie, Groupe Hospitalier Pitié-Salpêtrière, Paris, France.
J. Fraile M.D., Dept. of Cardiovascular Surgery, Clinica de la Concepcion, Madrid, Spain.
R. Frank M.D., Service de Cardiologie, Groupe Hospitalier Pitié-Salpêtrière, Paris, France.
G.E. Freud M.D., Dept. of Cardiologie, University Hospital Wilhelmina Gasthuis, Amsterdam, The Netherlands.
S. Furman M.D., Dept. of Surgery, Cardiothoracic Division, Montefiore Hospital and Medical Center, Bronx, N.Y., U.S.A.

F. Gallais-Hamonno M.D., Service de Cardiologie, Groupe Hospitalier Pitié – Salpêtrière, Paris, France.
U. Gebhardt, Bio-Electronic Laboratory, Dept. of Internal Medicine I, R.W. Technical University, Aachen, F.R. Germany.
H. de Geest M.D., Div. of Cardiology, Dept. of Internal Medicine, Univ. Clinic St. Raphael, Leuven, Belgium.
R.G. Gold M.D., Shotley Bridge Hospital, Newcastle, England.
B.S. Goldman M.D., Div. of Cardiologic Surgery, Toronto General Hospital, University of Toronto, Toronto, Canada.
A.L. Graulle M.D., C.H.U. Rangueil, Toulouse, France.
W. Greatbatch FIEEC, Dept. of Physiology, Houghton College, Houghton, U.S.A.
G.D. Green B.Sc., Dept. of Clinical Physics and Bio-Engineering, West of Scotland Health Boards, Glasgow, Scotland.
P. Greenberg M.D., Div. of Clinical Physiology and Sect. of Cardiology, Memorial Hospital Medical Center, Long Beach, California, U.S.A.
Y. Grosgogeat M.D., Service de Cardiologie, Groupe Hospitalier Pitié – Salpêtrière, Paris, France.
R. Hardjowyono M.D., Dept. of Thoracic Surgery, University Hospital, Groningen, The Netherlands.
J.W. Harthorne M.D., Cardiac Unit, Massachusetts General Hospital Harvard Medical School, Boston, U.S.A.
R.A. Heinle M.D., Div. of Cardiology, Dept. of Medicine, Genesee Hospital and University of Rochester, School of Medicine and Dentistry, Rochester, U.S.A.
P.A. van der Heyden Ph.D., Compliance Dept., Vitatron Medical, Dieren, The Netherlands.
Ch. Himmler M.D., Dept. of Cardiology, I. Med. Klinik, Technical University of Munich, Munich, F.R. Germany.
J.N. Homan van der Heide M.D., Dept. of Thoracic Surgery, University Hospital, Groningen, The Netherlands.
W.B. Hood M.D., Cardiol. Div., Thorndike Mem. Lab. and Dept. of Medicine, Boston City Hospital, Boston University, Boston, U.S.A.
D. Hunt M.D., Dept. of Cardiology, Royal Melbourne Hospital, University of Melbourne, Melbourne, Australia.
W. Irnich Ph.D., Bio-Electronic Laboratory, Dept. of Internal Medicine I, R.W. Technical University, Aachen, F.R. Germany.
G. Joskowicz, Dept. of Cardiology, University of Vienna, Vienna, Austria.
M. Kleinert M.D., First Medical Department, General Hospital Hamburg, Hamburg, F.R. Germany.
J.W. Kozlowski M.D., Institute of Cardiology, Medical Academy, Lodz, Poland.
T. Kraska M.D., Dept. of Cardiology, Medical Academy of Warsaw, Warsaw, Poland.
J. Kreuzer, Dept. of Thoracic Surgery, Univ. Hospital, Frankfurt on Main, F.R. Germany.
L. Kubler, Clinique des Maladies Cardiovasculaires, Université de Nancy, Nancy, France.
H. Kuhn M.D., I. Med. Klinik B, Univ. of Düsseldorf, Düsseldorf, F.R. Germany.
H. Kulbertus M.D., Div. of Cardiology, Institute of Medicine, Univ. of Liège, Liège, Belgium.
A. Laczkovics, Dept. of Cardiology, University of Vienna, Vienna, Austria.
M.S. Lampadius Dipl. Ing., Munich Institute of Technology, Munich, F.R. Germany.
S. Larsson M.D., Dept. of Thoracic Surgery, Sahlgrenska Hospital, University of Göteborg, Göteborg, Sweden.
M.F. Lefèbvre M.D., Centre Hospitalier Régional, Lille, France.
G. Lehmann, Battery Department, Saft, Poitiers, France.
P. Lenfant, Battery Department, Saft, Poitiers, France.
M. Levander-Lindgren M.D. Pacemaker unit, Karolinska Sjukhuset, Stockholm, Sweden.
L.P. Lolkema Ing., Compliance Dept., Vitatron Medical, Dieren, The Netherlands.
J.E. Madias M.D., Cardiol. Div. Thorndike Mem. Lab. and Dept. of Medicine, Boston City Hospital, Boston University, Boston, U.S.A.
J. Maragno M.D., Div. of Cardiology, Dept. of Clinical Medicine, Medical School and Padova General Hospital, Padova, Italy.
C. Meere M.D., Montreal Heart Institute, Montreal, Canada.
J. Meibom M.D., Dept. of Cardiology, Rigshospital, Copenhagen, Denmark.
W.E. Meier M.D., Surgical Clinic A, Kantonsspital, Zürich, Switzerland.
G. Myers Ph.D., Dept. of Surgery, Beth Israel Medical Center, Newark, U.S.A.
W. du Mesnil de Rochemont M.D., Dept. of Radiology, Univ. of Cologne, Cologne, F.R. Germany.

J. Messenger M.D., Div. of Clinical Physiology and Sect. of Cardiology, Memorial Hospital Medical Center, Long Beach, California, U.S.A.
U. Mödder M.D., Dept. of Radiology, Univ. of Cologne, Cologne, F.R. Germany.
H.G. Mond M.D., Dept. of Cardiology, Royal Melbourne Hospital, University of Melbourne, Melbourne, Australia.
T. Moreno M.D., Cardiol. Div. Thorndike Mem. Lab. and Dept. of Medicine, Boston City Hospital, Boston University, Boston, U.S.A.
K. Muckus M.D., Dept. of Cardiovascular Surgery, Kaunas Med. Institute, Kaunas, Lithuania, U.S.S.R.
J.R. Muir M.D., Dept. of Cardiology, The Welsh Nat. School of Medicine, University of Wales, Cardiff, England.
M. Murtra M.D., Dept. of Surgery, Centro Quirurgico San Jorge, University of Barcelona, Barcelona, Spain.
O.S. Narula M.D., Div. of Cardiology, The Chicago Medical School, Univ. of Health Sciences, North Chicago, Illinois, U.S.A.
A. Nava M.D., Div. of Cardiology, Dept. of Clinical Medicine, Medical School and Padova General Hospital, Padova, Italy.
J. Nieveen M.D., Dept. of Cardiology, University Hospital, Groningen, The Netherlands.
L.S. Ong M.D., Div. of Cardiology, Dept. of Medicine, Genesee Hospital and University of Rochester, School of Medicine and Dentistry, Rochester, U.S.A.
Opolski M.D., Dept. of Cardiology, Medical Academy of Warsaw, Warsaw, Poland.
V. Parsonnet M.D., Dept. of Surgery, Beth Israel Medical Center, Newark, U.S.A.
J.C. Petitot M.D., Service de Cardiologie, Groupe Hospitalier Pitié – Salpêtrière, Paris, France.
M. Pieniak M.D., Dept. of Cardiology, Medical Academy of Warsaw, Warsaw, Poland.
I.J. Pinto M.D., Dept. of Cardiology, Univ. of Calcutta, Calcutta, India.
G. Pioger M.D., Cardiac Stimulation Center, Clinique d'Alleray, Paris, France.
F.A. Pirzada M.D., Cardiol. Div., Thorndike Med. Lab. and Dept. of Medicine, Boston City Hospital, Boston University, Boston, U.S.A.
H. Pour Kalbassi M.D., Queen Pahlavi Foundation, Cardiac Medical Center, Tehran, Iran.
H.W. Präuer M.D., Dept, of Cardiology, I. Med. Klinik, Technical University, Munich, F.R. Germany.
T.A. Preston M.D., FACC., Div. of Cardiology, U.S. Public Health Service Hospital and Pacemaker Center, University of Washington, Seattle, Washington, U.S.A.
P.F. Puel M.D., C.H.U. Rangueil, Toulouse, France.
G. Rabago M.D., Dept. of Cardiovascular Surgery, Clinica de la Concepcion, Madrid, Spain.
Radecki M.D., Dept. of Cardiology, Medical Academy of Warsaw, Warsaw, Poland.
A.C.M. Renirie Inc., Research and Development Dept. Vitatron Medical, Dieren, The Netherlands.
A.F. Rickards M.D., The National Heart Hospital, London, England.
A. Rio, Clinique des Maladies Cardiovasculaires, Université de Nancy, Nancy, France.
F.A. Rodrigo Ph.D., Dept. of Cardiology, Univ. Hospital, Leyden, The Netherlands.
P. Satter M.D., Dept. of Thoracic Surgery, Univ. Hospital, Frankfurt on Main, F.R. Germany.
A. Schaudig M.D., Chir. Klinik, University of Munich, Munich, F.R. Germany.
A.A. Schneider Ph.D., Catalyst Research Corporation, Baltimore, U.S.A.
K.F. Seidl, M.D., Dept. of Cardiology, I. Med. Klinik, Technical University, Munich, F.R. Germany.
L. Seipel M.D., I. Med. Klinik B, Univ. of Düsseldorf, Düsseldorf, F.R. Germany.
A. Senning M.D., Surgical Clinic A, Kantonsspital, Zürich, Switzerland.
A.H. Sheikh-Zadeh M.D., Queen Pahlavi Foundation, Cardiac Medical Center, Tehran, Iran.
J.G. Sloman M.D., Dept. of Cardiology, Royal Melbourne Hospital, University of Melbourne, Melbourne, Australia.
G. Soots, Centre Hospitalier Régional, Lille, France.
R.A.J. Spurrell M.D., Dept. of Cardiology, St. Bartholomew's Hospital, London, England.
K. Steinbach M.D., Dept. of Cardiology, University of Vienna, Vienna, Austria.
P. Stirbys M.D., Dept. of Cardiovascular Surgery, Kaunas Medical Institute, Kaunas, Lithuania, U.S.S.R.
M.J. Stopczyk M.D., Institute of Biocybern. and Biomedical Engineering, Polish Academy of Science, Warsaw, Poland.
R. Sutton M.D., Dept. of Cardiology, Westminster Hospital, London, England.
M.J. Tabaee-Zadeh M.D., Queen Pahlavi Foundation, Cardiac Medical Center, Tehran, Iran.
F. Tepper M.S., Catalyst Research Corporation, Baltimore, U.S.A.
H.J.Th. Thalen M.D., Dept. of Cardiology, University Hospital, Groningen, The Netherlands.

G. Thompson B.Sc., Computer Appl. Unit, Greater Glasgow Health Board, Glasgow, Scotland.
R. Thurmayer, Chir. Klinik, University of Munich, Munich, F.R. Germany.
N.G. de Vega M.D., Dept. of Cardiovascular Surgery, Clinica de la Concepcion, Madrid, Spain.
K. Venkataraman M.D., Cardiol. Div., Thorndike Mem. Lab. and Dept. of Medicine, Boston City Hospital, Boston University, Boston, U.S.A.
J.K. Vohra M.D., Dept. of Cardiology, Royal Melbourne Hospital, University of Melbourne, Melbourne, Australia.
S. dalla Volta M.D., Div. of Cardiology, Dept. of Clinical Medicine, University of Padova, Medical School and Padova General Hospital, Padova, Italy.
H.J.J. Wellens M.D., Dept. of Cardiology, University of Limburg, Annadal Hospital, Maastricht, The Netherlands.
C.J. Westerholm M.D., Thoracic Dept. University Hospital, Uppsala, Sweden.
A. Wirtzfeld M.D., Dept. of Cardiology, I. Med. Klinik, Technical University of Munich, Munich, F.R. Germany.
M. Zimmermann, Chir. Klinik, University of Munich, Munich, F.R. Germany.
R.J. Zochowski M.D., Ph.D., Dept. of Cardiology, Medical Academy of Warsaw, Warsaw, Poland.
P.M. Zoll M.D., Dept. of Medicine, Harvard Medical School and Beth Israel Hospital, Boston, U.S.A.

OPENING

INTRODUCTION

A.J. Blankestijn, Ing.

The introduction of advanced electronic devices and lithium power sources has continued to increase both the reliability and lifetime of pacemaker systems. This has led not only to their greater acceptance by the medical profession but also to their use for a wider variety of disorders, and as a result of this more and more physicians and medical technicians are entering this expanding branch of medicine.

In the light of these circumstances Vitatron Medical decided to hold a Second European Pacemaker Colloquium in Brussels, following the first one in Arnhem in 1975. In this way we hoped to be able to continue with our aim of providing the medical practitioner, the research worker and the pacemaker manufacturer with an opportunity of exchanging ideas and experiences.

We were very pleased to be able to welcome as chairman Professor Homan van der Heide of The University of Groningen, and as opening speaker Professor Denolin, President of the European Society of Cardiology and Professor of Cardiology in our host city Brussels.

From the list of prominent speakers and participants we knew that all the ingredients were available for a successful meeting. It was an honour for Vitatron Medical to act as host to all those who helped to make this Second Pacemaker Colloquium a great success.

OPENING ADDRESSS

PROF. DR. J.N. HOMAN VAN DER HEIDE
Chairman of the Colloquium

As a pacemaker manufacturer, Vitatron Medical has induced by now millions of carefully-regulated, life-saving impulses in many sick hearts outside their plant territory in Dieren.

When Van den Berg, Nieveen and I developed the first pacemaker in Groningen in the '60s, we never dreamed of the developments Vitatron has made possible today, after they took over from us. We continued, however, our medical interest in the development of better and safer ways of electro-stimulation of the heart.

Because of the close and happy cooperation in the past years – and I sincerely hope in the years to come – it is a great pleasure for me to be invited to take the chair in the second Colloquium on Cardiac Pacing organized by Vitatron.

Now that for nearly 50% of our patients, by the use of a lithium energy source, low-output electrodes, and sophisticated integrated circuits, the implantation of a lifetime pacemaker has become daily practice, we have reached one of our goals set in earlier years. Only one year after the pacemaker congress held in Tokyo in '76, we have assembled again to discuss new developments: a vital sign of life and a tribute to the inventiveness and cooperation of the electronic industry and the medical profession. General Eisenhower, once President of the United States, has said it more clearly: "Guns and dollars are no substitute for brains and willpower."

Many problems remain to be solved; i.e. the development of a dependable, easy-to-implant atrial electrode and the development introduction and acceptance by all manufacturers of a standardized lead-to stimulator connector. The organization of a standardized follow-up system is slowly progressing, but a simple, effective computer system is still lacking. The ultimate goal of health care is that every patient who needs a pacemaker can get one implanted. To achieve this, we have to bring the pacemaker to the patient, and not the patient to the pacemaker or a large, complicated medical center. For this, we do not need to choose between simple or complicated pacemakers, but we must depend on a reliable stimulator, easy to implant and interchangeable without the need to replace the myocardial electrode.

The development of pacemaker stimulation started in large medical centers. Some years later, we saw a healthy shift of pacemaker implantations done in smaller local hospitals. Today, as the pacemakers become more complicated and the indications for pacemaker implantation multiply, we see a large number of patients returning to the larger medical centers. I sincerely hope this picture will be reversed in the near future and it must change, otherwise we will never reach our ultimate goal.

I hope the colloquium will contribute to this purpose.

OFFICIAL OPENING

PROF. DR. H. DENOLIN
President of the European Society of Cardiology

It is a great pleasure for the President of the European Society of Cardiology to welcome to Brussels the participants of this Colloquium on Pacemakers and to wish them a fruitful work session. The increasing number of patients with pacemakers indicates the importance of the problem and the necessity of constantly renewed discussion on this important aspect of therapy. Techniques of resuscitation with electrical stimulation have been mainly developed since Zoll's publication in 1952. However, other works had already prepared the ground, among these, the work of our compatriot, Wegria from Liège, in collaboration with Wiggers in 1940 comes to mind. Since then, cardiologists, surgeons and engineers have contributed greatly to the development of cardiac pacing, both in determining the indications and refining techniques. It was Stokes and Adams in Dublin who, during the first part of the 19th century, reported the primary cardiac cause of severe bradycardia and its complications. The electro-physiological work of Gaskell followed by the observations of His in 1893 permitted the identification of the mechanism of bradycardia as an atricular-ventricular dissociation.

However since that time, the indications for cardiac pacing have become numerous and at the same time, anatomo-pathological aspects have been developed parallel to the concurrent considerable technical evolution. You have many things to discuss during these days concerning the fields of cardiology, technology and perhaps also the socio-economic points of view. I wish you therefore great success in your discussions and I declare open this Second Colloquium on Pacemakers.

Section I

CONDUCTION SYSTEM

INTRODUCTION

SALOMÃO SEQUERRA AMRAM

The fact that the Organizing Committee of this Second European Colloquium on Pacemakers has planned that its first Session should deal with Conduction, as studied by electrophysiologic technics, reveals the present state of pacing as a science. Also the circumstance that, in the scope of the future International Society of Pacing and of our Journal PACE, the diagnostic and therapeutic stimulation of the cardiovascular system, pacemaker technology and also cardiac electrophysiology are included, is symptomatic of the present trends in the field.

At our Hospital in Lisbon we have a combined Medical-Surgical Unit for Cardiac Pacing and Electrophysiology, and the recordings of endocardial potentials of the specialized conduction system and other electrophysiologic studies, temporary pacemaker insertion and permanent endocardial implantation are done in the same Laboratory.

We have the privilege to have as participants at this Session world-known authorities responsible for many of the achievements in the field of cardiac electrophysiology. It is therefore understandable that my Introduction should be a brief one.

It is our belief that the issue on the program "to Pace or not to Pace" is in a not small measure influenced by the results of the electrophysiologic studies of the kind that will be presented by the participants. The recording of His bundle potentials has diagnostic value and prognostic significance and may therefore be important when one is faced with the issue of prophylactic pacing therapy, and also in preventing unnecessary pacemaker implantation.

At this time I will only mention some of the data related to cardiac conduction that have proved to be of prognostic value and therapeutic relevance to the indication and mode of pacing.

Insofar as the sino-atrial node is concerned it is conceptually important to consider it always in relation with the remaining specialized conduction system of the heart. It is accepted that its dysfunction can lead to electrophysiologic disturbances in a previously normal atrio-ventricular conduction and to changes in the morphology of the QRS complexes. It is also known that a significant number of patients with sino-atrial disease, have pathologic lesions of the intraventricular conduction. We can, this way, look at the specialized electrical networks of the heart as being a single, overall and probably highly synchronized conduction system. The methodologic protocol for the diagnosis of sino-atrial node dysfunction, including the conduction disturbances into and out of this important structure, and the mechanism of reentry in sinus node reciprocating tachycardia will be discussed.

Regarding atrio-ventricular conduction, the detection by electrophysiologic studies, of incomplete bilateral bundle branch block, in cases where the conventional electrocardiogram shows only a pattern of right or left monofascicular block or a bifascicular block is a matter of great interest (and debate). What is the prognostic meaning of the finding, in some of these cases, of a prolonged H-V conduction interval, attesting to a more generalized involvement of the specialized intraventricular conduction system? Drs. Narula, Seipel and Kulbertus will give us the results of their long-term follow-up studies in cases of right bundle branch block with and without axis deviation of the QRS on the frontal plane and also in cases of left bundle branch block, and their bearance to the subject of prophylactic pacing.

Of great interest in this regard, is the role of His bundle recordings in recent myocardial infarction complicated by incomplete bilateral bundle branch block, and its value in the immediate and long-term prognosis and in the indication for a permanent pacemaker implant.

The study in the electrophysiology laboratory of antegrade and retrograde ventriculo-atrial conduction, the demonstration of concealed conduction, and the analysis of reentry through normal and accessory conduction pathways has shown its clinical relevance, and may be essential for the rational choice of stimulation mode, in cases of sick sinus syndrome and paroxysmal tachycardias.

The results of studies on the body surface recording of His-Purkinje activity, in man, by the use of a signal averaging technic, a complex method, but simple for the patient will be presented.

As our knowledge of the basic mechanisms of cardiac conduction and arrhythmias derived from electrophysiologic studies is expanded, the field of pacing as a therapeutic tool will find an even more solid implantation in the clinical practice of Cardiology.

THE NORMAL ANATOMY OF THE SINUS NODE AND ITS PATHOLOGY

J.CL. DEMOULIN AND H.E. KULBERTUS

Normal anatomy of the sinus node

The heartbeat normally originates from the sinus node. This structure is oval-shaped, measures approximately 15 × 5 × 1.5 mm, and lies at the junction between the superior vena cava and the lateral border of the right atrium. The sinus node is located under the epicardium and is composed of small (5 × 10 u) pale, poorly striated cells with large, well stained nuclei. These cells are embedded in a framework consisting of collagenous elastic and reticular fibrils (1, 2, 3, 4, 5, 6, 7, 8, 9, 10, 11). The specific elements of the sinus node of dog and man have been described by James et al. (12) at the electronic microscope; they have been designated "P cells" and hypothesized to possess the pacemaker function. The relative content in connective tissue progressively increases with age until the age of 50 to 60 when collagenous fibers and nodal cells are present in approximately equal amounts.

The richness of the sinus node in nervous structures has been unanimously acknowledged (6, 8). It is so striking that the node has frequently been considered as a neuromyocardial entity rather than a specific myocardial one (8). Several studies indeed confirmed that the nodal area is high in catecholamine content and has strong anticholinesterase reactions (7, 13, 14). Large and numerous nerves are seen to reach the external surface of the node whereas isolated or grouped ganglion cells can be found within the nodal boundaries. This richness in nervous structures is undoubtedly of extreme importance for the physiological functioning and adaptation of the nodal pacemaker.

The sinus node is centered by a large artery which runs parallel to its major axis. This artery frequently originates from the right main coronary vessel (65% of cases), but sometimes arises from the left circumflex artery (35%). Besides this major artery, the node is surrounded by a circle of smaller vessels fed by branches of the left and right coronary trees. They show multiple anastomoses which may be intracoronary, intercoronary, or even extracoronary, for example with bronchial connections (15, 16).

Several investigators have described preferential pathways of conduction connections, within the atrium, the sino-atrial to the atrio-ventricular node. Like many others (11, 13), we have always been unable to demonstrate, on a morphological basis, the presence of specialized atrial internodal pathways in the human heart. It is true, however, that areas of nodo-atrial continuity are consistently seen along the margins of the compact sinus node (11). Such areas of blending of nodal and atrial cells are notably found in the regions presumed to be the site of origin of the bundles described by Bachmann (anterior aspect of the head of the node); Thorell (tail of the node) and Wenckebach (endocardial margin of the body of the node).

Methods of investigation

The sino-atrial region can be obtained for histological examination by using the following method. The heart being removed, a first cut is made from the orifice of the inferior vena cava to the upper part of the right atrial appendage. The second cut passes posterior to the right atrial appendage and is directed towards the orifice of the superior vena cava. The third cut goes from the superior to the inferior vena cava and thus separates a block of atrial myocardium which is fixed and embedded in paraffin. 10 u thick sections are prepared parallel to the long axis of the sinus node. Each fortieth section is stained by hematoxylin-eosin, Azan-Heidenhaim's solution or Masson's trichrome. Twenty to forty sections are also stained by orcein or Congo red with a view to study the pathological changes of elastic fibers and to search for amyloid deposits. Finally, Bodian's staining is used to analyze the nervous structures.

The ageing sinus node and the sinus node in cardiac patients

It has already been mentioned that the fibrous stroma of the sinus node progressively increases with age while the total number of specific cells diminishes (18, 19, 20). In diseased hearts, it is sometimes difficult to demonstrate more than a few nodal cells embedded in "a sea of collagen tissue" (11). In a recent report, we (21) described the histopathological findings in the sino-atrial region of 14 patients with overt cardiac disease but whose atria remained under sinus control. Nine patients had coronary artery disease, 4 showed complete heart block and 1 simultaneously had both. Among these patients, three were found to have a sinus node almost completely destroyed by fibrosis. In two of them, the nodo-atrial muscle cell junctions were largely replaced by intranodal and perinodal fibrosis. Diseased nerves or ganglia were observed in 4 hearts. Seven subjects had alterations of the atrial muscle wall. These data demonstrate that some patients whose sinus node is destroyed, who fail to show any clear zone of nodo-atrial continuity, who have pathological alterations of the perinodal nerves and ganglia and of the right atrial wall may still remain in normal sinus rhythm. These observations raise the question of how many nodal cells are needed to ensure a proper sinus impulse and of whether the impulse can be generated outside the geographic limits of the node, for example, towards the region of the crista terminalis.

The sinus node in atrial fibrillation

In his classical study, Hudson (22) reported that patients with sustained atrial fibrillation nearly always had lesions of the sinus node. He went as far as stating that he would be able, from the histological appearance of the sinus node, to guess whether atrial fibrillation had been present during life, or not.

We have confirmed this opinion in a limited number of cases (21) and showed that sustained atrial fibrillation was commonly associated with 1) fibrosis of the sinus node; 2) alterations of the perinodal nerves and ganglia; 3) and lesions of the atrial wall. It seems reasonable to believe that a poor sinus node function is a predisposing factor or, even, a prerequisite for the development of chronic atrial fibrillation.

The sinus node in the so-called sino-atrial disease

The sino-atrial rhythm disorders are generally agreed to consist of 1) bradycardic arrhythmias with episodes of sinus bradycardia, sinus arrest or pauses, and/or sino-atrial block; 2) a reluctance of escape junctional pacemakers to emerge and 3) in about 2/3 of cases, episodes of supraventricular, mainly atrial, rapid dysrhythmias.

In a recent report (21), we were able to describe the pathological findings in 6 instances of sino-atrial rhythm disorders occurring three times in the setting of a chronic sinus node disease, twice during an acute episode of myocardial infarction, and once in a case of diphtheritic myocarditis.

The alterations which were most consistently observed can be summarized as follows:

a) total or subtotal destruction of the sino-atrial node (5 cases)
b) total or subtotal interruption of the areas of nodo-atrial continuity (5 cases).
c) inflammatory or degenerative changes of the nerves and ganglia surrounding the node (4 cases).
d) pathological alterations of the atrial wall generally characterized by large areas of loss of muscle mass or architecture (5 cases).

These alterations were nearly always associated with chronic or acute lesions involving the node of Tawara, the bundle of His, its branches, or their distal subdivisions. These pathological alterations may probably explain the various physiological disorders observed in this disease.

The bradycardic episodes may reflect deficiency of sinus node automaticity or impaired conduction from the center of the node to its periphery or from the node itself to the atrial myocardium. These disorders can be accounted for by the severe changes observed within the node, along the areas of nodo-atrial continuity and, finally, in the perinodal nervous structures.

The reluctance of satisfactory escape junctional pacemakers to emerge might be accounted for by two different mechanisms. First of all, the atrio-ventricular junction is quite commonly the site of pathological alterations in the setting of sinoatrial disease. In addition, a normal sympathetic input is mandatory to ensure a proper automatic function of the junctional pacemaker and the changes of the intracardiac ganglia probably play a significant role in this respect.

The pathological observations may also offer a satisfactory explanation for the occurrence of tachycardic rhythm disorders. The lesions seen along the sino-atrial junctions as well as at the level of the approaches to the atrio-ventricular node may favour the genesis of reentrant beats or tachycardias. The same holds true for the alterations of the atrial wall which delinate, at this level, ideal paths for circus movement and reentrant excitation.

Conclusions

The sinus node is an oval-shaped structure composed of a mixture of nodal muscle cells and connective tissue. The relative content in connective tissue gradually increases with age. In diseased hearts it is sometimes difficult to demonstrate more than a few nodal cells embedded in collagen. The nodal-atrial muscle cell junctions are also largely replaced by intranodal and perinodal fibrosis. This pathologic appearance of the sino-atrial node region is generally found in patients who have shown antemortem the so-called sino-atrial rhythm disorders. It is also commonly encountered in the heart from subjects with sustained atrial fibrillation. It may surprisingly be depicted in some individuals with overt cardiac disease in whom the atria have constantly remained under normal sinus node control.

References

1. Keith, A. & Flack, M.W., The form and nature of the muscular connections between the primary divisions of the vertebrate heart. *J. of Anatom. and Physiol.*, 41, 172 (1907).
2. Blair, D.M. & Davies, F., Observations on the conducting system of the heart. *J. of Anatom.*, 69, 303 (1907).
3. Copenhaver, W.M. & Truex, R.C., Histology of the atrial portion of the cardiac conduction system in man and other mammals. *Anatom. Record.*, 114, 601 (1952).
4. Lev, M. & Watne, A.L., Method for routine histopathologic study of human sino-atrial node. *Archiv. of Pathol.* 57, 168 (1954).
5. James, T.N., Anatomy of the human sinus node. *Anatom. Record.* 141, 109 (1961).
6. Hudson, R.E.B., *Cardiovascular pathology*. London, E. Arnold. (1965).
7. Lev, M. *The conduction system in Pathology of the Heart and Blood Vessels.* 3rd Edition. Springfield, Illinois. (1968).
8. Rossi, L., *Histopathologic features of cardiac arrhythmias.* Milano, 1969.
9. Titus, J.L., Anatomy of the conduction system. *Circulation*, 47, 170 (1973).
10. Kulbertus, H.E. & Demoulin, J.C. The conduction system: Anatomical and Pathological Aspects. In: *Cardiac Arrhythmias. The modern electrophysiological approach.* Krikler D.M. and Goodwin, J.F., London, 1975.
11. Truex, R.C., The sino-atrial node and its connections with the atrial tissues. In: Wellens, H.J.J. et al. (ed). *The conduction system of the heart*, Leiden 1976.
12. James, T.N., Sherf, L., Fine, G. & Morales, A.R., Comparative ultrastructure of the sinus node in dog and man. *Circulation*, 34, 139 (1966).
13. James, T.N. & Spence, C.A., Distribution of cholinesterase within the sinus node and the A-V node of the human heart. *Anatom. Record.*, 155, 151 (1966).
14. Shendler, R., Harakal, C., Sevy, R.W., Catecholamine content of the sino-atrial node and common right atrial tissue. *Proceedings of the Society of Experimental Biology and Medicine*, 128, 798 (1968).
15. Verhaege, L. & Van der Hauwaert, L., Arterial blood supply of the human sinus node. *Brit. Heart J.*, 29, 801 (1967).
16. Kennel, A.J. & Titus, J.L., The vasculature of the human sinus node. *Mayo Clinic Proceedings*, 47, 556, (1972).
17. Janse, M.J., Anderson, R.H., Specialized internodal atrial pathways; fact or fiction? *European J. of Cardiol.*, 2, 117 (1974).
18. Davies, M.T., Pomerance, A., Quantitative study of ageing changes in the human sinoatrial node and internodal tract. *Brit. Heart J.*, 34, 150 (1972).
19. Lev, M., Ageing changes in the human sinoatrial node. *J. Gerontol.* 9, 1, (1954).
20. Sims, B.A., Pathogenesis of atrial arrhythmias. *Brit. Heart J.*, 34, 336, (1972).
21. Demoulin, J.C., & Kulbertus, H.E., Pathological correlates of atrial arrhythmias. In: *Reentrant Arrhythmias, Mechanisms and Treatment.* H.E. Kulbertus, Ed., Baltimore, University Park Press, 1977.
22. Hudson, R.E.B., The human pacemaker of the heart and its pathology. *Brit. Heart J.*, 22, 152 (1960).

EVALUATION OF THE CARDIAC CONDUCTION SYSTEM BY HIS BUNDLE RECORDINGS

ONKAR S. NARULA

Introduction

Intracardiac catheter recordings of the specialized conducting tissue have greatly enhanced diagnostic acumen in A-V conduction disorders and disturbances of cardiac rhythm (1-9). His bundle (BH) recordings in conjunction with stimulation studies are now a clinical diagnostic tool available in an increasing number of cardiac catheterization laboratories. Such recordings of the specialized conduction system in man have both diagnostic value and are of clinical therapeutic and prognostic significance (10, 11). His bundle recordings permit a breakdown of the P-R interval into its three component conduction intervals, i.e., intra-atrial (P-A), A-V nodal (A-H), and His-Purkinje system (H-V) (12). The therapy and prognosis of A-V conduction defects may depend on the site of the lesion which cannot always be localized on the basis of the standard surface electrocardiogram. The range of a normal P-R interval is very wide (0.12-0.20 sec.) as compared to the narrow range of conduction time through the His-Purkinje system (H-V = 0.035 to 0.045 sec.) or the BH (0.015 to 0.020 sec.). The P-R interval or the QRS complex may remain within normal limits despite significant delays in the BH (even up to 200%).

The purpose of this chapter is to discuss the normal and abnormal electrophysiology of the human cardiac conduction and clinical application of the newer techniques.

I. Technique

His bundle electrograms are usually obtained from the right side of the heart, although an approach via the left heart may be utilized. An ordinary bipolar pacing catheter, preferably 5F in size, with ring electrodes 1 c.m. apart is introduced percutaneously into a femoral vein (right or left) and placed under fluoroscopic control and electrographic monitoring in the BH region or in apposition with the septal leaflet of the tricuspid valve. The catheter terminals are connected to the input of a DC pre-amplifier. Recordings are obtained at filter settings of 40-200 Hz and at paper speeds of 100-200 mm/sec. A second similar bipolar or a quadripolar pacing catheter is introduced via an arm vein into the high right atrium (HRA) for stimulation purposes and/or recordings of HRA electrograms. Multiple surface ECG leads (representing the three planes) are recorded simultaneous with the intracardiac leads so as to enable precise and accurate measurements of H-V time.

The various conduction times are measured as follows: P-A = from the earliest onset on the P wave on any of the multiple surface ECG leads or from the first rapid deflection of the high right atrium (HRA) to the first rapid atrial deflection recorded on the His bundle lead. A-H = from the first rapid deflection of the atrial electrogram recorded on the His bundle lead to the *onset* of the BH deflection. H-V = from the onset of BH deflection (slow or rapid components) to the onset of the earliest ventricular activation noted on either of the surface ECG leads or the His bundle lead.

II. Normal conduction times

In our laboratory the normal range and mean standard deviation of conduction intervals is: P-A = 25 to 45 milliseconds (37 ± 7); A-H = 50 to 120 milliseconds (77 ± 16); H-V = 35-45 milliseconds (40 ± 3); and BH = 15 to 20 milliseconds (17). These values are almost similar to those published by others, except for a slightly longer range of normal H-V time (35-55) quoted by others (3, 18, 19). The reasons for this discrepancy have been discussed in detail in a previous communication (17). In patients with normal A-V conduction, during atrial pacing 1:1 A-V conduction is generally seen at rates $\leqq$ 130/minute, and at higher rates, physiologic second degree (Type 1 A-V block) may be manifested in the A-V node. Contrary to an isolated report the present author believes that the development of second degree A-V block distal to the His bundle at rates $\leqq$ 150/minute is an abnormal finding (20).

III. Value of His bundle recordings

Various clinical settings in which His bundle recordings may be of diagnostic, therapeutic, and prognostic value are discussed below:

A. Atrio-Ventricular Block

Previous reports have demonstrated that all three degrees of A-V block may occur due to lesions in any portion of the A-V conducting system except the atrium. Only first and second degree (Type I) block have been documented in the latter (5, 21, 22). The incidence of chronic 2° and 3° A-V block at various sites in the A-V conduction system is given in Table 1. In clinical practice the documentation of A-V block alone is not sufficient as the prognosis and therapy are dependent both on the site and the degree of block. This information can be precisely obtained only by BH recordings as the standard ECG has its inherent limitations (5, 21).

Table 1. Site of block (From ref. 21)

	No. of	*Site of block*			
Block	*cases*	*P-A*	*A-H*	*BH*	*H-V*
Second degree					—
Type I	19	–	14 (74%)	1 (5%)	4 (21%)
Type II	23	–	–	8 (35%)	15 (65%)
2:1 or 3:1 (Fixed)	20	–	7 (35%)	3 (15%)	10 150%)
Third degree	81	–	13 (16%)	13 (16%)	55 (68%)

1. Intra-atrial Lesions:

Cases with first degree A-V block due to intra-atrial conduction delays are usually associated with multiple supraventricular arrhythmias i.e., atrial fibrillation, flutter, or at times may present with a (pseudo) silent atria (10, 17). Since complete A-V block due to intra-atrial lesions has not been documented, such cases may not progress to third degree A-V block. In addition, in these cases digitalis may be safely given for the management of multiple supraventricular arrhythmias.

2. A-V Nodal Lesions:

In contrast to intra-atrial lesions, digitalis glycosides should be administered with caution in patients with A-V nodal delays. Although chronic first degree or type I second degree A-V nodal block may eventually progress to higher degree of A-V block, the rate of progression is usually relatively slow and is rarely sudden or unpredictable (Figure 1). Therefore, in the absence of any symptoms, patients with first degree or type I second degree A-V nodal block may be clinically followed without a fear of unexpected Adams-Stokes attacks. The existence of type II second degree A-V nodal block has not been proven to date although some controversy exists in this area.

During complete heart block (CHB) the QRS morphology, the heart rate, and/or the response of the rhythm to drugs cannot be relied upon to determine

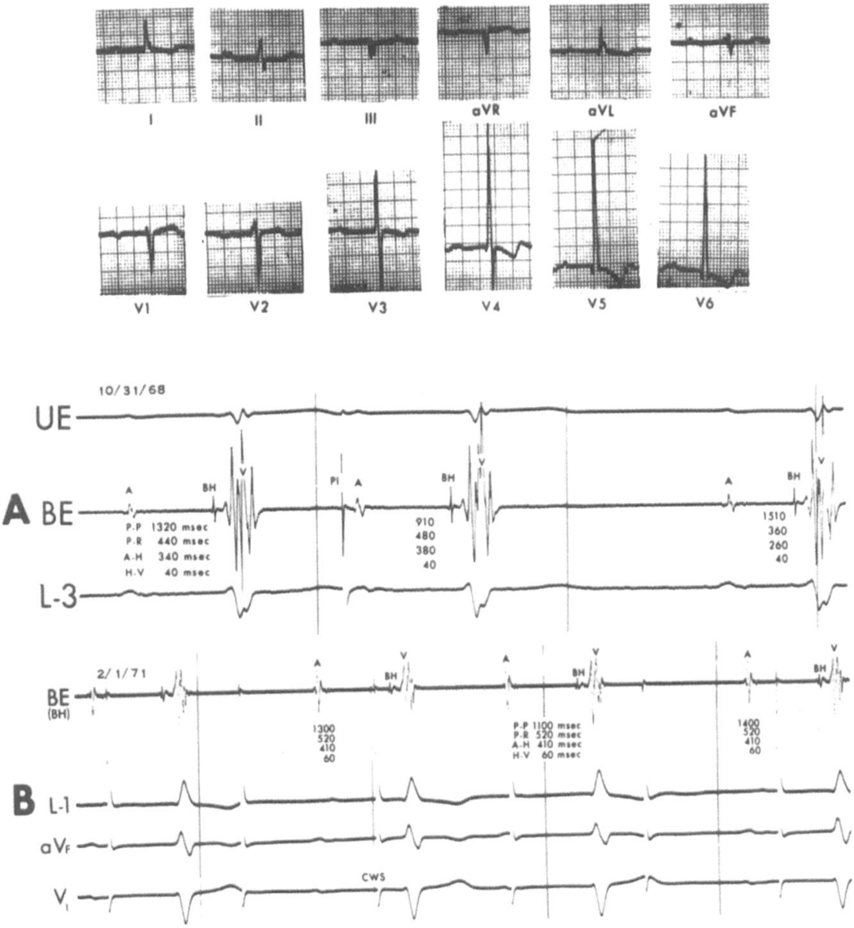

Figure 1. Follow-up observation in a patient with first degree A-V block due to severe A-V nodal delay.

A. Recordings on 10/30/68 showed that the P-R interval (440 msec.) was prolonged due to a severe prolongation of the A-H time (340 msec.). The H-V time (40 msec.) was normal.

B. Subsequent recordings on 2/1/71 show the persistence of first-degree A-V block as the permanent ventricular standby pacemaker is suppressed by external chest wall stimuli (CWS). The A-H time has lengthened slightly over this period (from 340 to 410 msec.). The H-V time also shows a slight lengthening (40 to 60 msec.). Note the absence of progression to second-degree A-V block despite severe A-V nodal delays.

the site of block. Recent investigations by this author suggest that localization of block and the site of origin of a subsidiary escape pacemaker, by BH recordings, is not a reliable criterion to distinguish the patients prone to syncope or dizziness from the asymptomatic group (23). Frequently patients with CHB (chronic or acute) localized in the A-V node, may have syncope due to an unstable subsidiary junctional pacemaker and may require management with an artificial pacemaker. Patients with CHB despite an acceleration in heart rate up to $\geq$ 72/min with atropine or exercise, are not immune to asystole and syncope. However, the presence or absence of symptoms may be correlated to the response: a) to overdrive suppression or the recovery time of the escape pacemakers and b) autonomic influences, in patients with CHB. Patients with corrected junctional recovery time of $\leq$ 200 msec, especially after atropine are not likely to have syncope or dizziness (23).

3. His-Purkinje System (HPS):

Progression of first degree or second degree blocks in the HPS to higher degrees of A-V block (second degree or third degree) and to total ventricular asystole are often not predictable. In cases with lesions in the HPS, 1:1 A-V conduction may change to CHB or vice versa within a few minutes without any obvious reasons (6, 21). Digitalis may be administered safely to patients with first degree delay in the HPS. Procainamide and Quinidine prolong the HPS conduction time and should be given with caution in patients with an abnormal H-V time (24).

For clinical purposes, whenever possible, the ECG pattern of second degree A-V block should be classified into type I or type II. The reason is that the classical type II block (with a constant P-R interval throughout) is always localized in the HPS, and type I block may occur due to lesions anywhere in the A-V conduction system (25). Type I block, in the majority of the cases, is localized in the A-V node, and in a small number of cases in the HPS (21). Despite type I block the prognosis of the latter cases is not different from that of type II at a similar lesion site, i.e., HPS. Type I or II second degree block in the HPS often progress unpredictably to CHB and Adams-Stokes attacks. During CHB the escape subsidiary pacemakers located distal to the block in the HPS are in the long run unreliable and unstable. In view of the above facts, others as well as the present author recommend that serious consideration be given to prophylactic permanent pacemaker implantation even in asymptomatic patients with type I or type II second degree HPS block (26, 27). Asymptomatic patients with permanent established stable complete A-V block due to HPS lesions are not recommended for permanent pacer implant unless the rate is $\leq$ 40/min or the response to overdrive suppression shows a prolonged recovery time.

B. Intraventricular Conduction Defects

Intraventricular conduction defects (IVCD) are comprised of abnormalities in one or more segments of the His-Purkinje system, i.e., the main His bundle, right and left bundle branches, and anterior and posterior subdivisions of the left bundle branch, and the peripheral Purkinje system. During normal A-V conduction the impulse arrives simultaneously at the terminals of both bundle branches or at all three fascicles (right bundle branch, anterior and posterior divisions of left bundle branch) (6, 15, 21). Block in one or two fascicles in any combination should not delay ventricular depolarization as the impulse is transmitted without any delay through the remaining intact fascicle. Therefore, in cases with unifascicular or bifascicular block a normal H-V time indicates that the remaining fascicles are intact, whereas a prolonged H-V time suggests that all the three fascicles and/or the His bundle are also diseased in addition to the block obvious on the surface ECG.

The various ECG features, i.e., the shape, duration, and the axis of the QRS complex may suggest the site of dominant delay or block in the HPS. However, the severity of delay and the number of sites involved in the HPS often cannot be completely determined on the basis of a standard ECG. Isolated intra-His bundle lesions are even harder to detect on the surface ECG as the QRS complex may remain unaltered or completely normal. Furthermore, a recent report by this author indicates that various types of ECG bundle branch block patterns may result from selective intra-His lesions alone due to asynchronous conduction (or longitudinal dissociation) within the BH in patients with normal bundle branches (28). Such cases may be detected by intracardiac recordings and BH stimulation studies.

In patients with various types of IVCD, His bundle recordings are useful in evaluating the severity of delay and the number of sites involved in the His-Purkinje system. Table 2 shows the frequency of a prolonged H-V time with various types of ECG patterns (29). The data in Table 2 also explain why some patients with similar ECG patterns, i.e., right bundle branch block (RBBB) and a left axis deviation (LAD) may progress to complete heart block and syncope

Table 2. H-V Abnormalities in 451 patients with intraventricular conduction defects (From ref. 29)

No. of cases	*Conduction defect*	*Prolonged H-V*
123	LBBB	79%
8	Int. LBBB	63%
5	RAD	40%
76	LAD	30%
62	RBBB	32%
131	RBBB + LAD	72%
30	RBBB + RAD	87%
16	GIVCD	87%

within a short time whereas others do not. Despite similar ECGs, different degrees of delay may exist in the remainder of the functioning His-Purkinje system and normal or abnormal H-V intervals may be seen in these cases (Figure 2).

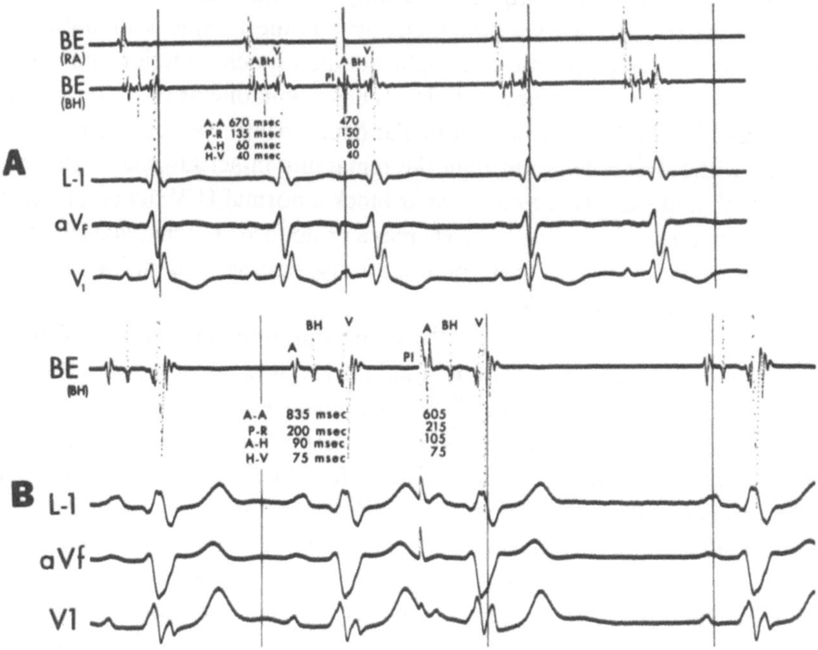

Figure 2. Despite similar ECG patterns i.e., right bundle branch block and left axis duration, in two different patients His bundle recordings show normal (45 msec) and abnormal (60 msec) H-V times in Panels A and B, respectively.

Table 2 shows a prolonged H-V time in 30% of the cases with isolated LAD and 32% of cases with isolated RBBB. The prolonged H-V time in these groups is presumably due to an intra His bundle lesion, in addition to the obvious LAD or RBBB pattern on the ECG. These data further explain why some patients may directly progress to complete heart block without a change in QRS duration and/or an axis shift.

The prognostic value of H-V intervals is suggested by several recent reports based on retrospective or prospective observations in patients with bundle branch block patterns (11, 30, 31). Follow-up observations by the author, ranging over from 2 to 8 years, in 95 patients with RBBB and LAD show that in the group of patients with a normal H-V time and without a permanent pacemaker, irrespective of the symptoms of syncope or dizziness, the mortality per year of follow-up was almost identical and equal to that of in general population for that age group (Table 3) (11). In the group of patients with a prolonged H-V time and without a pacemaker (asymptomatic) the mortality was 200% greater than those with a permanent pacemaker (symptomatic). It is probable (but not proven) that the difference in mortality between the two groups of patients, is due to the development of sudden complete A-V block. In view of these observations, this

Table 3. Prospective study of RBBB and LAD, Narula et al. (Jun. 68-Jan. 76)

Mean age 72

95

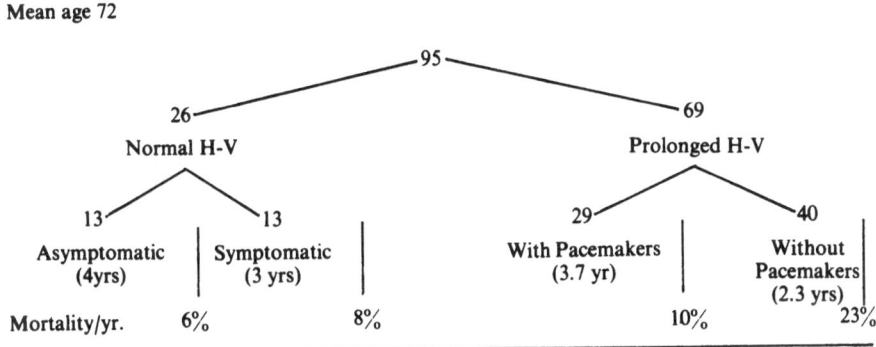

	Normal H-V		Prolonged H-V	
	26		69	
	13	13	29	40
	Asymptomatic (4yrs)	Symptomatic (3 yrs)	With Pacemakers (3.7 yr)	Without Pacemakers (2.3 yrs)
Mortality/yr.	6%	8%	10%	23%

author and others have recommended prophylactic pacing in selected asymptomatic elderly patients with H-V > 70 msec and an ECG pattern of RBBB and LAD (11, 30). However, at the present time some controversy exists pertaining to the indications for prophylactic pacing (32). Observations over a longer follow-up period and studies from several centers hopefully should clarify the validity of these preliminary observations.

C. A-V Block During Acute Myocardial Infarction

Several studies have reported a very high incidence of mortality in patients developing a fresh bifascicular block (RBBB and LAD) during acute myocardial infarction (33, 34). Lichstein et al. have reported that in their series of cases with acute myocardial infarction and associated fresh bundle branch block the mortality was 72% versus 25% in patients with abnormal and normal H-V times, respectively (33). Atkins et al. have reported sudden death in some patients, during the follow-up period, despite recovery from A-V block associated with acute myocardial infarction (34). It was suggested that a significant residual conduction defect persisted despite restoration of 1:1 A-V conduction and was probably responsible for subsequent progression to complete A-V block and sudden death. These authors further suggested that in the latter patients a permanent pacemaker implantation should be considered on a prophylactic basis after recovery from an infarction and prior to discharge from the hospital (34). Preliminary observations by the present author substantiate the persistence of a residual conduction defect, indicated by a prolonged H-V time, in patients with acute block localized in the His-Purkinje system (35). The above discussion suggests that in selected patients with myocardial infarction, His bundle recordings may be useful from prognostic and therapeutic viewpoints.

D. Disorders of Impulse Generation

The function of sinus node (SN) as an impulse generator can be evaluated by measurement of sinus node recovery time (SRT) following overdrive suppression (36, 37). The sinus node may be suppressed by right atrial pacing (AP) at rates ranging from 120 to 200 beats/minute for periods of 2 minutes at each level. SRT is defined as the interval from the last paced P wave to the succeeding spontaneous sinus P wave. Overdrive suppression of the sinus node is seen in normal cases as well as in those with sinus node dysfunction. The diagnosis of the latter depends upon the degree of depression. The normal range of SRT is equal to control sinus cycle length $+ \leqq$ 525 msec. (36). In normal cases the SRT is essentially independent of the rate and duration of AP, whereas in patients with SN dysfunction, the SRT is usually proportional within limits to the rate and duration of AP.

The SRT may not be prolonged in all patients with sinus bradycardia (SB) and the symptoms of syncope or dizziness may not always be due to SB. Therefore, symptomatic cases with or without SB and suspected of sinus node dysfunction may be evaluated by measuring SRT. Since atropine may enhance sino-atrial conduction, it is recommended that the SRT be re-evaluated following atropine administration (2-2.5 mg), in cases suspected of sinus node dysfunction (Figure 3), but with a normal SRT before atropine (37). Changes in circulating catecholamines or basal state may alter the measurements of SRT. Preliminary studies suggest that administration of propranolol may unmask sinus node dysfunction in patients with a normal SRT due to increased amounts of circulating catecholamines at the time of the study (38).

In patients presenting with paroxysmal supraventricular arrhythmias or atrial fibrillation and symptoms of syncope or dizziness, sinus node dysfunction may be diagnosed by measurement of SRT during periods of spontaneous sinus rhythm. Patients with SB or borderline heart rates may be considered for evaluation of sinus node function by measurement of SRT prior to the institution of propranolol therapy for management of angina. Patients with sinus node dysfunction may require pacemaker implantation so as to enable safe administration of propranolol therapy.

Some workers have claimed that Sino-atrial (S-A) conduction can be evaluated by premature atrial beats induced in the middle portion of the resting sinus cycle (39). Our observations and those of others suggest that the use of PAB's for estimation of SACT is usually not reliable or useful for evaluation of sinus node function (Fig. 4) (36, 37, 40).

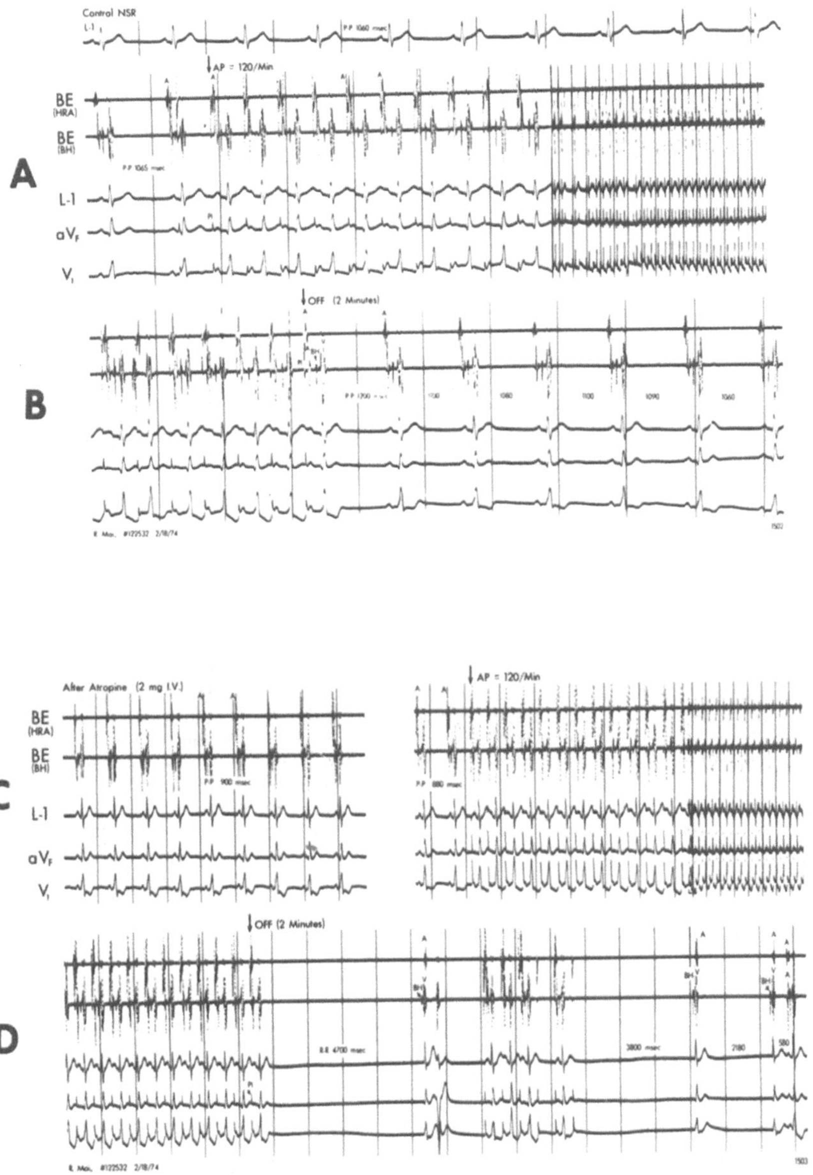

Figure 3. Sinus node recovery time (SRT) for evaluation of etiology of syncopal attacks in a patient with a normal ECG and heart rates approximately 60/minutes. His bundle recordings showed a normal A-H and H-V conduction. (From ref. 37)

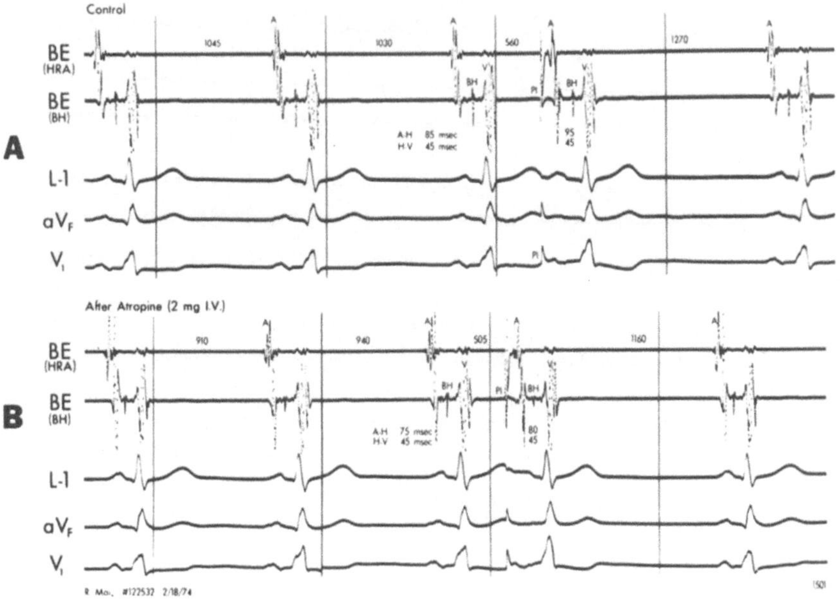

Figure 4. Premature beats before and after atropine in the same patient as in Figure 3.

A. The control sinus cycle is 1030 msec. An induced Premature Atrial Beat (PAB) at a coupling interval of 560 msec is followed by a return cycle of 1270 msec. The return cycle is equal to the control sinus cycle and the sum of the atrio-Sinus-sinoatrial conduction times. The S-A conduction time is 120 msec. (Half of the difference between 1270 and 1030 = 240 msec).

B. After intravenous atropine (2 mg), the basic sinus cycle shortens to 940 msec. An induced PAB (coupling interval = 505 msec) is followed by a return cycle of 1160 msec. The S-A conduction time (110 msec) is essentially similar to that in A and within the normal range. The above data, along with Figure 3, show the inadequacy of PABs in determining sinus node dysfunction. (From ref. 37)

E. Arrhythmias

His bundle recordings are useful in cases with Wolff-Parkinson-White syndrome and those with arrhythmias in the following clinical settings:

1. To differentiate between a premature ventricular contraction (PVC) and aberrant conduction when abnormal QRS complexes ($\geqq$ .12 sec.) are seen during atrial fibrillation especially in patients receiving digitalis. Demonstration of the presence of a BH deflection (with an H-V time $\geqq$ than that in the normal beats) or the absence of a BH preceding the abnormal QRS complexes indicates a supraventricular beat with aberrant conduction or a PVC, respectively.

2. BH recordings may permit differentiation between ventricular tachycardia (VT) and supraventricular or junction tachycardia with aberrant conduction. This differentiation is clinically significant in relation to digitalis administration. Absence of a BH deflection preceding the aberrant QRS complexes is suggestive of ventricular origin of the tachycardia whereas the demonstration of a BH

deflection, preceding each QRS complex, especially when associated with a normal or a prolonged H-V time, is suggestive of supraventricular origin. In the latter case the possibility of ventricular origin of the tachycardia cannot be mathematically excluded. In patients with VT a His bundle deflection may rarely precede the QRS complexes at a normal or prolonged H-V time. However, it is to be pointed out that in the latter case the control H-V time, i.e., during normal sinus rhythm, must be greater than the H-V time recorded during VT. During VT, the His bundle may be activated in a retrograde fashion and may precede the QRS complex at an interval shorter than the control.

3. His bundle recordings in conjunction with the atrial and ventricular stimulation studies are clinically useful in patients with paroxysmal tachycardia:

a) to elucidate the mechanism of an arrhythmia by controlled initiation and termination of the tachycardia.

b) in patients with a history of an arrhythmia, but without any documentation, the diagnosis may be confirmed by stimulation studies (Fig. 5, 6).

c) In patients with a previous electrocardiographic demonstration of tachycardia but without a documentation of its origin (SVT or VT), and following a spontaneous or a controlled conversion, electrical stimulation studies may enable documentation of its origin and mechanism (Fig. 7, 8). Electrophysiological studies under these settings are useful during considerations for drug or pacer therapy in patients with arrhythmias.

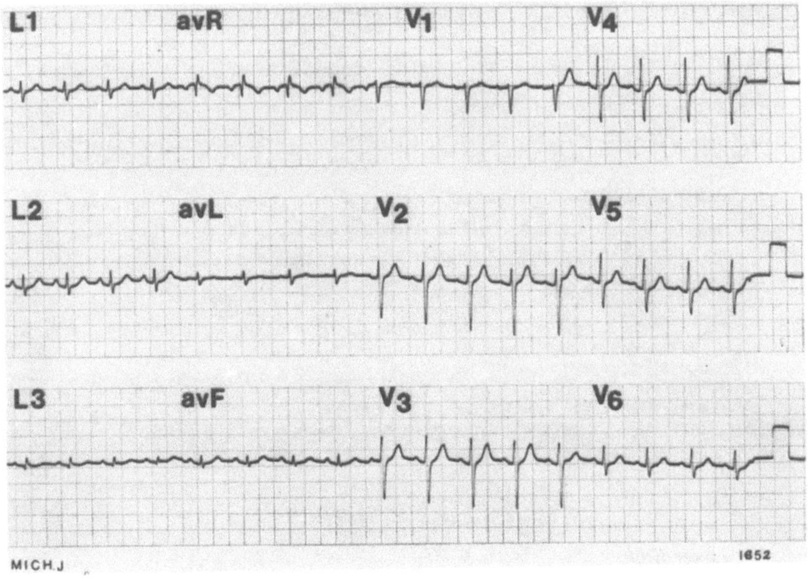

Figure 5. Twelve lead ECG shows normal findings in a patient with a history of palpitations and rapid heart beat without any ECG documentation either during several hospital admissions or on 24 Holter monitor recordings.

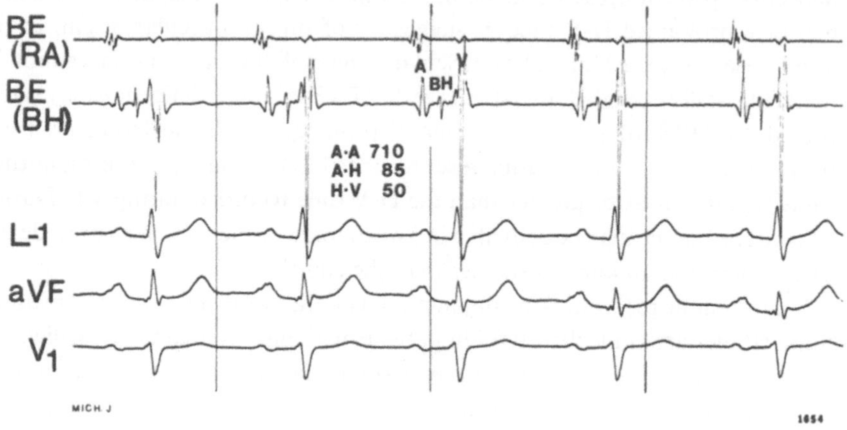

Figure 6. Shows usefulness of Electrophysiologic studies in unmasking the nature and mechanism of the palpitations in the same patient as in Fig. 5.

Upper Half: His bundle recordings during NSR show normal A-V conduction and without any evidence of bypass tracts functioning in antegrade direction.

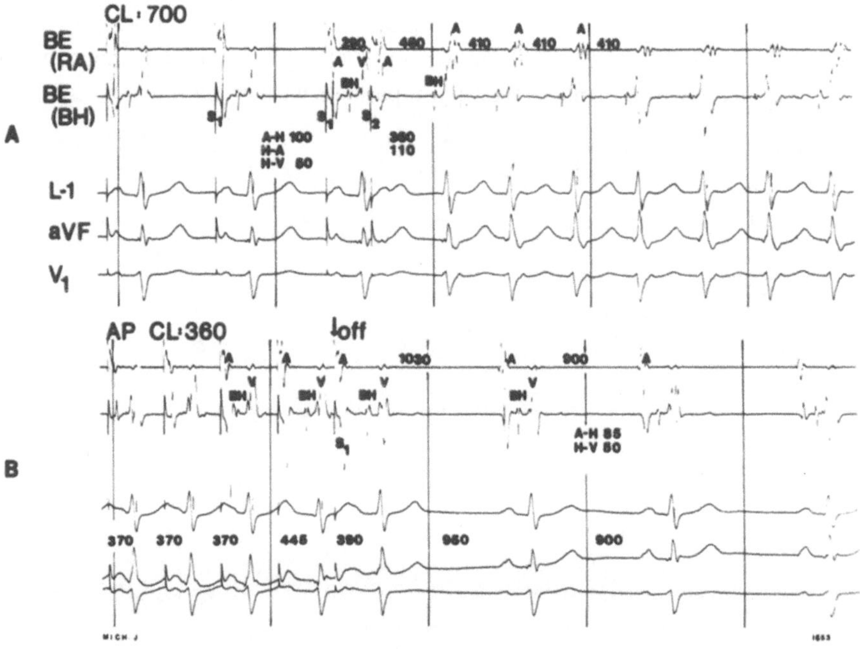

Figure 6. Lower Half:

A. Shows initiation of a supraventricular tachycardia (SVT) with a single premature beat during atrial pacing (AP) at a basic cycle length (CL) of 700 msec. The site of re-entry is localized in the A-V node.

B. Shows termination of SVT by AP at a CL of 360 msec.

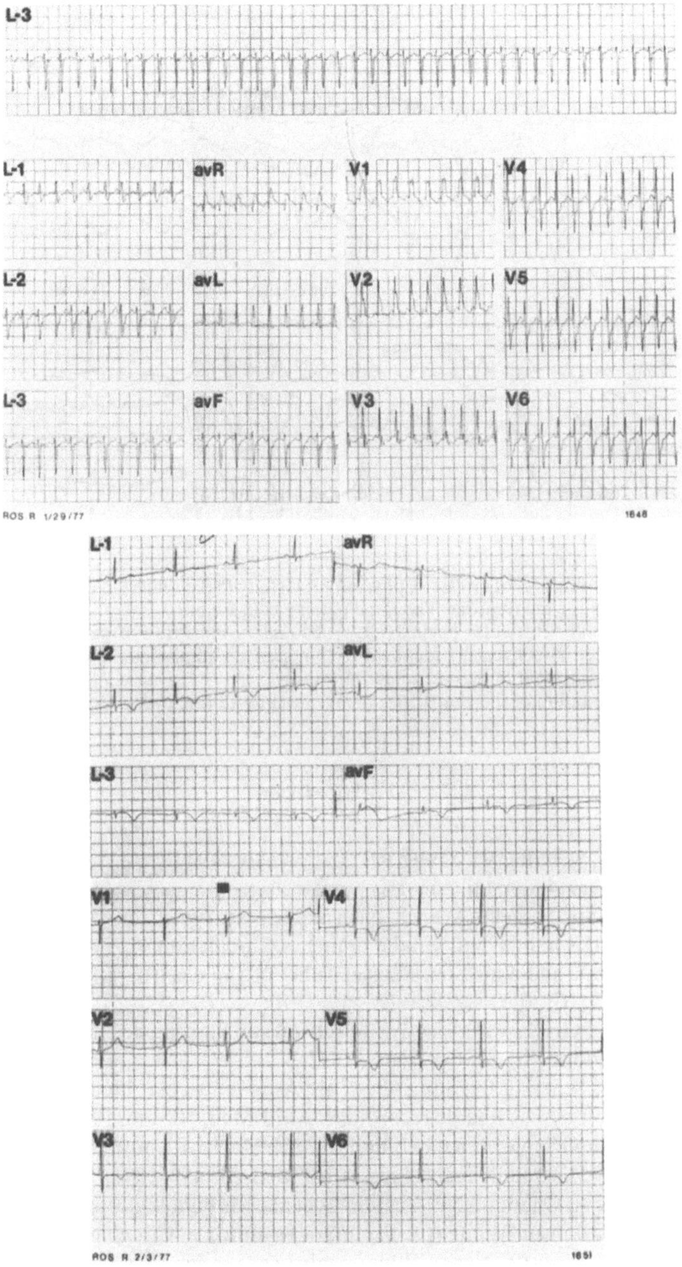

Figure 7. Upper Half:
Twelve lead ECG on admission in an 18 year old female patient shows tachycardia of unknown origin (Ventricular or supraventricular).
Lower Half:
Five days later and after spontaneous conversion a 12 lead ECG shows NSR with non specific T-wave changes.

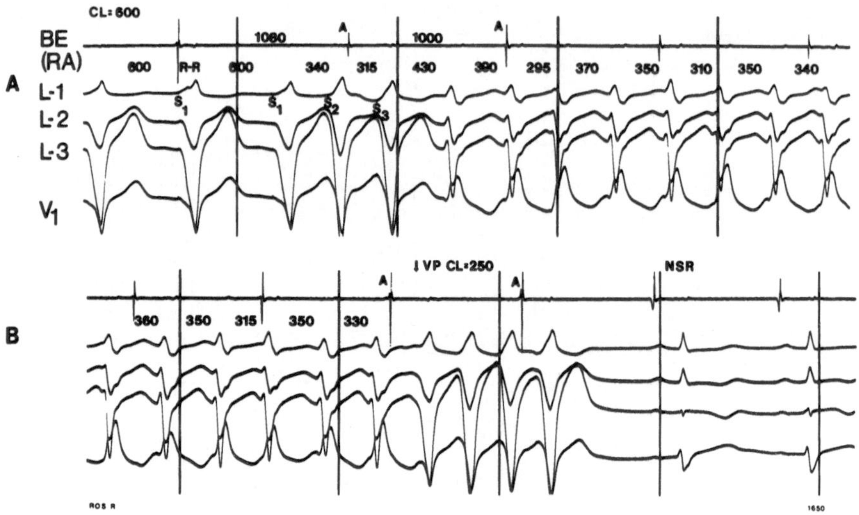

Figure 8. Shows usefulness of an electrophysiological study (5 days later) in documenting the nature and mechanism of the tachycardia. The same patient as in Figure 7.

A. During regular ventricular pacing (CL = 600 msec) induction of paired premature stimuli (S_2S_3) induced a tachycardia identical to that seen on admission. A-V dissociation and BH recordings indicate it to be ventricular in origin.

B. Shows termination of the ventricular tachycardia by ventricular stimulation.

References

1. Narula OS, Scherlag BJ, Javier RP et al., Analysis of the A-V conduction defect in complete heart block utilizing His bundle electrograms. Circulation 41: 437, 1970.
2. Narula OS and Samet P: Wenckebach and Mobitz type II A-V blocks due to lesions within the His bundle and bundle branches. Circulation 41: 947, 1970.
3. Damato, AN and Lau SH: Clinical value of the electrogram of the conduction system. Prog. Cardiovasc. Dis. 13: 119, 1970.
4. Puech P and Grolleau R: L'activité électrique du faisceau de His, normale et pathologique. Sandoz Pharm. Co., Paris, 1972.
5. Narula OS, Scherlag BJ, Samet P, et al.: Atrioventricular block: Localization and classification by His bundle recordings. Am J Med, 50: 146, 1971.
6. Narula OS and Samet P: Right bundle branch block with normal, left axis deviation: Analysis by His bundle recordings. Am J Med, 51: 432, 1971.
7. Castellanos A, Chapunoff E, Castillo C, et al.: His bundle electrograms in two cases of Wolff-Parkinson-White (pre-excitation) syndrome. Circulation, 41: 399, 1970.
8. Narula OS: Wolff-Parkinson-White syndrome (a review). Circulation, 47: 872, 1973.
9. Rosen KM, Rahimtoola SH, Chuquimia R, et al.: Electrophysiological significance of first degree atrioventricular conduction disturbance. Circulation 43: 491, 1971.
10. Narula OS: The value of His bundle electrocardiography in cardiac diagnosis, in Fowler No (ed): Diagnostic methods in cardiology. F.A. Davis Co., Philadelphia, 1975, p. 133.

11. Narula OS, Gann D, and Samet P: Prognostic value of H-V intervals, in Narula OS (ed): His bundle electrocardiography and clinical electrophysiology. F.A. Davis, Co., Philadelphia, 1975, p. 437.
12. Narula OS, Cohen LS, Scherlag BJ, et al.: Localization of A-V conduction defects in man by recording of His bundle electrogram. Am J Cardiol, 25: 228, 1970.
13. Scherlag BJ, Lau SH, Helfant RH, et al.: Catheter technique for recording His bundle activity in man. Circulation, 39: 13, 1969.
14. Narula OS, Scherlag BJ and Samet P: Prevenous pacing of the specialized conducting system in man: His bundle and A-V nodal stimulation. Circulation, 41: 77, 1970.
15. Narula OS, Javier RP, Samet P, et al.: Significance of His and left bundle recordings from the left heart in man. Circulation 42: 385, 1970.
16. Narula OS, Runge M and Samet P: A new catheter technique for His bundle recordings via the arm veins. Br Heart J, 45: 1226, 1973.
17. Narula OS: Validation of His bundle recordings: Limitations of the catheter technique, in Narula, OS (ed.): His Bundle electrocardiography and clinical electrophysiology, F.A. Davis Co., Philadelphia, 1975, p. 65.
18. Dhingra RL, Rosen KC, and Rahimtoola SH: Normal conduction intervals and responses in sixty-one patients using His bundle recording and atrial pacing. Chest 64: 55, 1973.
19. Castillo C, Castellanos S, and Agha AS: Significance of His bundle recordings with short H-V intervals. Chest 60: 142, 1971.
20. Damato AN, Varghese PJ, Caracta AR, Akhtar M, and Lau SH: Functional 2:1 A-V block within the His-Purkinje system: Simulation of type II second degree A-V block. Circulation 47: 534, 1973.
21. Narula OS: Current concepts of A-V block, in Narula OS (ed.): His bundle electrocardiography and clinical electrophysiology. F.A. Davis Co., Philadelphia, 1975, p. 139.
22. Narula OS, Runge M and Samet P: Second degree Wenckebach type A-V block due to block within the atrium. Br. Heart J, 34: 1127, 1972.
23. Narula OS, Narula JT: Junctional pacemakers in man: Response to overdrive suppression with and without parasympathetic blockade. Circulation 57: May, 1978.
24. Damato AN, Caracta AR, Akhtar M, and Lau SH: The effects of commonly used cardiovascular drugs on A-V- conduction and refractoriness, in Narula OS (ed): His bundle electrocardiography and clinical electrophysiology. F.A. Davis Co., Philadelphia, 1975, p. 105.
25. Narula OS: Wenckebach type I and type II atrioventricular block (revisited). Cardiovasc Clin, 6 (1): 138, 1974.
26. Haft JI: His bundle electrogram. Circulation 47: 897, 1973.
27. Rosen KM: Evaluation of cardiac conduction in the cardiac catheterization laboratory. Am J Cardiol, 30: 701, 1972.
28. Narula OS: Longitudinal dissociation in the His bundle: Bundle branch block due to asynchronous conduction within the His bundle in man. Circulation 56: 996, 1977.
29. Narula OS: Intraventricular conduction defects, in Narula OS (ed.): His Bundle electrocardiography and clinical electrophysiology, F.A. Davis Co., 1975, p. 177.
30. Vera Z, Mason DT, Fletcher RD, Awan NA, Massumi RA: Prolonged His-Q interval in chronic bifascicular block. Relation to impending complete heart block. Circulation 53: 47, 1976.
31. Scheinman MM, Peters RW, Modin G, Brennan M, Mies C, Young JO: Prognostic

value of intra nodal conduction time in patients with bundle branch block. Circulation 56: 240, 1977.
32. Denes P, Dhnigra RC, Wu D, Chuquimia R, Amat-y-leon F, Wyndham C, Rosen KM: H-V interval in patients with bifascicular block (right bundle branch and anterior hemiblock). Am J Cardiol, 35: 23, 1975.
33. Lichstein E, Gupter PK, Chadda KD, Lin H, and Sayeed M: Findings of prognostic value in patients with incomplete bilateral bundle branch block completing acute myocardial infarction. Am J Card, 32: 913, 1973.
34. Atkins JM, Leshin SJ, Blomquist G, et al.: Ventricular conduction blocks and sudden death in acute myocardial infarction. N. Engl. J Med, 288: 281, 1973.
35. Narula OS and Javier RP: Sequelae of A-V block in acute myocardial infarction. Circulation (Suppl. II) 45: 197, 1972.
36. Narula OS, Samet P, and Javier RP: Significance of the sinus node recovery time. Circulation 45: 140, 1972.
37. Narula OS: Disorders of Sinus node function: Electrophysiologic evaluation, in Narula OS (ed): His Bundle electrocardiography and clinical electrophysiology. F.A. Davis Co., Philadelphia, 1975, p. 275.
38. Chuquimia R, Vasquez M, Qureshi T, Khan M, Towne WD, Narula OS: Effect of Propranolol on sinus node recovery time and sino-atrial conduction time. Clinical Research, 25: 3, 1977.
39. Strauss HC, Saroff AL, Bigger JT, Jr., et al.: Premature atrial stimulation as a key to the understanding of sino-atrial conduction in man. Circulation 47: 86, 1973.
40. Breithardt G, Seipel L, and Loogen F: Sinus node recovery time and calculated sinoatrial conduction time in normal subjects and patients with sinus node dysfunction. Circulation 56: 43, 1977.

SIGNIFICANCE OF HIS BUNDLE RECORDING IN BUNDLE BRANCH BLOCK*

LUDGER SEIPEL, GÜNTER BREITHARDT AND HORST KUHN

His bundle studies in patients with bundle branch block (BBB) have revealed abnormal intraventricular conduction in many patients especially with left bundle branch block (LBBB). The electrophysiological explanation and the clinical significance of a prolonged His-ventricle (H-V) time is controversial. Therefore, we compared the electrophysiological data with the clinical, hemodynamic and morphological findings in patients with BBB as well as the outcome during follow-up.

Method and material

His bundle electrography was performed in the conventional technique according to Scherlag et al. (1). His bundle recording was performed with a special 4 F bipolar catheter for single use (Cordis). Our normal value for the A-H interval is $89 \pm 17{,}2$ ms, and for the H-V interval $43 \pm 6{,}9$ ms ($\bar{x} \pm$ s.d.) (2). The V-RVA time was measured according to Castellanos et al. (3), our normal value being 5-25 ms. For determination of the different refractory periods the definitions of Wit et al. (4) were used. In addition to His bundle studies long-term ECG tape recordings were done. Nearly all patients with LBBB underwent heart catheterization including coronary arteriography, left ventricular angiography as well as pulmonary arterial pressure measurement at rest and during exercise. The exception of the rule were only four very old patients with LBBB and documented myocardial infarction. In 31 patients with LBBB without coronary heart disease (CHD) or rheumatic valvular lesions endomyocardial biopsy from the right ventricle using a Konno biotome (5) was performed. For quantitation of the electron microscopic findings a semi-quantitative morphological score was used. In this score degenerative changes, alterations of mitochondria, myofibrillar changes, interstitial fibrosis, and hypertrophy of the muscle fibers were assessed according to their frequency and severity (6). Statistical analysis was done by the Wilcoxon test.

* Supported in part by grant of Landesamt für Forschung NRW.

Seventy-three cases with LBBB were studied (Tab. 1). There were 27 female and 46 male patients. Fourteen of these patients had CHD, six rheumatic valvular lesions. Twenty-two patients suffered from congestive cardiomyopathy (CCM). In 10 patients a so-called latent cardiomyopathy (LCM) was suspected which has previously been defined (7). These patients had normal clinical and hemodynamic findings at rest. However, during exercise an elevation of the pulmonary arterial pressure was observed indicating an abnormal left ventricular function. In some of these patients a CCM developed during follow-up (7). In three patients the LBBB pattern appeared after heart operation. In 18 patients all findings during rest and exercise were normal. Therefore, the LBBB was declared as of unknown etiology. Sixteen patients with LBBB had a history of attacks of dizziness or syncope.

Nineteen patients with complete right bundle branch block (RBBB) and normal QRS axis were studied. There were four female and 15 male cases. The mean age was 45.4 years. In five of them the RBBB pattern appeared after heart operation. The mean age of this subgroup was 28.4 years. In all patients with RBBB His bundle studies were done because of a history of dizziness or syncope.

Table 1. H-V interval in 92 patients with bundle branch block

LBBB	*age*	*H-V normal*		*H-V prolonged*		*Total*		
Etiology	*y.*	*n*	*H-V ms*	*n*	*H-V ms*	*n*	*H-V ms*	
CHD	63.1	2	50.0 ± 8.5	12	78.5 ± 13.4	14	74.4 ± 16.3	CHD vs Rheum. HD: $p < 0.05$
Rheum. HD	52.7	2	51.0 ± 1.4	4	67.8 ± 12.3	6	62.2 ± 12.9	
postop.	52.7	2	51.0 ± 7.1	1	62.0	3	54.7 ± 8.1	CHD vs postop.: $p < 0.10$
CCM	44.0	1	56.0	21	79.6 ± 28.1	22	78.8 ± 27.8	CCM vs LCM, unknown: $p < 0.02$
LCM	47.7	4	49.0 ± 4.2	6	70.3 ± 12.0	10	61.8 ± 14.4	
unknown	44.9	5	50.4 ± 4.8	13	69.2 ± 10.0	18	63.9 ± 12.3	
total	48.9	16	50.5 ± 4.5	57	75.0 ± 19.7	73	69.6 ± 20.2	total vs RBBB: $p < 0.05$
RBBB	45.4	14	43.8 ± 5.9	5	77.8 ± 16.0	19	52.7 ± 17.9	

Results

From the 73 patients with LBBB 65 had sinus rhythm, 8 atrial fibrillation. Two of the patients with sinus rhythm showed abnormal sinus node function. Twenty-nine patients with sinus rhythm had a P-R interval of 0.20 s or longer. In 12 of these patients with first degree A-V block the A-H interval was prolonged.

The H-V interval in patients with LBBB ranged from 44 ms to 190 ms. The mean value of all patients was 69.6 ± 20.2 ms. In 11 of 19 patients with intermittent LBBB the H-V interval was constant during normal and abnormal QRS pattern. In the remaining 8 cases the H-V interval showed a sudden prolongation when the bundle branch block appeared. There was no difference in H-V time in patients with LBBB and normal axis or left axis deviation (LAD). The with first degree A-V block (P-R $\geq$ 0.20 s) showed a significantly longer H-V time (79.8 $\pm$ 26.2 ms) than patients with normal P-R interval (62.7 $\pm$ 10.9 ms) (p < 140 ms duration (63.8 $\pm$ 15.3 ms). The difference was not significant. Patients with first degree A-V block (P-R $\geq$ 0.20 s) showed a significant longer H-V time (79.8 $\pm$ 26.2 ms) than patients with normal P-R interval (62.7 $\pm$ 10.9 ms) ($p < 0.005$). However, even in patients with normal A-V conduction time in the ECG abnormal H-V intervals were found. In the 16 patients with syncope the H-V time was somewhat longer (78.8 $\pm$ 34.5 ms) than in the remaining patients (63.3 $\pm$ 14.6 ms). The difference was not significant.

Tab. 1 shows the frequency of normal and abnormal H-V intervals in subgroups of patients with LBBB of different etiology. With one exception, only abnormal H-V intervals were found in patients with CCM, whereas in the other groups normal and abnormal values were measured. Even in patients with LBBB

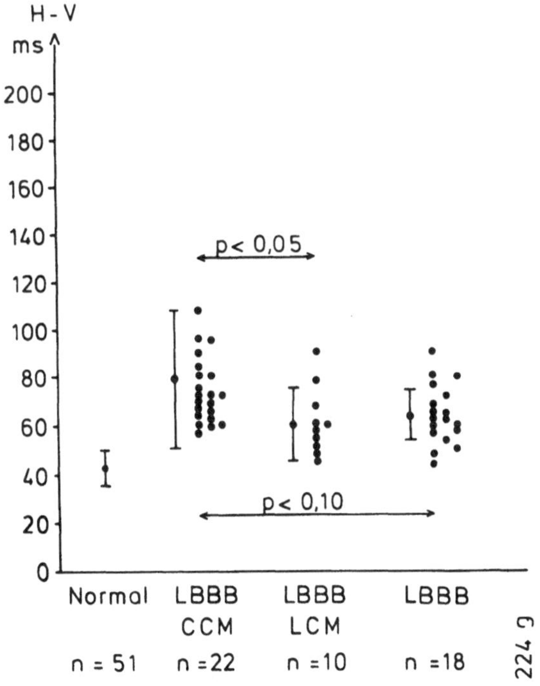

Figure 1. H-V interval in normals, in patients with LBBB and congestive cardiomyopathy (CCM), with LBBB and latent cardiomyopathy (LCM), and with LBBB without other abnormal findings.

of unknown etiology abnormal H-V intervals were seen. The mean H-V interval in patients with CCM (78.8 ± 27.7 ms) on the one hand was significantly longer than in the groups of patients with LCM and LBBB of unknown etiology (63.2 ± 12.9 ms) on the other ($p < 0.02$). However, there was an overlapping of the single values as shown in Fig. 1. Therefore, the differences between the mean H-V interval in patients with CCM and in patients with LBBB of unknown etiology as a single group was not significant. There was no difference in the H-V time between patients with CCM and CHD.

The V-RVA interval in 10 patients with LBBB and normal H-V time in whom the parameter was measured ranged from 16 ms to 20 ms. The mean value was 18.4 ± 2.2 ms. Nine patients with a prolonged H-V time showed a V-RVA interval between 12 ms and 42 ms (Fig. 2). The mean value of 28.0 ± 13.9 ms was not significantly different from the former group due to the small number of patients.

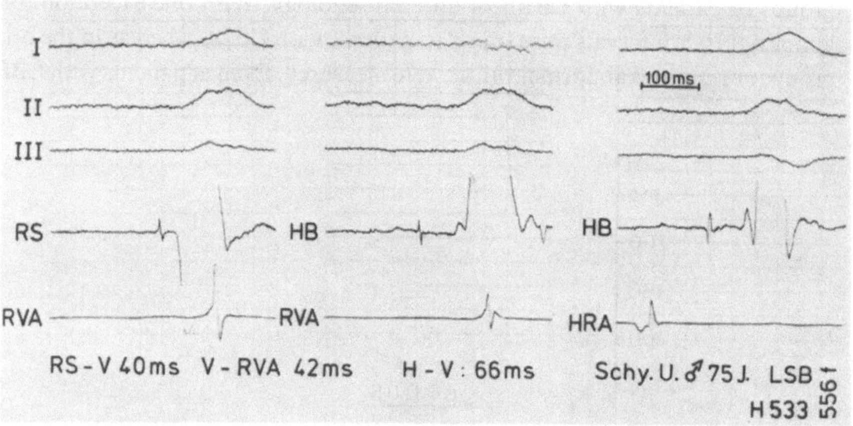

Figure 2. Recordings of the ECG (lead D I-III), the right bundle branch (RS) and the His bundle (HB) potentials simultaneously with the activation of the right ventricular apex (RVA) and high right atrial potentials (HRA). In this patient with LBBB the H-V interval is prolonged as well as the V-RVA time.

The electron microscopic evaluation of the biopsy specimen revealed in all 31 patients with LBBB without CHD or rheumatic lesions an abnormal morphology of the ordinary right ventricular myocardium. Even in patients with LBBB and completely normal clinical and hemodynamic findings myocardial hypertrophy, degenerative changes, and alterations of the mitochondria were seen. Plotting the H-V time versus the morphological score no strong correlation was found (Fig. 3). However, the five patients with a normal H-V interval all had low scores between one and four points, whereas all patients with a high morphological score had a prolonged H-V time. In contrast, some patients with a low score had very abnormal H-V intervals.

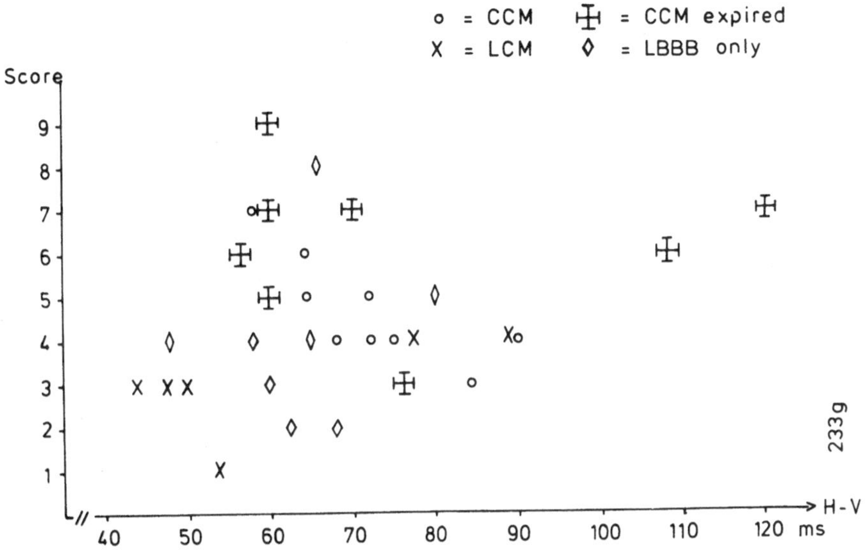

Figure 3. Correlation between H-V intervals and electron microscopic findings (Morphological score) in 31 with LBBB.

In three patients with LBBB a higher degree A-V block occurred during introduction of the very stiff biotome. The block was always located distal to the His potential. In all three cases a one-to-one conduction resumed some hours later. No complication was seen during His bundle recording.

All patients with RBBB had sinus rhythm at the time of study. Nine of these patients showed abnormal sinus node function. Four patients had a first degree A-V block, one of them due to A-H prolongation, the remaining three due to H-V delay with or without A-H prolongation. The H-V time in the group of patients with RBBB ranged from 36 ms to 112 ms. The mean value of 52.7 ± 17.9 ms was significantly shorter than the mean H-V time in the patients with LBBB (Tab. 1). The V-RVA interval was measured in 5 patients with RBBB ranging form 34 ms to 68 ms. The mean value of the V-RVA time in this group was 47.6 ± 12.8 ms.

In 10 patients with BBB an intermittent higher degree A-V block was documented during long-term monitoring. Seven cases had LBBB, three RBBB. In all patients His bundle study revealed a very abnormal atrioventricular conduction (Tab. 2). Two patients (H 109, H 508) had extremely long A-H intervals with block above the level of His at very low frequencies during atrial pacing. The other eight patients had a critically prolonged H-V time ranging from 72 ms to 190 ms. In seven of these patients with a prolonged H-V time atrial pacing was performed. In five of them a block distal to the His occurred at rates between

Table 2. Electrophysiological findings in 10 pts. with BBB and documented intermittent A-V block (all values in ms). For explanation see text.

pts.		*sinus rhythm*		*programme atrial pacing ($S_1S_1$750)*		*high rate test*	
		A-H	*H-V*	*ERPAVN*	*ERPHPS*	*S-S block*	
H 109	LBBB	220	44	> 750	-	750	AVN
H 122	LBBB	130	190	300	540	600	HPS
H 166	LBBB	88	94	1 : 1 ERPA 200		429	HPS
H 344	LBBB	88	80	325	410 RBBB	429 333	RBBB AVN
H 432	LBBB	64	72	210	440	600	HPS
H 445	LBBB	152	80	-	-	-	
H 493	LBBB	130	80	1 : 1 ERPA 260		300	AVN
H 101	RBBB	110	70	-	-	750	HPS
H 508	RBBB	500	52	> 750	-	750	AVN
H 590	RBBB	145	85	650	-	600	HPS

80/min and 140/min. In one additional patient (H 344) a RBBB pattern appeared at a pacing rate of 140/min in addition to the LBBB without A-V block. In this patient a block proximal to His occurred at a rate of 180/min. One patient had a one-to-one conduction during high rate test until block distal His occurred at a rate of 200/min. Only in two of the patients (H 122, H 432) with a block distal to the His potential during high rate test the effective refractory period of the His-Purkinje system (ERP HPS) could be measured during programmed atrial stimulation. In the other patients the block during programmed atrial stimulation occurred first in the A-V node or there was a one-to-one conduction up to the ERP of the atrium (A) was reached. All ten patients received a pacemaker.

The follow-up period of the patients ranged from a few months up to five years. During this period seven patients died. All patients who died had a prolonged H-V interval. However, death was always due to congestive heart failure. In one patient a complete A-V block occurred. This patient with LBBB had a H-V time of 72 ms at the time of the His bundle study in 1972. He received a pacemaker. In 1976 a complete A-V block was documented at the first time when the pacemaker was switched off by chest wall stimulation in the pacemaker clinic (Fig. 4).

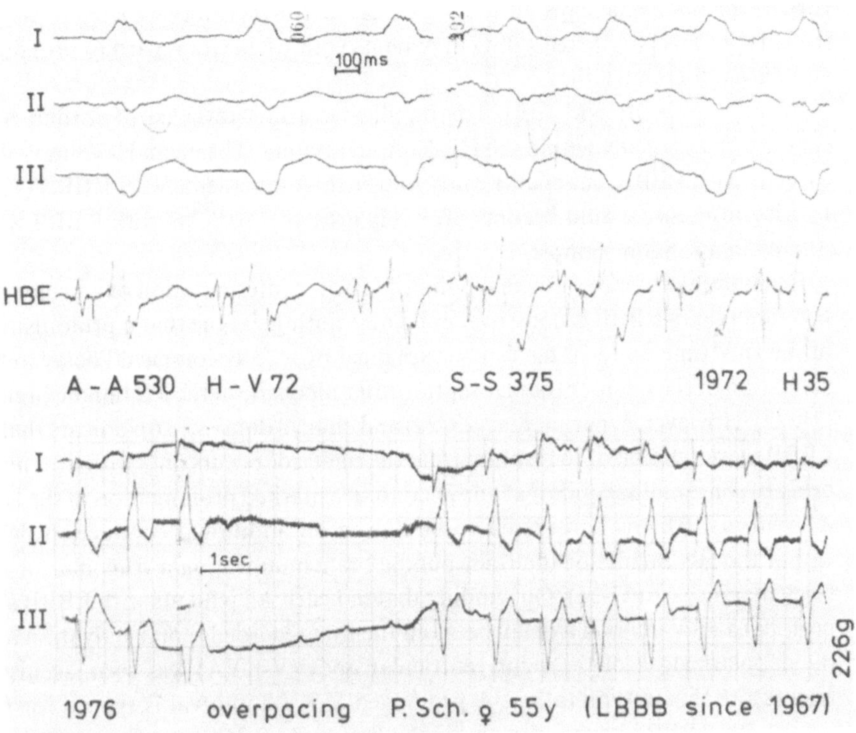

Figure 4. Development of complete A-V block in a patient with LBBB and prolonged H-V time four years after His bundle study. The upper panel shows the His bundle electrogram during sinus rhythm and atrial pacing in 1972. In the lower panel a complete A-V block is documented after switching off the pacemaker by chest wall stimulation in 1976

Discussion

Left bundle branch block has a bad prognosis. Some long-term studies have found a mean survival time of less than five years after documentation of LBBB (8, 9). Many of these patients develop congestive heart failure due to cardiomyopathy (10-13). In some patients the LBBB seems to be the first manifestation of heart disease whereas a CCM is developing some years later (11). In addition, the occurrence of complete A-V block in patients with LBBB was observed (11, 14) which may cause sudden death. However, other patients with LBBB seem to have a good prognosis not differing from those with RBBB (15-18). Even in some groups of patients with RBBB the prognosis is serious. Some studies (19, 20) have found a high incidence of sudden death in patients with surgically induced RBBB after heart operation. The purpose of our study was to find out possible clinical, electrophysiological or morphological differences in patients with

LBBB which may have prognostic significance. Furthermore we tried to clarify the value of His bundle recording in patients with BBB with regard to prognosis and pacemaker indication.

In many patients with BBB His bundle recording revealed abnormal A-V conduction especially within the His-Purkinje system. The mean H-V interval in patients with LBBB was significantly longer than in patients with RBBB (Tab. 1). The difference would become probably greater if patients with RBBB were studied in a random sample.

From the electrophysiological point of view the interpretation of a prolonged H-V interval in LBBB is controversial. Some authors argue that a prolongation of the H-V time up to 20 ms can be explained by a "physiological" delay in the activation of the interventricular septum after blockade of the left bundle branch (21, 22). However, experimental (23, 24) and clinical data (25, 26) indicate that in LBBB the activation of the septum from the right side occurs only with a minimal delay of some milliseconds if at all. Therefore, a marked prolongation of the H-V interval in LBBB is considered to be due to an additional conduction delay within the His bundle or the right bundle branch indicating a truncular or trifascicular disease (27-35). Our finding that in nearly all patients with LBBB and prolonged H-V interval a delay between the first recorded septal activation and the depolarization of the right ventricular apex (V-RVA) was seen, seems to underscore this interpretation. A prolonged V-RVA interval is typical for patients with RBBB in our series and in the literature (3,36). Castellanos et al. (3) found normal V-RVA interval in their patients with LBBB, but the authors did not give any comment on the H-V times in their patients. In addition, the constant normal H-V time in some patients with intermittent LBBB as observed in our study and by others (37, 38) demonstrates that the occurrence of block within the left bundle branch does not necessarily prolong H-V time. In patients with RBBB a prolonged H-V time is always due to an additional delay in the His bundle or left bundle branch.

In patients with LBBB the surface ECG was not a good indicator of the duration of the H-V interval. According to previous findings (32) a prolonged H-V interval was often seen in patients with first degree A-V block. However, as in other studies (31, 39, 40) a normal P-R interval did not exclude an abnormal H-V time. Neither the QRS axis (41) nor duration (42) was a reliable predictor for the H-V time. The same was stated by others (31, 43).

Significant differences in H-V time were found in some subgroups of patients with LBBB of different etiology. In the group of patients with CCM nearly all patients had a prolonged H-V interval, whereas in the other groups normal and abnormal values were found. In contrast to other findings (42) there was no difference in the mean H-V interval between patients with CHD and CCM. However, the mean H-V interval in patients with CCM on the one hand was significantly longer than in patients with LCM and with LBBB of unknown etiology on the other. Even in patients with LBBB without any other sign of heart disease prolonged H-V times were found. The abnormal morphological findings in the right ventricular myocardium of these patients suggest that both the conduction system and the ordinary myocardium are involved in the same pathologic process. One can only speculate that perhaps these patients with a prolonged H-V interval will develop CCM in the future.

Postmortem histological examinations were performed only in a few cases with LBBB who underwent His bundle studies. In three patients with LBBB and a prolonged H-V time, Rosen et al. (42) found a severe damage of the bundle of His and/or the right bundle branch in addition to the left bundle alterations. From our study only a correlation between the findings from myocardial biopsy and the electrophysiological data is possible. It was very surprising to find in all patients with LBBB without CHD or rheumatic lesions abnormal morphological alterations in the right ventricular myocardium. This indicates that in LBBB the ordinary myocardium and the conduction system of the left and right ventricle are involved in the same process. This is in agreement with other clinical findings indicating that "LBBB is the result of heart disease and is evidence of cardiac disease" (44). If the morphological score of the electron microscopic studies is compared to the H-V time, no strong correlation exists. However, patients with a normal H-V interval had only one to four points, whereas each patient with a score greater than four points showed a prolonged H-V interval. The data may indicate that the progression of the morphological changes goes hand in hand with the impairment of intraventricular conduction. Further studies are needed to support this thesis.

In patients with syncope, the H-V time was somewhat longer than in the others, even if the differences were not significant. The problem is that we are not able to distinguish whether or not the syncope is due to higher degree A-V block. In 10 patients with documented intermittent higher degree A-V block extremely abnormal conduction times were found. Two patients had very long A-H intervals. In the remaining cases the H-V interval was delayed between 72 ms and 190 ms. With one exception, all these patients showed an abnormal behaviour during atrial pacing. It is interesting that in some patients with block distal to the His potential during high rate test, the ERP HPS could not be measured by programmed atrial stimulation. In these cases either the block first occurred distal to the A potential or there was a one-to-one conduction up to the ERP A. This phenomenon is favoured by the fact that in some cases with LBBB the refractory periods of the His-Purkinje System are paradoxically prolonged with increasing heart rate (38, 45). Even if the refractoriness is normal, a prolonged H-V time indicates an impairment of intraventricular conduction. Because of the possible functional dissociation of conduction time and refractoriness of the His-

Purkinje system a short ERP HPS does not exclude an intraventricular conduction defect (25). It is noteworthy that three patients with RBBB and normal axis developed higher degree A-V block in our series. In two of these patients the block appeared after surgical correction of a tetralogy of Fallot. This underscores previous observations that some of these patients have a serious prognosis (19, 20).

It is evident from our study and those of others (31, 46, 47) that the majority of patients with BBB showing higher degree block distal to the H potential have a prolonged H-V interval during orthograde conduction. We feel that a very long H-V interval is a potential precursor of intraventricular block. However, our follow-up studies indicate that even in patients with a prolonged H-V time the progression to complete block is a rare event. On the other hand, in our study as well as in the study of Dhingra et al. (46) many patients with a prolonged H-V interval died of their underlying heart disease. In most of these patients we cannot influence the bad prognosis by pacemaker implantation. In a given patient the significance of a prolonged H-V time remains unsettled.

It is noteworthy that no complication occurred during His bundle studies even in patients with LBBB. Stiff multipolar catheters may damage the His bundle or right bundle branch leading to A-V block in these patients (31). This complication documented in the literature (49-51) occurred in our laboratory only during the introduction of the stiff biotome into the right ventricle. Therefore, we use only small flexible electrodes for recording of His bundle potentials.

Summary

In 73 patients with left bundle branch block (LBBB) the result of His bundle recording was compared with the clinical and hemodynamic data including coronary arteriography, ventriculography, and pulmonary arterial pressure measurement during exercise. In 31 patients with LBBB without coronary heart disease (CHD) or rheumatic valvular lesions right ventricular endomyocardial biopsy was performed. In addition 19 patients with right bundle branch block (RBBB) and normal QRS axis were studied by His bundle electrography. The patients with LBBB had a significantly longer H-V time (69.6 ± 20.2 ms) than patients with RBBB (52.7 ± 17.9 ms). There were significant differences in H-V interval between patients with LBBB and congestive cardiomyopathy (CCM) or CHD (78.8 ± 27.8 ms and 74.4 ± 16.3 ms resp.) on the one hand and patients with suspected latent cardiomyopathy (LCM) and with LBBB of unknown etiology on the other (63.2 ± 12.9 ms). In all ten patients with documented intermittent A-V block prior to or at the time of the study His bundle recordings revealed a very abnormal atrioventricular conduction. Two patients had a very long A-H time, eight patients a H-V interval between 72 ms and 190 ms. Therefore, a critically prolonged H-V time seems to be a potential precursor of intraventricular block.

The electron microscopic analysis of the specimen obtained by biopsy showed abnormal morphological changes of the ordinary myocardium in all patients with LBBB studied. This indicates that LBBB is the result of heart disease even in clinically normal patients.

During the follow-up period seven patients died. All patients had a prolonged H-V interval but death was due to congestive heart failure. One additional patient with a prolonged H-V interval developed complete A-V block. The data indicate that patients with a prolonged H-V interval have a bad prognosis, but the bad prognosis is due to the underlying myocardial disease. In a given patient the prognostic significance of a prolonged H-V interval remains unsettled.

References

1. Scherlag, B.J., Lau, S.H., Helfant, R.H., Berkowitz, W.D., Stein, E. & Damato, A.N., Catheter technique for recording His bundle activity in man. *Circulation* 39, 13 (1969).
2. Seipel, L., Both, A. & Loogen, F., Klinische Bedeutung der His-Bündel Elektrographie. *Klin. Wschr.* 53, 499 (1975).
3. Castellanos, A., Agha, A.S., Befeler, B., Castillo, C.A. & Berkovitz, B.V., A study of arrival of excitation at selected ventricular sites during human bundle branch block using close bipolar catheter electrodes. *Chest* 63, 208 (1973).
4. Wit, A.L., Wiss, M.B., Berkowitz, W.D., Rosen, K.M., Steiner, C. & Damato, A.N., Patterns of atrioventricular conduction in the human heart. *Circulation Res.* 27, 345 (1970).
5. Konno, S. & Sakakibara, S., Endomyocardial biopsy. *Dis. Chest* 50, 345 (1963).
6. Kuhn, H., Breithardt, G., Knieriem, H-J., Loogen, F., Endomyocardial catheter biopsy in heart disease of unknown etiology.
In: Kaltenbach, M. et al. (ed.) *Cardiomyopathies and myocardial biopsy*, Berlin 1977.
7. Loogen, F., Kuhn, H., Classification and natural history of primary cardiomyopathies. In: Riecker, G. et al. (ed.), *Myocardial failure*, Berlin 1977.
8. Johnson, R.P., Messer, A.D., Shreenivas & White, P.D., Prognosis in bundle branch block. II. Factors influencing the survival period in left bundle branch block. *Amer. Heart J.* 41, 225 (1951).
9. Smith, S., & Hayes, W.L., The prognosis of complete left bundle branch block. *Amer. Heart J.* 70, 157 (1965).
10. Blondeau, M., Le bloc complet de la branche gauche avec forte déviation axiale gauche de QRS. I Etude clinique. *Arch. Mal. Coeur* 67, 621 (1974).
11. Kuhn, H., Breithardt, L.K., Breithardt, G., Seipel, L., & Loogen, F., Die Bedeutung des Elektrokardiograms für die Diagnose und Verlaufsbeobachtung von Patienten mit kongestiver Kardiomyopathie. *Z. Kardiol.* 63, 916 (1974).
12. Schneider, J.F., Thomas, H.E., Kreger, B., McNamara, P., Left bundle branch block in Framingham. *Circulation Suppl.* 53-54/II, 128 (1976).

13. Wiberg, T., Gobel, F.L., & Richman, H.G., The significance and prognosis of bundle branch block. *Circulation suppl.* 49-50/III, 57 (1974).
14. Snyder, J.W., Basta, L.L., & Woolson, R.F., The relative risk of spontaneous complete atrioventricular block in elderly patients with impaired intraventricular conduction. *J. Electrocardiol.* 8, 95 (1975).
15. Messer, A.L., Johnson, R.P., & White, P.S., Prognosis in bundle branch block. III. Comparison of right and left bundle branch block with a note on the relative incidence of each. *Amer. Heart J.* 41, 239 (1951).
16. Rodstein, M., Gubner, R., Mills, J.P., Lovell, J.F., & Ungerleider, H.E., Mortality study in bundle branch block. *Arch. intern. Med.* 87, 663 (1951).
17. Rotman, M., & Triebwasser, J.H., A clinical and follow-up study of right and left bundle branch block. *Circulation* 51, 477 (1975).
18. Smith, R.F., Jackson, D.H., Harthorne, J.W., & Sanders, C.A., Acquired bundle branch block in a healthy population. *Amer. Heart J.* 80, 746 (1970).
19. Quattlebaum, T.G., Varghese, P.J., Neill, C.A., & Donahoo, J.S., Sudden death among postoperative patients with tetralogy of Fallot. *Circulation* 54, 289 (1976).
20. Wolff, G.S., Rowland, T.W., & Ellison, R.C., Surgically induced right bundle-branch block with left anterior hemiblock. *Circulation* 46, 587 (1972).
21. Haft, J.I., Weinstock. M., DeGuia, R., Gupta, P.K., Fano, A., Assessment of atrioventricular conduction in left and right bundle branch block using His bundle electrograms and atrial pacing. *Amer. J. Cardiol.* 27, 474 (1971).
22. Castellanos, A., H-V intervals in LBBB (Letter). *Circulation* 47, 1133 (1973).
23. Amer, N.S., Stukey, J.M., Hoffman, B.F., Cappelletti, R.R., & Domingo, R.T., Activation of the interventricular septal myocardium studied during cardiopulmonary bypass. *Amer. Heart J.* 59, 224 (1960).
24. Durrer, D., van Dam, T., Freud, G.E., Janse, M.J., Meijler, F.L., & Arzbacher, R.C., Total excitation of the isolated human heart. *Circulation* 41, 899 (1970).
25. Rosen, K.M., Rahimtoola, S.H., Sinno, M.Z., & Gunnar, R.M., Bundle branch and ventricular activation in man. *Circulation* 43, 193 (1971).
26. Narula, O.S., Javier, R.P., Samet, P (& Maramba, L.C., Significance of His and left bundle recordings from the left heart in man. *Circulation* 42, 385 (1970).
27. Berkowitz, W.D., Lau, S.H., Patton, R.D., Rosen, K.M., & Damato, A.N., The use of His bundle recordings in the analysis of unilateral and bilateral bundle branch block. *Amer. Heart J.* 81, 340 (1971).
28. Cannom, D.S., Goldreyer, B.N., & Damato, A.N., Atrioventricular conduction system in left bundle branch block with normal QRS axis. *Circulation* 46, 129 (1972).
29. Fleischmann, D., Mathey, D., Bleifeld, W., Irnich, W., & Effert, S., His-Bündel-Elektrographie bei Patienten mit intraventrikulären Leitungsstörungen. *Klin. Wschr.* 51, 1066 (1973).
30. Guérot, C., Coste, A., Valere, P.E., Motté, G., & Tricot, R., Enregistrement de l'activité du tronc du faisceau de His et de ses branches dans les troubles de conduction intraventriculaire. *Arch., Mal. Coeur* 66, 269 (1973).
31. Narula, O.S., Intraventricular conduction defects. In: Narula, O.S. (ed.), *His bundle electrocardiography and clinical electrophysiology*, Philadelphia 1975, p. 177.
32. Rosen, K.M., Rahimtoola, S.H., Chuquimia, R., Loeb, H.S., & Gunnar, R.M., Electrophysiological significance of first degree atrioventricular block with intraventricular conduction disturbance. *Circulation* 43, 491 (1971).
33. Scheinman, M., Weiss, A., & Kunkel, F., His bundle recordings in patients with bundle branch block and transient neurologic symptoms. *Circulation* 48, 322 (1973).

34. Vera, Z., Mason, D.T., Fletcher, R.D., Awan, N.A., & Massumi, R.A., Prolonged His-Q interval in chronic bifascicular block. *Circulation* 53, 46 (1976).
35. Wong, B.Y.S., & Dunn, M., Transient unifascicular, bifascicular and trifascicular block: Electrophysiologic correlation in a patient with rate-dependent left bundle branch block and transient right bundle branch block. *Amer. J. Cardiol.* 39, 116 (1977).
36. Kastor, J.A., Goldreyer, B.N., Moore, E.N., Shelburne, J.C., & Manchester, J.H., Intraventricular conduction in man studied with an endocardial electrode catheter mapping technique. *Circulation* 51, 786 (1975).
37. Cannom, D.S., Goodman, D.J., & Harrison, D.C., Electrophysiological studies in patients with rate-related intermittent left bundle branch block. *Brit. Heart J.* 36, 653 (1974).
38. Denes, P., Wu, D., Dhingra, R.C., Amat-y-Leon, F., Wyndham, C., & Rosen K.M., Electrophysiological observations in patients with rate-dependent bundle branch block. *Circulation* 51, 244 (1975).
39. Lang, K., Klinik der AV-Überleitungsstörungen. *Herz-Kreisl.* 9 82 (1977).
40. Puech, P., Corrélations entre les enregistrements de surface et l'électrogramme hisien. In: Seipel, L. et al. (ed.) *His-Bündel Elektrographie*, Stuttgart 1975, p. 91.
41. Spurrell, R.A.J., Krikler, D.M., & Sowton, E., Study of intraventricular conduction times in patients with left bundle-branch block and left axis deviation and in patients with left bundle branch block and normal QRS axis using His bundle electrograms. *Brit. Heart J.* 34, 1244 (1972).
42. Rosen, K.M., Ehsani, A., & Rahimtoola, S.H., H-V intervals in left bundle-branch block. *Circulation* 46, 717 (1972).
43. Waisser, E., Gaasch, W.H., Quinones, M.A., & Alexander, J.K., His bundle electrograms in patients with congestive cardiomyopathy. *Europ. J. Cardiol.* 2, 343 (1975).
44. Lamb, L.E., Kable, K.D., & Averill, K.H., Electrocardiographic findings in 67375 asymptomatic subjects V. Left bundle branch block. *Amer. J. Cardiol.* 6, 130 (1960).
45. Neuss, H., Thormann, J., & Schlepper, M., Electrophysiologic findings in frequency-dependent left bundle-branch block. *Brit. Heart J.* 36, 888 (1974).
46. Gupta, P.K., Chadda, L.D., Lichstein, E., Liu, H., & Sayeed, M., Intraventricular conduction time in patients with bundle branch block. *J. Electrocardiol.* 6, 181 (1973).
47. Ranganathan, N., Dhurandher, R., Philips, J.P., & Wigle, E.D., His bundle electrogram in bundle-branch block. *Circulation* 45, 282 (1972).
48. Dhingra, R.C., Denes, P., Wu, D., Wyndham, C.R., Amat-y-Leon, F., Town, W.D., & Rosen, K.M., Prospective observations in patients with chronic bundle branch block and marked H-V prolongation. *Circulation* 53, 600 (1976).
49. Jacobson, L.B., & Scheinman, M., Catheter-induced intra-Hisian and intrafascicular block during recording of His bundle electrogram. *Circulation* 49, 579 (1974).
50. Kimbris, D., Dreifus, L.S., & Linhart, J.W., Complete heart block occurring during cardiac catheterization in patients with preexisting bundle branch block. *Chest* 65, 95 (1974).
51. Levites, R., Toor, M., & Haft, J.I., Progressive improvement of His-Purkinje conduction during recovery from catheter-induced heart block. *Amer. Heart, J.* 91, 79 (1976).

SATRAP: A COMPUTER STUDY OF HIS BUNDLE POTENTIALS OBTAINED BY A NON-INVASIVE METHOD*

G. Fontaine, F. Gallais-Hamonno, R. Frank
and Y. Grosgogeat

His bundle recording, an essential element of modern clinical electrophysiology, has been the subject of much research in recent years (7, 8). The depolarisation of the Bundle of His is usually recorded with the use of transvenous endocavitary bipolar pacing catheters.

His bundle potentials are reduced to several microvolts during transmission to the surface. As a result, His bundle electrocardiography is very difficult, these potentials being of the same order as those originating from skeletal muscle depolarisation (1, 9).

The use of summation and averaging techniques introduced simultaneously by Berbari (1) and Stopczyk (10) has been a great advance in this field. This technique is applicable as the signal is in phase with ventricular depolarisation, while the muscle artefacts are random deflections. The same method has since been developed upon by several groups (3, 5, 6, 9).

A computer programme has been developed in our department to study electrophysiological signals by the averaging technique on a PDP 11 mini-computer. The programme, originally conceived to study the morphology of delayed potentials obtained with chest wall electrodes in patients with chronic ventricular tachycardia who had already undergone epicardial mapping (4), is also used in recording His bundle electrocardiogram.

The bipolar chest lead derivation of the ECG is fed into an amplifier fitted with a large gain control (G = 10000) and passive filters (15-100 Hz). A threshold detector synchronises the computer which displays the processed signal on a Tektronix 4010 console.

In summation averaging techniques, the problem of whether the signal recorded is the depolarisation of an atrio-ventricular structure or an artefact produced by muscular potentials often arises. Like Berbari (2), we have found by experience that the most reliable criterion is the reproducibility of the phenomena recorded. For this reason, four independent consecutive averaging series of 100 complexes have been included in our programme. The signals correspond-

* Supported in part by:
L'Association de Recherche et d'Entraide Cardiologique et Angéiologique (A.R.E.C.A.). La Caisse Régionale d'Assurances Maladie de Paris (C.R.A.M.P.).

ing to these four averaging series are presented in phase on the Tektronix 4010 screen on the same time scale.

The atrio-ventricular junctional activation observed is not the brief deflection of the His bundle electrogramme recorded by the endocavitary bipolar catheter but a wider deflection which may last tens of milliseconds. A typical example obtained from a patient with a long P-R interval is illustrated (Fig. 1).

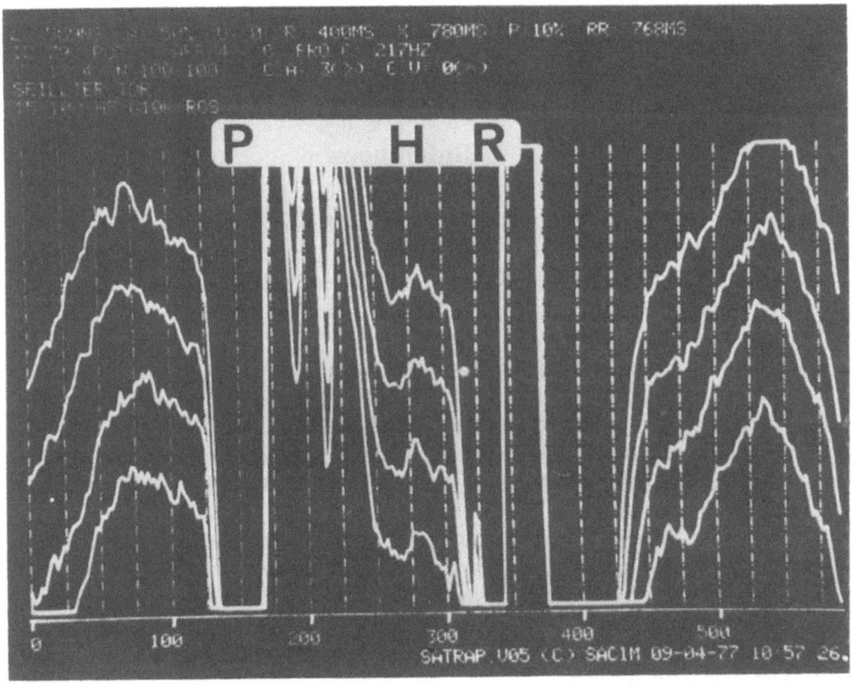

Figure 1. Four independent consecutive averaging series of surface potentials recorded from a bipolar sagittal lead in a 71 year old patient with normal P-R (0,18 s). The other items displayed on the picture document:

- Patient's name and arrhythmia. Filter setting and gain adjustment.
- Date, hour, minutes, seconds at the time of the display.
- Length of the display 589 ms.
- Adjustment of fiducial point with display 400 ms.
- Beat to beat interval at the time of the display 768 ms.
- Selection window for further upcoming beats. 780 ms ± 10% (Rejection of PVCS or change in the rhythm).
- Identification of the picture (No 79).
- Channel frequency 217 hertz.
- Number of beats in a series (100).
- Number of series on the display (4).
- Parameters for display adjustment.

When the first series is inscribed the remaining part of the display occurs automatically.

This technique is still at an experimental stage and not yet in routine use. The programme was conceived as a modular system and all parameters of signal treatment and display may be controlled during examination. They are initially set at standard default values. In its present version ventricular extrasystoles in phase with the QRS complexes or runs of muscular interference may upset the averaging process. The reliability of triggering also affects the quality of the result. Nevertheless, the development of the programme is still in progress and new modules will be added.

It would appear possible to develop in the near future a non-invasive device to monitor the evolution of atrio-ventricular conduction defects in ambulant patients.

References

1. Berbari E.J., Lazarra R., Samet P., Scherlag B.J., Non-invasive technique for detection of electrical activity during the P-R segment. Circulation 1973: 48, 1005.
2. Berbari E.J., Scherlag B.J., El-Sherif N., Befeler B., Aranda J.M., Lazarra R., The His Purkinje electrocardiogram in man: an initial assessment of its uses and limitations. Circulation 1976: 54, 219.
3. Damato A.N., Non-invasive methods for recording bundle of HIS activity. Amer. J. Cardiol. 1974: 33, 444.
4. Fontaine G., Guirandon G., Frank R., Vedel J., Grosgogeat Y., Cabrol C., Facquet J., Stimulation studies and epicardial mapping in ventricular tachycardia: study of mechanisms and selection for surgery. In: Reentrant arrhythmias, H. Kulbertus ed. MTP pub. Lancaster 1977.
5. Furness A., Sharratt G.P., Carson P. The feasibility of detecting HIS bundle activity from the body surface. Cardiovasc. res. 1975: 9, 390.
6. Hishimoto Y., Sawayama I., Non-invasive recording of HIS bundle potential in man, simplified method. Brit. Heart J. 1975: 37, 635.
7. Narula O.S., HIS bundle electrocardiography and clinical electrophysiology. F.A. Davis pub. Philadelphia 1975.
8. Puech P., Grolleau R., L'activité du faisceau de HIS normale et pathologique. Sandoz Pub. Paris 1972.
9. Ros H.H., Non-invasive detection of HIS bundle activity, thesis Amsterdam 1976.
10. Stopczyk M.J., Kope J., Zochowski R.J., Pieniak M., Surface recording of electrical heart activity during the PR segment in man by a computer averaging technique. IRCS Int. Res. Comm. System 1973.

A TECHNIQUE FOR NON-INVASIVE HIS-PURKINJE SYSTEM (HPS) RECORDING

J.K. Cywinski,* J.R. Mniece,* G.J. Ledee* and J. Ruskin**

Summary

Electrocardiograms were recorded from human volunteers using bipolar chest electrodes and standard leads I, II and III. The chest lead signals were amplified approx. 10^5 times, filtered and time-averaged over 128 consecutive beats. For signal conditioning and averaging, an analog- and digital microprocessor-based system was employed. The noise reduction resulting from the averaging technique permitted extraction of microvolt-range activity in the P-Q segment of the heart cycle otherwise regarded as silent. The recorded waveforms were triangular, approx. 5 msec in duration and 3-6 microvolts in amplitude. They preceded the ventricular depolarization complexes by 25-45 msec. On some volunteer patients, the externally-recorded waveform was compared with an internal electrogram recorded from an indwelling catheter. The correlation of events corresponding with internally-recorded His bundle activity was promising.

Introduction

Clinical recording of His-Purkinje System (HPS) activity by means of heart catheterization and pacing has opened a broad field of investigation into the origins and sites of rhythm disturbances. The heart catheterization procedure, however, is not usually done repeatedly, as would be necessary for trend analysis. Catheterization study results thus remain questionable as to whether findings are truly representative or changeable in time. Non-invasive recording methods are very attractive, as they permit harmless examinations to be carried out and allow studies to be repeated as often as desirable. Moreover, they would probably reduce catheterization work if capable of clarifying questionable situations. It is, therefore, not surprising that in several centers all over the world, non-invasive HPS recording has been under investigation since it was first reported by Berbari (1) and Stopczyk (2) in 1973. The aims of our study were to demonstrate the

* Dept of Medical Engineering, Massachusetts General Hospital, Boston, Mass.
** Cardiac Unit, Massachusetts General Hospital, Boston, Mass.

feasibility of developing a simple, portable, microprocessor-based instrument to serve this purpose routinely and to assess the correlation of externally recorded waveform events with corresponding simultaneous intracavitary recording from catheterized patients.

The electrical potentials resulting from HPS activity are present on the human body surface. Their amplitude is very small, experimentally recorded by Berbari (3) and theoretically predicted by Ross (4) to be in the order of a few microvolts. Such small amplitudes are usually obscured by electrical noise, which is in the order of 20 to 100 microvolts. By band-pass frequency filtering and coherent time-averaging, it is possible to improve the signal-to-noise ratio to distinguish HPS voltages from background noise.

Methods and instrumentation

Body surface HPS activity signals were recorded from bipolar nonstandard chest leads. Self-adhesive long-term monitoring pregelled disposable electrodes made of silver-silver chloride and manufactured by NDM[1] were used. In most cases, lead placement was as follows: (–)–anterior, 2 cm below mediasternal notch; RL, ground; (+)–anterior, 15 cm left of the sternum at the level of the 4th intercostal space. The signals from these electrodes were fed into a preamplifier (battery powered Ortec-Brookdeal Mod. 5001, low-noise) with a gain of 500. After being passed through an isolation amplifier (AD273K) and a bandpass single-pole filter, 5-1250 Hz (-3dB, 20 db/decade), the resulting signal was fed into a low-gain channel on an FM tape recorder (Vetter Model A). Simultaneously, the signal was further amplified by a factor of 100 using an LM 741 operational amplifier and fed into a high-gain channel on the same tape recorder. Recording was done at a speed of 7½ ips which resulted in signal high frequency cutoff at 700 Hz.

With catheterized patients, a His bundle electrogram was tape-recorded along with the standard three-lead electrocardiogram. An intracardiac bipolar catheter with two ring electrodes 1 cm apart was used. The multichannel E for M Mod. VR6 recorder with V1203/V1251 and V1201 ECG preamplifiers performed conditioning of the respective signals.

After acquiring analog data from 9 catheterized patients and approx. 25 non-catheterized volunteers (surface leads only) and storing it on magnetic tape in the above-mentioned fashion, the signals were played back for further filtration, digitization and averaging, and display. The high gain recorded signals were band-pass (5-300 Hz) filtered by a Mod. 330 MR Krohn-Hite four-pole electronic filter (24 dB/octave) and then fed to a 12 bit analog-to-digital converter interfaced with an Intel 8080 microprocessor system. The digital sampling rate

[1] NDM Corporation, Dayton, Ohio.

was 2 kHz, corresponding to .5 msec per sample. In order to coherently average HPS activity, it was essential to trigger from the QRS waveform consistently and accurately. Signals recorded in the low-gain channels were used for this purpose. Jitter and detrimental effects of baseline shifts when using analog triggers, as described by Brandon & Brady and referenced by Berbari (3), led us to devise a digital QRS-trigger program within the microprocessor system itself. This also helped to reduce slightly the amount of auxiliary hardware in the playback/analysis system. HPS signals were then averaged for 128 consecutive heart beats.

Basically, our QRS digital detection scheme mimics the visual recognition of QRS onset. The processor interpolates the baseline and the first slope of the R-wave and then identifies the intersection of the two lines as the onset of QRS and the digital triggering point.

Specifically, the microprocessor QRS detection program first searches for 8 consecutive steps of the same sign and greater than a predetermined value. After finding such a sequence, it calculates the average slope per sample (ASR) from the last four samples and identifies the last sample as the rough QRS detection point (RQRS). The program then averages the values from 64 samples to 32 samples before RQRS (16 msec) and labels this the baseline (BLL). It then takes the value of the sample at RQRS and iteratively subtracts ASR until the value is less than BLL. The number of iterations is subtracted from RQRS and this point is labelled the accurate QRS (AQRS) and serves as the fiducial marker for subsequent coherent time averaging of all data stored in the circular buffer for the 236 msec preceding AQRS and 20 msec after that event. Such a digital QRS detection scheme produces negligible jitter, although its extent has not yet been evaluated.

Results and discussion

Representative recordings from one catheterized patient are shown in Figure 1. The bottom trace represents an HPS surface recording taken simultaneously with an HBE intracardiac recording (middle trace). The intracardiac catheter was positioned along the septum in the right ventricle while being confirmed radiologically. Although the HPS waveform is not easily interpretable, it clearly shows electrical activity slightly preceding, then coinciding, and then following the intracardiac HBE spike. Further complexity of HPS waveform interpretation is added by a relatively irreproducible morphology from one patient to another. A representative recording from another patient, markedly different from that in Figure 1, is shown in Figure 2. This patient had complete P-wave dissociation, so P-activity is not visible on the tracing. Both cases, though differ-

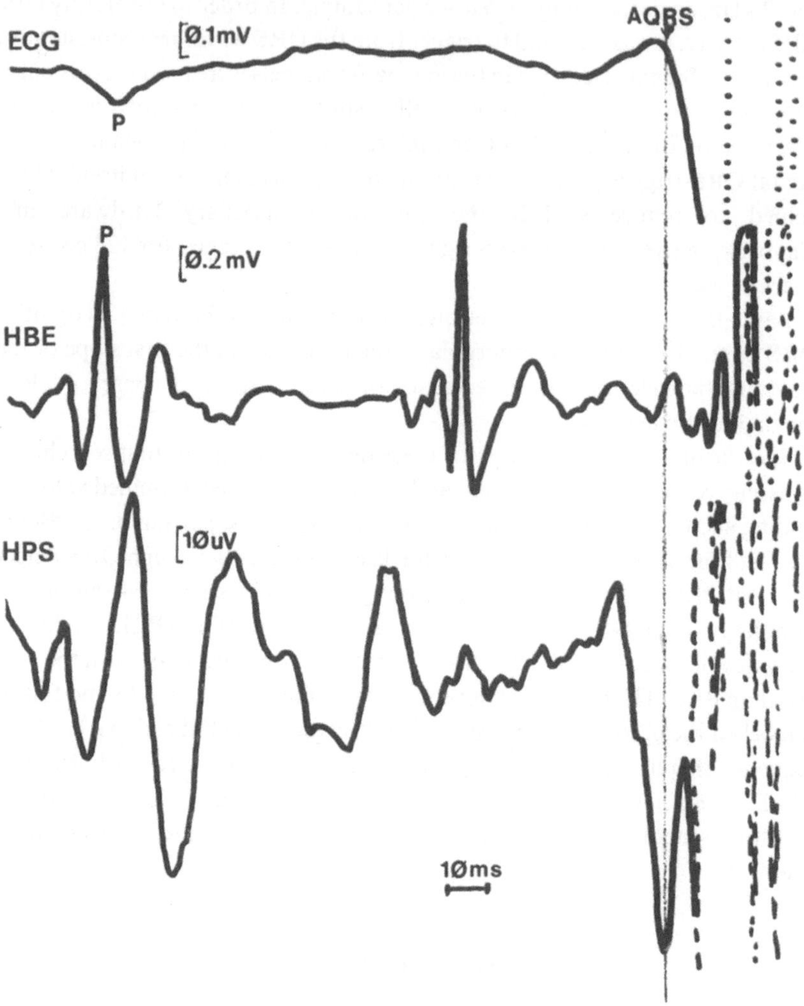

Figure 1. Simultaneous high gain (HPS) and low gain (ECG) surface and intracavitary (HBE) recording in man. AQRS-trigger point (see text).

ing remarkably, have a common characteristic, as evident in the HPS tracings: There is electrical activity, in the microvolt amplitude range, coinciding with, and slightly preceding and following the electrical activity recorded intracavitally as the His bundle electrogram.

Further studies on lead placement, noise reduction techniques and clinical correlations are in progress, as the results obtained thus far are promising. Furthermore, the use of an inexpensive microprocessor-based system, as reported by Dennis & Cywinski (5) for future HPS studies has proven its feasibility and may make this method a valuable clinical tool, aiding the diagnosis of heart rhythm disturbances.

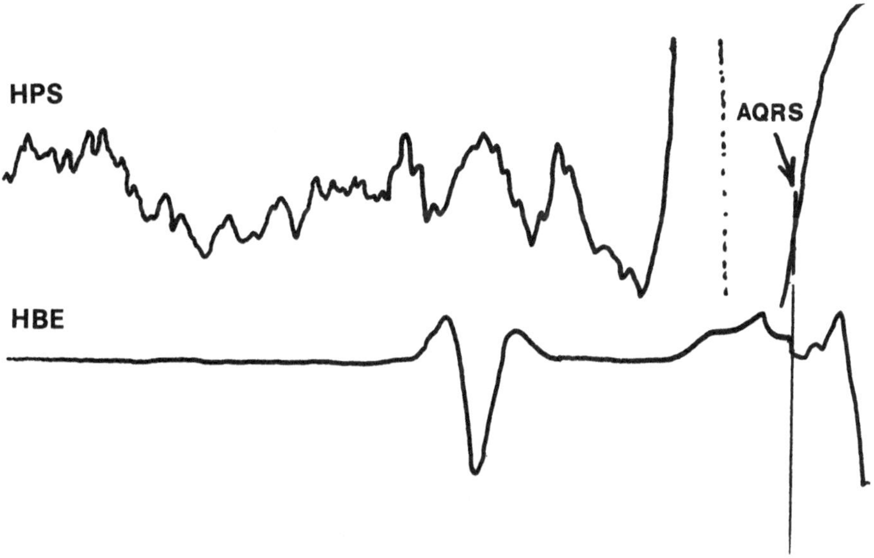

Figure 2. Simultaneous high gain (HPS) surface and intracavitary (HBE) recording in man with P-dissociation. Scale and legend same as on Fig. 1.

References

1. Berbari, E.J., Lazzara, R., Samet, P., Scherlag, B.J. Non-invasive technique for detection of electrical activity during the P-R segment. *Circulation* 48: 1005-1013 (1973).
2. Stopczyk, M.J., Kopec, J., Zochowski, R.J., Pieniak, M. Surface recording of electrical heart activity during the P-R segment in man by a computer averaging technique. *International Research Communication System*, August, 1973.
3. Berbari, E.J., Scherlag, B.J., El-Sherif, N., Befeler, B., Aranda, J.M., Lazzara, R. The His-Purkinje electrocardiogram in man: An initial assessment of its uses and limitations. *Circulation* 54: 219-224 (1976).
4. Ross, H.H. *Non-invasive detection of His bundle activity.* Vrije Universiteit te Amsterdam, 1976.
5. Dennis, J.H., Cywinski, J.K. The use of microprocessor for non-invasive recording of electrical activity from the conduction system of the heart. In: *Proc. 29th Ann. Conf. Engineering in Med. & Biol.*, Nov., 1976.

DISCUSSION I. CONDUCTION SYSTEM

Chairman: S. Sequerra Amram *(Lisbon, Portugal)*

J.G. Sloman *(Melbourne, Australia)*: Mr. Chairman, I would like to say that I think this morning's session has been really a very excellent exposition of the state of the art of His Bundle Recording and its value in clinical cardiology. I would like to just very briefly emphasize the point that Dr. Narula made about the fact that we can only use the information if we are entirely certain that the study has been carried out adequately. I make this point because, on a number of figures we have seen this morning, the multiple-channel technique – which I think we all accept must be used – has not been utilized to the greatest extent. I think it is very, very important that there must be multiple external ECG leads, three at least and preferably four, five or six, so that you get the right time for your ventricular depolarization. I also saw – and perhaps this is rude of me to say it – a number of His Bundle Recordings this morning where you have only one channel of the His Bundle at one frequency response.

If we are going to develop this technique more, I think that we also must have many more, perhaps two, three or four different frequency recordings of our His Bundle potential. If you are to measure things accurately, this is absolutely essential. I bring this to your attention because I think we in this group and in the International Society on Cardiac Pacing and Electrophysiology must set the standards for correct adequate scientific recording of intra-cardiac potentials.

L. Seipel *(Düsseldorf, E.R. Germany)*: I cannot see any value in recording the His Bundle Potential at different frequencies. What is the value of these recordings? I cannot see this from the clinical viewpoint. If we have a good His potential and you are recording this with a usual frequency, then I cannot see any advantage of multiply recordings of the His Potential at different frequencies.

O.S. Narula *(Chicago, U.S.A.)*: I am glad to hear the comment of Dr. Sloman, because that has been my biggest beef all these years: that we will destroy the technique if it is not used meticulously. I think if you are going to do these recordings for diagnostic purposes and to decide about a patient's fate, it must be done properly and multiple ECG leads must be used as everybody has accepted, I assume. This morning I wanted to stress the point that if you let a trainee perform a His Bundle study, without supervision of an expert, he is simply excited to find a potential on the screen and may not explore the region further. A large amplitude of a potential does not always mean that we have the proximal portion of the His Bundle; the anatomic area of the His Bundle must be explored thoroughly. His Bundle pacing must be used to validate the H potential. I think you have a better chance of getting an appropriate recording if you do not use a pre-formed catheter. Every heart has a variable anatomy and if you use a non-pre-formed catheter it will adapt to the curvature of the heart in a given patient. True, it does make life easier with a pre-formed catheter to go from the right atrium to the right ventricle, but it certainly ruins the study.

S. SEQUERRA AMRAM *(Lisbon, Portugal):* Could you be more specific about the point that Dr. Sloman made; do you think it is really important to have multiple His Bundle electrograms at different frequencies?

O.S. NARULA *(Chicago, U.S.A.):* Dr. Scherlag has done quite a bit of work in this area and we have also explored the possibility of using different filter settings to find if the H-V does vary. We did not find any differences in H-V at different frequencies. I have to agree with Dr. Kulbertus – that using different frequency ranges does not offer any advantage. I want to stress again, however, that the most crucial part is exploration and the recording of the most proximal portion of the His Bundle.

S. SEQUERRA AMRAM *(Lisbon, Portugal):* Thank you, that is also what we have found in our laboratory. The use of different frequencies for the His Bundle recordings can give cleaner tracings, but without significant changes in the H-V intervals. On the other hand the importance of recording simultaneously at least 4 surface leads deserves to be emphasized.

DR. S. FURMAN *(New York, U.S.A.):* May I support some of the statements made by Dr. Narula. For the past three years we have carefully studied patients with symptoms suggestive of Stokes-Adams Syndrome but who have had no evidence of fixed or intermittent heart block, sick sinus syndrome or any other cardiac or neurologic basis for syncope. Though some of the patients had electrocardiographic evidence of fascicular block, none had any demonstrated periods of tachycardia or bradycardia to account for the neurologic manifestations during any non-invasive examinations including observation in a monitored unit and prolonged Holter monitoring. In the absence of these findings a thorough, exacting His bundle study was performed.

If A-V block was demonstrated during the study a pacemaker was implanted. If block was not demonstrated the patients were implanted at the discretion of the referring cardiologist, as we could not recommend pacer implant on the duration of the H-V interval alone. Both those implanted and not were divided into five groups according to the duration of the H-V time; under 55 msec. (no implants); 55-60 msec. and 65 msec. and above.

Of the patients with an H-V interval of 55 msec. or less all have survived and none have shown late heart block. Of those with an H-V of 55-60 msec., half were implanted and half not. Of the unpaced, one third died suddenly or showed progression to heart block. Of the paced, none died suddenly. Of the groups with an H-V interval of 65 msec. or over the results were more striking. In the unpaced group half died suddenly or progressed to heart block, in the paced group there were no sudden deaths. All differences were statistically significant.

We now feel that the His Bundle study is very valuable in the symptomatic patient without documented heart block to determine which are at risk. The presence of fascicular block could not assist in making a decision about implant before the His Bundle study.

S. Sequerra Amram *(Lisbon, Portugal):* Thank you Dr. Furman for this additional information. I would like to ask Dr. Kulbertus if he has found A-V or intra-ventricular conduction disturbances in sino-atrial disease, in the absence of pathologic lesions at the junctional region and below.

H. Kulbertus *(Liège, Belgium):* As it has been pointed out, the number of patients with so-called sinus node disease who come to autopsy is very small.

Another difficulty is that we did not have electro-physiological studies before death in the six cases that I have shown this morning. So, I really cannot answer your question.

K. Lang *(Mainz, F.R. Germany):* I would like to ask Dr. Narula and the members of the panel about carotid sinus pressure. If you do carotid sinus pressure and you find that it produces marked sinus arrest or A-V block, do you then think that this does not mean that the cardiac conduction system is diseased or do you think that it has some bearing on this process?

O.S. Narula *(Chicago, U.S.A.):* My comments pertaining to carotid sinus stimulation were meant for sinus nodes alone, and not to evaluate the A-V conduction system. The problem which I have addressed myself to many times is: What is the degree of carotid sinus stimulation we must apply to say "This is the period of asystole which is enough." It will vary from individual to individual; some physician may be more aggressive and may even in a normal person produce an asystole. So it is complicated, but if you can give the gentlest stimulation and find a long period of asystole, and if atropine asystole cannot be reproduced, with the same degree of carotid sinus stimulation, in my opinion that would definitely confirm the diagnosis of hypersensitive sinus node. I do not think we can evaluate atrio-ventricular conduction with carotid sinus stimulation.

M. Bilitch *(Los Angeles, U.S.A.):* Dr. Narula pointed out in one figure that he had an H-V interval ranging from 35 to 65 and he said that, in his opinion the right H-V each time was 65. What was your criterion for your selection that time? Did you do His Bundle pacing to find this answer? Because from the slide it looked as if it also could have been atrial potentials.

O.S. Narula *(Chicago, U.S.A.):* The time did not permit me to show slides on every patient. However, in every single patient, atrial pacing must be done to separate "A" and His potentials. So the one in which we measured an H-V time of 65 milliseconds, there was nothing between His and the "A" potential. As the "A" potential was differentiated by pacing, the other potential had to be the His potential. I am a firm believer and proponent of performing His pacing for validation of His potentials. In all our patients we do His pacing. The H-V of 65 was validated by His pacing in the patient referred to by Dr. Bilitch.

S. Sequerra Amram *(Lisbon, Portugal):* Unfortunately we do not have time for more questions. But before we finish, I would like to ask Dr. Seipel the following. He mentioned that the prognosis in fascicular block with a prolonged H-V time was related to the underlying cardiac disease of pathology. Does he mean that death is specifically related to the occurrence of syncopal episodes or other manifestations of heart disease?

L. Seipel *(Düsseldorf, F.R. Germany):* I can only say from the patients we have studied, that all patients who died did so from congestive heart failure and not from A-V block. We have never seen a sudden death in any patient. We have seen some patients with a left bundle branch block and further complete normal findings who developed a cardiomyopathy some years later. I think that left bundle branch block is a potential precursor of cardiomyopathy in many patients and the bad prognosis at these patients is due to the myocardial disease.

It is also demonstrated in the Framingham study, as presented last year in Miami, that follow-up of patients with left bundle branch block, showed congestive heart failure in many patients. I think these are in principle the same results. Our electron microscopic studies also show the same results, i.e., that patients with left bundle branch block have extremely abnormal morphological findings. I think the reports in which it is stated that the left bundle branch blocks have a very bad prognosis – 3.3 up to 5 years – is due to cardiomyopathy in these patients. But we also should be aware of the fact that there are other studies, for examplc by the U.S. Air Force, where these patients had a good prognosis of over 10 years. Therefore we have to be careful with final and overall conclusions.

S. Sequerra Amram *(Lisbon, Portugal):* Thank you Dr. Seipel. Dr. Kulbertus would you like to make any comment on this same subject?

H. KULBERTUS *(Liège, Belgium):* When you look for LBBB in population studies, its distribution curve appears to be double peaked when you have a sufficient number of cases. It seems that, in women, LBBB may more often be a simple concomitant of ageing than in men. But, between the ages of 50 and 60, you have a bump in the distribution curve which is due to the presence of male individuals with coronary heart disease or cardiomyopathy. I therefore agree with Dr. Seipel that the group with LBBB shows an overall higher mortality rate possibly due to the presence of cases with coronary disease, or myocardial disease. When it is related to ageing, LBBB is likely to be of better prognosis.

S. SEQUERRA AMRAM *(Lisbon, Portugal):* Thank you Dr. Kulbertus for this additional information. We have to close this section now. I thank you all for your most interesting contributions to the field of cardiac conduction.

Section II

TO PACE OR NOT TO PACE

CARDIAC PACING IN SICK SINUS SYNDROME

HILBERT J.TH. THALEN

Introduction

In a premier essay on ventricular fibrillation published in 1887, the famous physiologist John Mc.William (1) wrote:

"It may, in any case, be safely affirmed that the spontaneous contraction in the mammalian heart arises in the terminal (or ostial) portions of the great veins either exactly at their junction with the auricles, or in the walls of the veins at some little distance from the actual junction." In 1907 Keith and Flack (2), a medical student at that time, identified an aggregate of cells at the sino-atrial location exactly where Mc.William had predicted that the master pacemaker of the heart resided. They called it "the Primum mobile," the sino-atrial node (SAN) or pacemaker of the heart located at the antero-lateral junction of the superior vena cava with the base of the right atrial appendage.

Dysfunctions of this sino-atrial node like sino-atrial block and paroxysmal atrial fibrillation had already been described in 1916 by Levine (3), whereas Short (4) described the alternating sinus bradycardia-tachycardia phenomenon in 1954. Ten years ago Lown (5) reported that after cardioversion of atrial fibrillation certain patients showed a very slow sinus rhythm or no sinus rhythm at all. He called this abnormal response of the sinus node the "somnolent" or the "sick sinus." Ferrer (6, 7, 8) studied the sinus nodal dysfunctions more closely and reported in 1968 that these dysfunctions, referred to as the sick sinus syndrome (SSS), were not rare, but difficult to diagnose. The many publications (9, 10, 11) of the last decennia, especially Ferrer's monograph (6) published in 1974, have increased our knowledge on the sick sinus syndrome and indicated new diagnostic and therapeutic approaches. In this last respect cardiac pacing has found an increasing application and by now various centers report that arrhythmias of the sick sinus syndrome make up for 20-40% of their pacemaker indications (12, 13, 14, 15).

The sick sinus syndrome

The *arrhythmias of the sick sinus syndrome* can be classified in:

A. Generator failure of the sinus node, with:
1) intermittent or permanent sinus bradycardia;
2) intermittent or permanent cessation of sinus rhythm (sinus arrest) with or without atrial (a.o. flutter or fibrillation), junctional or ventricular escape rhythms;
3) combination of the above in the bradycardia-tachycardia syndrome;
4) permanent cessation of the sinus rhythm and replacement by atrial fibrillation often associated with a slow ventricular rate due to accompanying atrio-ventricular nodal disease; with
5) no or a very slow sinus rhythm after cardioversion.

B. Sino-atrial exit block, with or without atrial, junctional or ventricular escape rhythms.

In many instances the dysfunction of the sino-atrial node is associated with other conduction disorders like total atrio-ventricular heartblock (16, 17) about one third according to some authors (18, 19) – and intraventricular conduction defects.

For analysis of the *etiology of the sick sinus syndrome* certain influences should be excluded like primary vagotonia, high potassium levels, nicotine and drugs like digitalis and beta blockers.

The sick sinus syndrome itself is usually not caused by primary cell damage, but by secondary necrosis of the sino-atrial nodal cells commonly due to ischaemia caused by atherosclerotic lesions of the large coronary arteries. In this respect it is important to realize that the sino-atrial node receives its blood supply from the largest single atrial artery, which arises from the right (RCA) or left circumflex (CX) coronary arteries (20). Occlusion of the left anterior descending artery (LAD) with anteroseptal infarction is therefore seldom associated with arrhythmias of the sick sinus syndrome, but anterolateral infarction and especially inferior infarction are in many cases associated with sinus nodal arrhythmias. Rosketh and Hatle reported in 1971 that out of 32 patients with sick sinus syndrome 31 had experienced inferior infarctions (21).

Other vascular diseases, that affect the coronary arteries, can cause SSS arrhythmias like rheumatic and inflammatory conditions, acute and chronic coronary artery occlusions, myocarditis, pericarditis and cardiomyopathies. Ferrer (6) summarized also musculoskeletal diseases, infiltrative diseases (e.g. amyloïdosis) and diphtheria as causes.

Clinical manifestations of the sick sinus syndrome (6, 14, 17) originate from the intermittent or persistent arrhythmia, resulting in diminished cardiac output. Cerebral hypoperfusion manifests itself in dizziness, syncopal attacks or in less severe cases in personality changes, memory losses or periods of lightheadedness.

Other more general manifestations are fatigue, mild cardiac failure sometimes with episodes of respiratory distress due to pulmonary edema and changes in the pattern of micturition.

Diagnosis of the sick sinus syndrome may be difficult, due to its – many times intermittent – pattern. Special tests have been devised to provoke malfunctioning of the sinus node (22), viz.

1) administration of *atropine* intravenously in doses between 1 and 2 mgms. should not increase the slow sinus rate over 90/min.
2) administration of *isoproterenol* (1-2 mgr. in 500 ml. 5% dextrose (in water)) by intravenous drip (from 15 drips/min.) should not increase the sinus rate over 90-100/min.

Both methods have their disadvantages (a.o. arrhythmias from various origin) and do not provide very reliable answers. Sometimes the sinus rate may increase despite the fact that a dysfunctioning sinus node is involved.

3) The response to *atrial pacing with overdrive suppression* seems more promising (23, 24, 25).

With this test the atrium is stimulated for 2-4 minutes at rates between 120-140 imp./min. Then pacing is abruptly stopped and the delay until the first sinus beat is measured. The occasional atrial or junctional escape beat is not taken into account. The degree of overdrive suppression of the sinus node is correlated with the resting rate and can best be expressed as a percentage of the resting rate control cycle.

Probably due to an increase in the parasympathetic tone this overdrive suppression may also be seen in normals. Critical percentages exist for various control cycle frequencies. At low frequencies of 45/min. the critical percentage is somewhere around 120% of the control cycle; at frequencies of 60/min. and higher about 125%. Higher percentages indicate sinus nodal dysfunction. Some authors indicate an absolute time period despite the basic frequency. Escape intervals longer than this period of 1400 msec. suggest sinus nodal dysfunction. Sometimes they combine the test with the administration of atropine i.v. (26).

All of these tests do not, however, give a clear answer to the question of whether SSS is involved since many times the sino-atrial nodal dysfunction is temporary and can give normal responses during the periods in between.

4) The best method to diagnose sinus nodal dysfunction is to record the electrocardiogram during episodes of clinical symptoms (15, 27, 28). To get this

recording *electrocardiographic scanning* (Holter monitoring) or monitoring in the coronary care unit is our main diagnostic tool, except for patients who present themselves with severe sinus bradycardia or persistent atrial fibrillation with ventricular bradycardia, without direct causes like drug therapy or electrolyte imbalance.

The increase in the application of cardioscanning and the increase in the knowledge of the sick sinus syndrome has resulted in a still increasing number of SSS-patients, who needed treatment with cardiac stimulation.

Table 1. Indications for primary pacemaker-implantation during 1976 in the Pacemaker-clinic (Dept. of Cardiology and Dept. of Thoracic Surgery) University Hospital, Groningen (The Netherlands). Note the high incidence of Adams-Stokes attacks in the group with SSS.

		with Adams-Stokes attacks
Total AV Block	35 = 42%	45%
2nd degr. AV Block	7 = 9%	43%
Bundlebranch Block	12 = 15%	50%
RBBB	1	
RBBB + LAH	5	
RBBB + LAH + 1st degr. AV Block	3	
LBBB + 1st degr. AV Block	3	
Sick Sinus Syndrome	28 = 34%	65%
Sinus bradycardia	7	
SA Block	3	
Sinus Arrest	7	
Sinus Arrest + VES	3	
Sinus Arrest + 1st degr. AV Block	3	
Brady-Tachycardia	3	
Atrial Fibrillation	2	
Total	82 = 100%	

It can be seen from table I, which shows the indications for the first pacemaker implantations in 1976 in the Groningen clinic, that from the group with SSS, 2 out of every 3 patients had Adams-Stokes attacks. This means that mostly patients with severe clinical manifestations have been diagnosed. It seems reasonable to assume that sofar we have not identified the total group of patients with the SSS – such as patients with minor clinical manifestations – and that in the future this group of patients will further increase.

Therapy of the sick sinus syndrome

Although temporarily *pharmacological treatment* with drugs like atropine or isoproterenol may increase the heart rate moderately in emergency cases, the long-term use of drugs alone is mostly unsatisfactory (29).

At the present time, *cardiac pacing* is the treatment of choice for the bradyarrhythmias. When tachyarrhythmias occur long-term cardiac pacing is usually combined with digitalis and at the normal blood level (1.4 ± 0.7 ngm/ml) this is usually insufficient, also beta blockers (e.g. propranolol 4 × 10 or 20 mgm p.o. per day eventually higher) may be added till an acceptable result has been achieved (6, 13).

Complications with cardiac pacing in sick sinus syndrome

Cardiac pacing in sick sinus syndrome can produce two problems, one haemodynamic and the other an electrophysiologic complication.

1. *Haemodynamic complication*

In about one third of patients with SSS, other conduction defects like total AV block – caused by a double nodal disease – or intraventricular conduction defects can exist, as previously mentioned. Therefore and because of the intermittent pattern of the sinus nodal dysfunctions, the selected pacing mode is in most cases R-wave inhibited (or demand) ventricular pacing.

In these patients the sinus nodal frequency sometimes may be around the frequency of the implanted pacemaker. This can result in large changes of the blood pressure, caused by dysfunction of the atrio-ventricular heart valves due to the pacemaker electrical-induced depolarisation of the ventricles and sinus node induced depolarisation of the atria and to a lesser extent to the retrograde intraventricular depolarisation pattern (fig. 1A).

Due to this phenomenon Harthorne (31) could reproduce in one of his patients systolic blood pressure changes of about 120 mmHg. The patient experienced syncope even after the implantation of a ventricular R-wave inhibited pacemaker, that was proven to function properly. In the Boston series Harthorne found 3 patients with this complication. In our Groningen series we found 2 patients.

The *treatment* of the complication can be approached from two sides.

In the Boston group Harthorne changed the ventricular demand pacing system to an atrial demand pacing system (fig. 1B) or in the case of a complicating AV conduction defect in atrio-ventricular sequential pacing (32).

In our Groningen group we changed one temporary ventricular demand system for an atrial demand system. Our second patient, who complained of dizziness and not clear syncope and who demonstrated blood pressure changes of about 40-60 mmHg could be treated pharmacologically by decreasing the sinus rhythm with beta blockers (propranolol). The patient became asymptomatic on this therapy with a continuously stimulating pacemaker.

The ideal pacing system for these SSS patients would be an atrial demand – ventricular demand system, preferably with programmable frequencies, but this is not available at the moment in an implantable version (34).

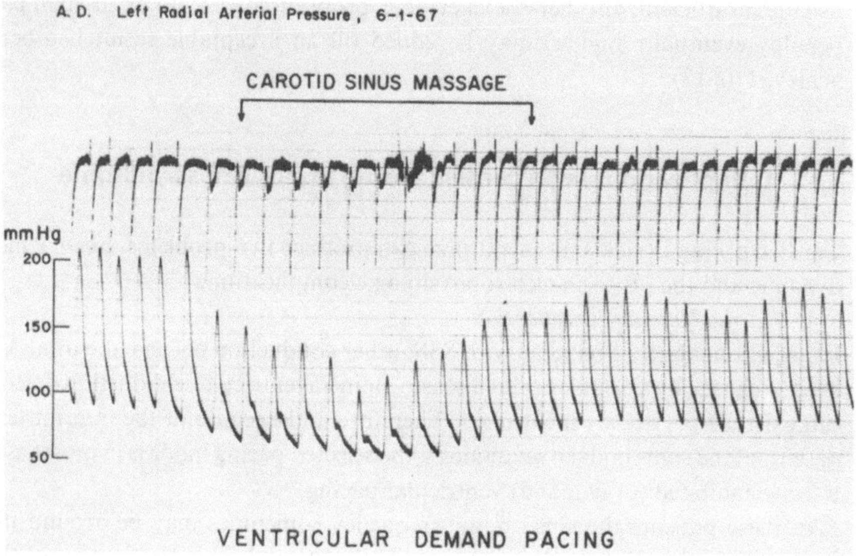

Figure 1A. Intra arterial recording of blood pressure with ventricular demand pacing in SSS. The recording with the patient lying supine shows pressure changes of over 120 mmHg.

2. *Electrophysiological complication*

The best treatment at the moment is therefore atrial or ventricular inhibited pacing with or without pharmacologic treatment or the more complicated atrio-ventricular sequential pacing.

All ventricular inhibited systems are not identical. Some systems are designed in such a way that atrial or ventricular tachycardias can initiate pacemaker malfunctioning. For an understanding of this complication we have to analyse the pacemaker sensing circuit and the anti-interference circuit. The sensing circuit has as its function the detection of the proper heart activity via the cardiac electrode. The electrophysiological signals of the heart depolarisation, in fact the depolarisation waves, R-waves, that pass along the electrode, have various configurations depending upon the localization of the electrode in the heart, the physiology of the myocardial tissue and the electrode applied. (33).

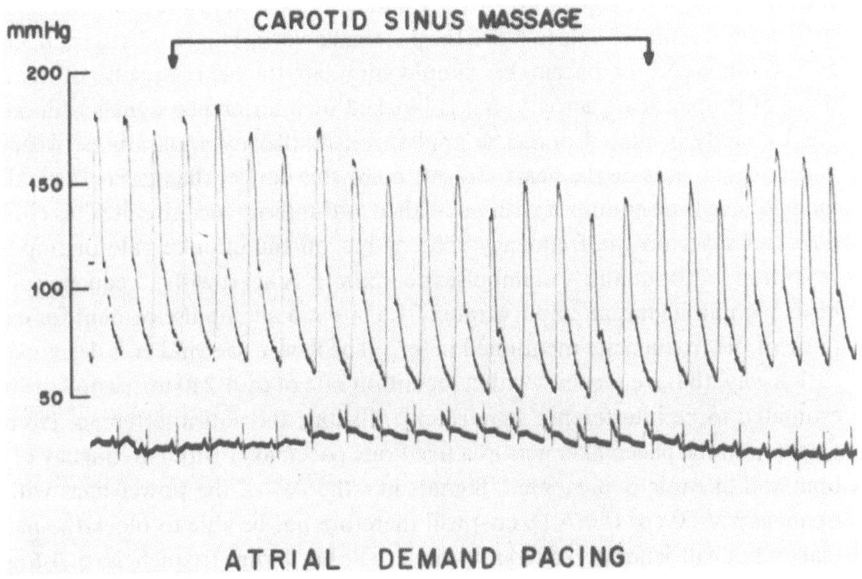

Figure 1B. Intra arterial recording of blood pressure in the same patient from fig. 1A during atrial demand pacing shows pressure changes of 40 mmHg due to the effect of the carotis massage on heart rate and peripheral resistance (courtesy Dr. Harthorne).

As pacemakers are made for general use, this means that the sensing circuit has to be able to detect a variety of signals for proper functioning. The most important part of the myocardial signal that is used for sensing, is the intrinsic deflection at the detecting electrode, that means the fast negative sweep. This negative sweep is determined by its frequency and its amplitude. (dv/dt)

The most frequently used frequency of this signal is estimated to be between 20-50 cps, but lower and higher frequencies have been recorded and scatterings between 10-100 cps are not uncommon e.g. in case of infarction lower frequencies have been found. The signal also has an amplitude, that varies with implantation time of the electrode (in reverse to the threshold it decreases after the initial implantation and then stabilises after some weeks) (34), electrode type (higher signals for intramural electrodes, lower for endocardial electrodes) and as has been demonstrated recently with the atrial frequency (a higher frequency entailing a higher amplitude) (35).

Because of these reasons the pacemaker manufacturer has to make a choice for the sensitivity frequency and amplitude. Signals above the characteristic line are sensed by the sensing circuit and are able to block the pacemaker.

It is clear that other signals above the frequency and amplitude characteristic of the sensing circuit are able to block the pacemaker also. This entails the danger of an asystole when the pacemaker should stimulate the heart because of the absence of proper heart activity, but is blocked by interference signals generated e.g. by badly insulated domestic appliances, diathermy apparatuses, weapon detectors etc. outside the heart. To overcome this danger the newer pacemaker models have been equipped with a so-called anti-interference circuit. This circuit does not react on the frequency content but on the impulse rate or impulse repetition i.e. the quantity of impulses per minute. A heart with a frequency of 90 beats per minute has an impulse rate of 1.5 cps and an impulse content for each pulse of the frequencies mentioned before. The newer pacemaker is designed in such a way, that frequencies with a repetition rate of over 240 m/sec or 4 cps are estimated to be interference signals and will start the anti-interference circuit, whereupon the pacemaker acts as a fixed rate pacemaker with a frequency of 70 bpm and asystole is prevented. Signals like the AC of the power lines with a frequency of 50 cps (USA 60 cps) will therefore not be able to block the pacemaker, but will generate a fixed rate mode. The borderline frequencies of 4-6 cps, where the interference circuit is started, generate sometimes a fixed rate frequency below the ordinary 70 bpm, due to the pacemaker circuit. (This same electronic borderline phenomenon is well known in another part of the pacemaker circuit when the proper heart frequency and the preset demand frequency are about the same, which can result in fusion beats).

The sick sinus syndrome poses a difficulty regarding its tachycardia. Sometimes this tachycardia can reach frequencies of over 200/min. This means that the R-waves present themselves to the detection circuit at repetition frequencies of 4 C.P.S. or higher. The pacemaker acts in these cases like it detects interference signals and starts functioning in its preset fixed rate mode.

We have not become aware of this complication from our own patients, but were shown an electrocardiogram (fig. 2) with this complication recorded by Dr. Porciello in Verona (Italy) (36). The various electrocardiographic tracings showed that the pacemaker (Vitatron MIP-R) functioned perfectly except during periods of high tachycardia. Analysis with a magnet proved that the pacemaker output circuitry was functioning properly. Thereupon the pacemaker was removed and the R-wave analyzed. The amplitude and frequency of the intrinsic signal were within the sensing range of the pacemaker involved. Unfortunately analysis during a period of an extreme tachycardia was not possible. With the assumption that the pacemaker circuit was defective the pacemaker was removed. Laboratory tests showed that the pacemaker circuits were all perfect. The only explanation that remained was the above mentioned phenomenon.

The problem has thereupon been solved from the technical side by a modification of the pacemaker anti-interference circuit. The modified pacemakers (Vitatron 40 RT and later models) received an anti-interference circuit that only starts to function for frequencies of 10 cps or higher or a repetition rate of the ventricular depolarisations above 600/min. This means that tachycardias below 600/min. will block the pacemaker and not start the anti-interference fixed rate mode.

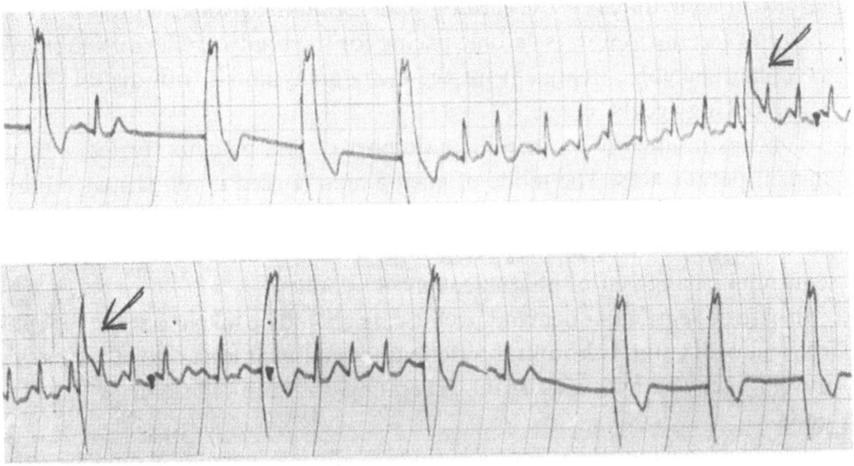

Figure 2. ECG recording in a patient with SSS. The pacemaker starts to function as a fixed rate unit when the tachycardia increases to ± 250/min. (upper recording). This phenomenon (see arrow) resembles pacemaker malfunction but is due to the low frequency response of the anti-interference circuit and is inherent to the pacemaker circuit. When the tachycardia stops (lower recording) the pacemaker starts to function normally again. Paper speed of the overlapping recordings 25 mm/sec. (courtesy dr. Porciello).

A disadvantage of this modification is that interference signals below 10 cps will have the same effect. However, most interference signals have far higher frequencies – most of them are related to the AC frequency of the power lines, and it seems reasonable to assume that the chance of interference signals falling in the range of 4-10 cps is smaller than heart frequencies, especially with tachycardia of the sick sinus syndrome.

After implantation of the modified unit the patient did not demonstrate the complication again. Although this case history may be an incidental case and the incidence of such an extreme tachycardia might be very low with sufficient pharmacological management, it seemed indicated to report this complication here, as it initiated an important modification in the pacemaker circuit.

Conclusion

Although some of the arrhythmias have already been reported over half a century ago, the broad scale of arrhythmias due to sino-atrial nodal dysfunction and summarized in the sick sinus syndrome have become more clear during the last decennia.

The best diagnostic approach for these sometimes persistent but mostly intermittent arrhythmias is the cardiographic scanning (Holter monitoring). The choice of treatment now is cardiac pacing for the bradycardias in combination with pharmacologic treatment for the tachy-arrhythmias with digitalis and/or beta blocking agents.

This has resulted in an increasing number of SSS patients treated with permanent pacemakers. The mode of pacing mostly used is ventricular inhibited stimulation. This may in some cases cause haemodynamic complications, which can be solved by changing the pacing mode to atrial demand or atrio-ventricular sequential pacing and/or pharmacological treatment.

In case of ventricular demand pacing care should be taken that the repetition frequency that starts the anti-interference circuit is at least above 5-6 c.p.s. to prevent tachy-arrhythmias from generating the anti-interference fixed rate mode.

The ideal pacing mode for sick sinus syndrome patients would be atrial-demand-ventricular-demand stimulation with programmable rate.

The ideal atrial electrode (33) and this ideal stimulation unit have not yet been produced in an implantable version. An attempt has been made to indicate with this survey the optimal therapy at this time, with some emphasis on its two complications.

References

1. Mc.William, J.A.: Fibrillar contraction of the heart. J. Physiol., 8: 296, 1887.
2. Keith, A. and Flack, M.W.: The form and nature of the muscular connections between the primary divisions of the vertebrate heart. J. Anat. and Physiol., 41: 172, 1906-1907.
3. Levine, S.A.: Observations on sino-auricular heart block. Arch. Intern. Med., 17: 153, 1916.
4. Short, D.S.: The syndrome of alternating bradycardia and tachycardia. Brit. Heart J., 16: 208, 1954.
5. Lown, B.E.: Electrical reversion of cardiac arrhythmias. Brit. Heart J., 29: 469, 1967.
6. Ferrer, M.I.: The sick sinus syndrome. Futura Publ. Comp. Inc., Mc. Kisco (N.Y.), USA, 1974.
7. Ferrer, M.I.: The sick sinus syndrome in atrial disease. J.A.M.A., 206: 645, 1968.
8. Ferrer, M.I.: The sick sinus syndrome. Circulation, 47: 635, 1973.

9. Bouvrain. Y., Slama, R., Temkine, J.: Le bloc sino-auriculaire et les "maladies du sinus." Arch. Mal. Coeur, 60: 753, 1967.
10. Bigger, J.T. and Strauss, H.C.: The evaluation of sino-atrial function in man. M.C.V. Quarterly, 9: 77, 1973.
11. Greenwood, R.J. and Finkelstein, D.: Sino-atrial heart block. Charles C. Thomas Publ., Springfield (Ill.) USA, 1964.
12. Joseph, S.P.: Energy thresholds in permanent atrial pacing via the coronary sinus. Proceedings Symp. Int. Troubles du rythme et électrostimulation – Toulouse (France) 1977. In press.
13. Bilitch, M.: Sick sinus node syndrome. Modern cardiac pacing, S. Furman and D.J.N. Escher, ed., Charles Press, Bowie (Maryl.) USA; p. 40-45, 1975.
14. Gurtner, H.P., Lenzinger, H.R. and Dolder, M.: Clinical aspects of the sick sinus syndrome. In Cardiac Pacing. B. Lüderlitz ed., Springer Verlag Berlin, F.R. Germany, p. 12-24, 1976.
15. Thalen, H.J.Th.: La choix de la méthode de surveillance des stimulateurs cardiaques pour un centre d'implantation. Proceedings Symp. Int. Troubles du rythme et électrostimulation – Toulouse (France) 1977. In press.
16. Brooks, C.Mc.C. and Lu, H.H.: The sino-atrial pacemaker of the heart. Charles C. Thomas Publ., Springfield (Ill.) USA 1972.
17. Rubenstein, J.J., Schulman, C.L., Yurchak, P.M. and De Sanctis, R.W.: Clinical spectrum of the sick sinus syndrome. Circulation, 46: 5, 1972.
18. Rosen, K.M., Loeb, H.S., Sinao, M.Z., Rahimtoola, S.H., Gunaar, R.M.: Cardiac conduction in patients with symptomatic sinus node disease. Circulation, 43: 836, 1971.
19. Narula, O.S.: Atrioventricular conduction defects in patients with sinus bradycardia. Circulation, 44: 1096, 1971.
20. James, H.N.: The coronary circulation and conduction system in acute myocardial infarction. Progr. Cardiovasc. Dis., 10: 410, 1968.
21. Rosketh, R. and Hatle, L.: Sinus arrest in myocardial infarction. Brit. Heart J., 33: 639, 1971.
22. Mandel, W.J., Hayakawa, H., Allen, H.N., Danzig, R. and Kermaier, A.I.: Assessment of sinus node function in patients with the sick sinus syndrome. Circulation, 46: 761, 1972.
23. Mandel, W.J., Hayakawa, H., Danzig, R. and Marcus, H.S.: Evaluation of sino-atrial node function in man by overdrive suppression. Circulation, 44: 59, 1971.
24. Narula, O.S., Samet, P., Javier, R.P.: Significance of the sinus node recovery time. Circulation, 45: 140, 1972.
25. Steinbeck, G. and Lüderlitz, B.: Sinus node recovery time and sino-atrial conduction time. In Cardiac Pacing. B. Lüderlitz ed., Springer Verlag Berlin, F.R. Germany. p. 45-58, 1976.
26. Delius, W. and Wirtzfeld, A.: The significance of the sinus node recovery time in the sick sinus syndrome. In Cardiac Pacing. B. Lüderlitz ed., Springer Verlag Berlin, F.R. Germany, p. 25-33, 1976.
27. Cannon, D.: The sick sinus syndrome. Grand Round presentation, Mass. Gen. Hosp., Boston, 1975.
28. Crook, B.R., Cashman, P.M.M., Stott, F.D., Raferty, E.B.: Tape monitoring of the electrocardiogram in ambulant patients with sino-atrial disease. Brit. Heart J., 35: 1009, 1973.
29. Cohen, H.E.: Sick sinus syndrome treatment. Circulation, 48: 671, 1973.

30. Wan, S.H., Lee, G.S., Toh, C.C.: The sick sinus syndrome. Brit. Heart J., 34: 942, 1972.
31. Harthorne, J.W.: Indications for various types of pacemakers. Boston Colloquium on Cardiac Pacing. J.W. Harthorne and H.J.Th. Thalen, ed. Martinus Nijhoff Med. Div. The Hague (The Netherlands) p. 33-47, 1977.
32. Harthorne, J.W.: Personal communication.
33. Thalen, H.J.Th.: Electrode design and new developments. Boston Colloquium on Cardiac Pacing. J.W. Harthorne and H.J.Th. Thalen, ed. Martinus Nijhoff Med. Div. The Hague (The Netherlands) p. 47-65, 1977.
34. Irnich, W.: The "Ideal" Pacemaker.*Ibidem*, p. 109-123.
35. Sutton, R.: The importance of the endocardial QRS for demand pacing in acute myocardial infarction. Proceedings IVth International Symposium on Cardiac Pacing, Groningen 1973. H.J.Th. Thalen, ed., Royal van Gorcum, Assen p. 421-424, 1974.
36. Porciello, P.I., Thalen, H.J.Th., Blankestijn, A.J., Renieri, A.C.M., Righetti, B. and Poppi, A.: Ritmo Competitivo indotto da elettrostimolatore a domanda ben funzionante in presenza di elevata tachicardia. Proc. V Congresso Nazionale di Ass. Naz. Medici Cardiologi Ospedalieri; Florence, p. 54-55, 1974.

CARDIAC PACING IN FASCICULAR BLOCK

Mariusz J. Stopczyk

Indication for permanent pacemaker insertion in cases of His-bundle-branch block is probably the most controversial among other indications in up-to-date state of pacemaking.

The problem of prophylactic pacemaker implantation in such cases arose with the observation of a high sudden death rate discovered in comparison of this group to patients revealing no particular conduction defects (1).

This fact was not confirmed by other authors during long-term follow-up studies (2, 3). Discussing this subject, we have first to differentiate strictly between the electrocardiographic definition of bi- and trifascicular block and data obtained from His-bundle studies. The last method is without doubt the only one that enables the introduction of the definition of distal and proximal site of conduction failure. As we may see from the already published data, these terms are not of the same value.

Distal heart block creates a very slow rate of escape rhythm, A-S attacks, high risk of sudden death, and, therefore, a clear indication exists for permanent pacing.

Ecg diagnosis of fascicular block does not always indicate a distal location of A-V pathways defect.

Bifascicular block with P-R time prolongation (called frequently "trifascicular disease") studied by His -bundle electrography revealed in fact only a low percentage of H-V prolongation (4). On the other hand, the same studies performed on syncopal patients by other authors, indicated one hundred per cent prolongation of H-V despite the fact that fascicular block or P-R prolongation existed only in a small percentage of the studied group (5).

Of course, there is theoretically and practically a higher chance for complete distal block to occur in patients with fascicular blocks. This fact can be easily explained, as the degenerative process, located in the conductive system is common in both situations. This general statement does not mean that in a particular case of bifascicular block a P-R prolongation can in fact not depend on A-V node malfunction parallel to partial distal conductive failure.

As a result of these findings a diagnosis based on His-bundle electrocardiography appears the most important for the final decision "to pace or not to pace." Although the method itself is not very difficult it cannot be applied for mass-screening tests for potential pacemaker candidates.

A noninvasive bloodless method for an out-patient clinic application is therefore needed.

Two principal ways of studies are now possible. The first one is the application of a stress test, mainly using atrial pacing. But atrial pacing with an endocardial electrode requires technically nearly the same procedure as HBE and therefore has to be excluded.

In our experience the atrial pacing test with transoesphageal electrodes fulfills in the majority of patients all needs as a basic screening test (7).

The measurement of ERP (effective refractory period) of the conduction system by synchronized pulses and continuous atrial pacing with gradual rate increase have the same significance as was indicated by Bisett et al. (8). The appearance of Wenckebach block is physiological at higher rates and can indicate junctional conduction failure, if it appears at a slower pacing rate at a range of 100 (Fig. 1a).

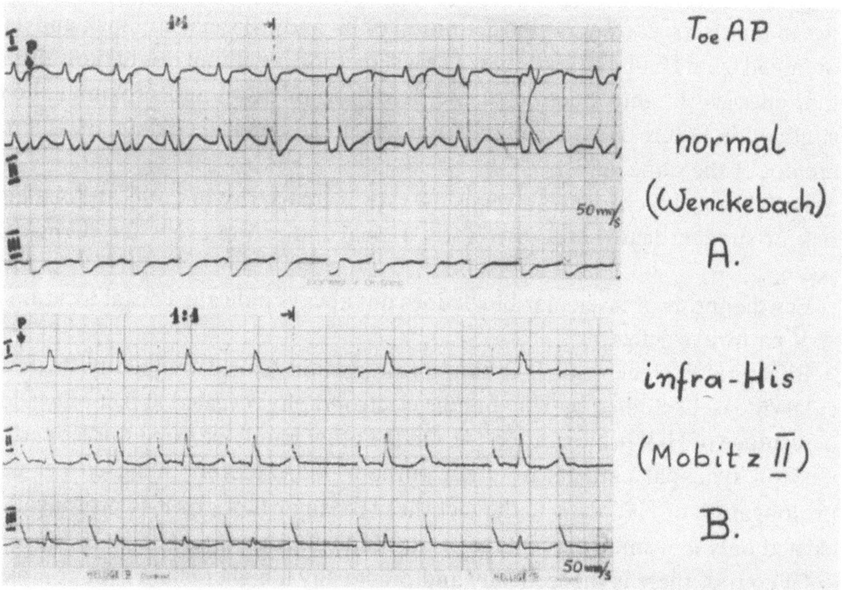

Figure 1.

Möbitz II type block appearing suddenly without preceding P-R delay is considered as a clear sign of distal block, with almost the same diagnostic value as the finding of H-V prolongation during HBE studies (9).

Our experiences confirmed the above observations (Fig. 1b). Transoesophageal atrial pacing tests are now routinely performed in several Polish centers.

In syncopal patients revealing no distal conduction failures as indicated by atrial pacing or HBE, other reasons of A-S attacks have to be considered. Bursts of ventricular ectopics, VT or VF are common; sometimes a paroxysmal conduction defect could be recorded during Holter's monitoring during continuous monitoring at rest and at exercise.

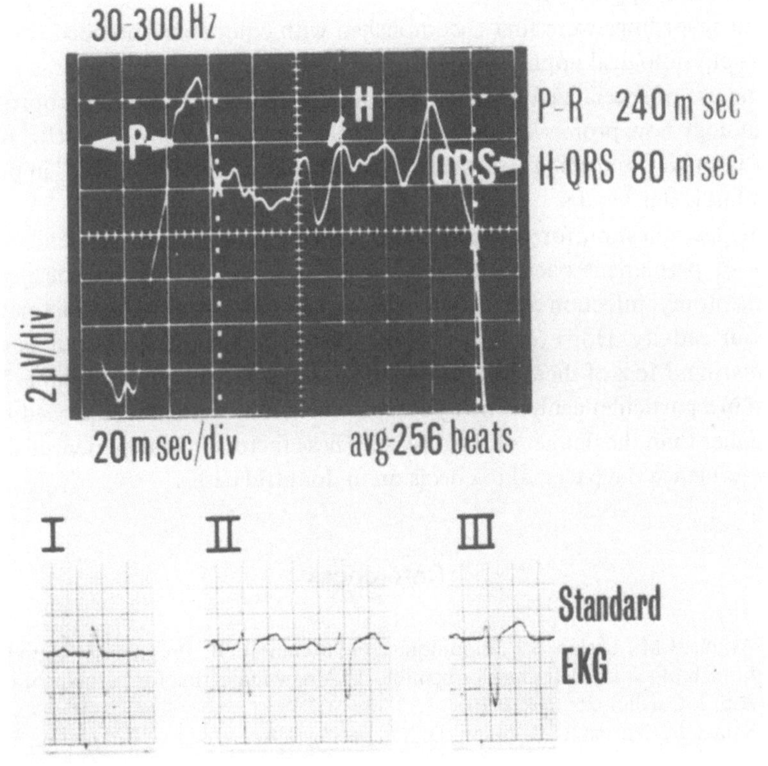

Figure 2. External HIS bundle recording 1 A-V infra-HIS block.

In the near future probably another method will be used widely for the differentiation of proximal or distal conduction failures mainly among patients with fascicular blocks.

I refer here to external, non-invasive studies of HB potentials from the chest skin-surface. This method has been presented by Cywinski during the preceding session. Since its early beginning we are enthusiastic about this method.

Starting in 1972 we recorded externally His-bundle potentials in man at the same time as Berbari and collaborators and Flowers and collaborators (10). Firstly, this method was not completely non-invasive because an overdriving pacemaker was needed for averaging synchronisation. Two years later we succeeded together with Dr. Wajszczuk in Detroit, in the recording of His-bundle signals with a spontaneous rhythm (11). An example of the application of this method in a case of an infra His block is shown in Fig. 2.

The application of large, general purpose, computers and an off-line procedure used in the early beginning made this technique very inconvenient for large clinical application.

Our recordings were first accomplished with equipment intended rather for neurophysiological application with hospitalized patients.

The use of specialized units constructed with very advanced microprocessor technology now promises an extensive application of non-invasive HBE recordings as an ideal screening test for the decision "to pace or not to pace" in patients with fascicular blocks.

The last question for prophylactic pacemaker implantation depends on the risks of permanent pacing. Displacement of endocardial electrodes, risk of thoracotomy, infection and technical complications are common factors limiting our activity. However the general trend of the complication rate is slowly decreasing. Most of them usually depend upon experience and available equipment in a particular center. In any case, the risk of the pacemaker procedure can be higher than the danger of the disease. These factors in unexperienced centers may influence the pacemaking decision in doubtful cases.

References

1. Atkins, J.M., Leshin, S.J., Bloomquist, G., Mellins, C.B., Prognosis of right bundle branch block and left anterior hemiblock: A new indication for permanent pacing. Am. J. Cardiol. 26: 624, 1970.
2. Samet, P., Narula, O.S., Gann, D., On pacing (letter to editor) Circulation 53: 204, 1976.
3. Dhingra, R.C., Denes, P., Wu, D., Chuquimia, R., Amat-Y-Leon, F., Wyndham, C., Rosen, K.M., Chronic RBBB and left posterior hemiblock. Clinical, electrophysiologic and prognostic observations. Am. J. Card. 36: 867, 1975.
4. Levites, R., Haft, J.J., Significance of first degree heart block/prolonged P-R interval in bifascicular block. Am. J. Cardiol. 34: 259, 1974.
5. Touboul, P., Ibrahim, M., Atrioventricular conduction defects in patients presenting with syncope and normal P-R interval. Brit. Heart J. 34: 1005, 1972.
6. Stopczyk, M., Lukasik, E., Pacing stress-tests of conductive system and His-bundle electrography; their significance for prophylactic pacemaker implantation. Kardiologia Polska 15: 483, 1972 (in Polish).

7. Stopczyk, M.J., Pieniak, M., Sadowski, Z., Zochowski, R.J., Transoesophageal atrial pacing as a simple diagnostic and therapeutic procedure. Proc. IV Int. Conf. on Med. Physics incl. Med. Eng. Göteborg, Sweden, 1972, 405.
8. Bisset, J.K., Kane, J.J., De Soyra, N., Murphy, M.L., Electrophysiological significance of rapid atrial pacing as a test of atrioventricular conduction. Cardiovasc. Res. 9: 593, 1975.
9. Akhtar, M., Damato, A.N., Clinical uses of His bundle electrocardiography. Part I. Am. Heart J. 91: 520, 1976.
10. Stopczyk, M.J., Kopeć, J., Zochowski, R.J., Pieniak, M., Surface recording of electrical heart activity during P-R segment in man by computer averaging technique. Int. Res. Com. Syst. 11 (21), 73-8, 1973.
11. Stoppyk, M.J.J., Pieniak, M., Wajszczuk, W.J., Rubenfire M., Sinus node activity in man and animal studies recorded by an on-line pre-memorized averaging technique. Proc. Vth Int. Symp. on Cardiac Pacing, Tokyo 1976, Excerpta Medica (in press).

CARDIAC PACING IN ACUTE MYOCARDIAL INFARCTION

J.P. van Durme, M.D.

Introduction

Before starting to review the indications for electrical stimulation during the acute phase of myocardial infarction, I would like to make two remarks. My premise will be that, in myocardial infarction, the use of electrical stimulation is an overall decision. I mean by that, that this decision is not to be made by looking at some isolated electrocardiographic findings, but that, in the acute phase, the same electrocardiographic appearance might very well be an indication for electrical stimulation in one patient – as we will see later on – whereas, in another patient, it will not be an indication. It means that you have to look not only at the electrocardiogram, but have to take into account also the hemodynamic situation of the patient who presents with some type of conduction defect.

The second remark I would like to make is that one has to make a very clear difference between *prophylactic* insertion of an electrode catheter – in which case only a small percentage of patients will need electrical stimulation – and instant electrical stimulation, which might be needed in patients with acute myocardial infarction.

Indications

Let us now review several possible indications for electrical stimulation in the acute phase of myocardial infarction. We have two major groups: on the one hand you have conduction defects, on the other hand you have tachyarrhythmia, be it at the ventricular or at the atrial level.

1. Conduction defects

Let us start with the conduction defects. A-V block, which goes together with slow heart rate, has in itself several good theoretical reasons for the use of electrical stimulation in the acute phase of myocardial infarction. Indeed, one knows actually that a certain percentage of patients who show a low degree of A-

V block in the acute stage will proceed to total A-V block; and that a certain percentage of these patients will have, at first appearance of total A-V block, a cardiac standstill. That is one good reason to use, eventually, electrical stimulation. Other good reasons, in the acute phase, are the fact that bradycardia in itself might harm the myocardium. It might harm it because the slower the heart, the higher the chances of origination of ectopic foci. It might harm the heart, for a second reason, because bradycardia in itself will lower the fibrillation threshold of the ventricle. Thirdly, when bradycardia is pronounced, usually it is associated with decreased cardiac output. So, here are several good theoretical reasons to pace the heart in the acute phase.

Let us now look at the practical situation. *First-degree heart block* will never be an indication even for prophylactic insertion of a pacing catheter. *Second-degree heart block* will be an indication for prophylactic insertion if one is dealing with Mobitz type 2, because one knows now that contrary patients with acute inferior infarction, in which they do have a Wenckebach phenomenon, patients with mobitz 2 block may progress rapidly to total A-V block and you do not have the intermediate stage of Mobitz I A-V block to pick them up. Second-degree A-V block will only be an indication if there is a progression of conduction disturbance. In cases of *total A-V block*, in acute myocardial infarction, the indication for pacing will depend on the location of the infarction. You all know that inferior wall infarction associated with total A-V block has a much better prognosis than when it is due to anterior wall infarction. This is due to the fact that the etiology of the *total A-V block* in an inferior wall infarction is completely different from the etiology of total A-V block in anterior wall infarction, when one looks upon it from an anatomical point of view. Thus, the practical standpoint will be: when *total A-V block is due to inferior wall infarction*, the indication for temporary pacing in the acute phase of myocardial infarction will only be applicable to those patients with slow heart rates which do not respond to intravenous injection of atropine. The situation is quite different in patients who develop *total A-V block due to anterior wall infarction*, where the total A-V block is due to extensive necrosis of the septum and of the anterior wall of the myocardium; in those patients, one will often see that the total A-V block is preceded by the development of bilateral bundle branch block: an association of complete right bundle branch block with left inferior hemi-block. The occurrence of anterior wall infarction with bilateral bundle branch block in the acute phase is an indication for prophylactic insertion of an electrode catheter. Whether or not one will impressively influence the ultimate prognosis is hard to define and one can certainly state that this ultimate prognosis will, in most cases, not depend on the fact that the patient has a heart block condition but on the extent of damage to myocardial contractility.

2. *Tachydysrhythmias*

Let us now turn to the indication of tachydysrhythmias in acute myocardial infarction. In some cases, especially in cases of *persistent ventricular dysrhythmias*, like recurrent ventricular tachycardia or recurrent ventricular fibrillation despite anti-dysrhythmic treatment, there might be an indication for combining electrical stimulation with this anti-arrhythmic treatment.

The ideal way to stimulate the heart is to use atrial pacing. But, this is not always possible. We treated a patient with an acute inferior wall infarction, who developed frequent ventricular ectopic beats in this way. In this patient there had been a problem of recurrent ventricular fibrillation, despite adequate anti-dysrhythmic treatment. We decided to stimulate this patient in order to try to prevent ventricular fibrillation. We started with atrial pacing, but due to the impairment of atrial-ventricular conduction a sequence of functional Wenckebach phenomena resulted. This Wenckebach sequence in this patient had as its result that the ventricular rate did not increase enough so that ventricular ectopic beats were still present. In this case, the only possibility was to switch to ventricular pacing.

To summarize the indications for ventricular tachydysrhythmias: any case of recurrent ventricular tachycardia and ventricular fibrillation, which does not respond to adequate medical treatment, is an indication for combined electrical stimulation and anti-dysrhythmic treatment in my opinion.

Finally there are a few instances of *supraventricular tachyarrhythmia* which are infrequent, where electrical stimulation might be useful.

There is – at least in the acute phase of myocardial infarction – almost never an indication for instant electrical stimulation. But, when you have an electrode positioned in a patient, and when he develops a supraventricular tachyarrhythmia, it is in many cases very easy to convert the tachyarrhythmia to normal sinus rhythm by over-driving the frequency of the heart by fast atrial stimulation, or by inducing temporary atrial fibrillation in the patient.

3. *Diagnosis of tachycardia*

I would like to finish with a last indication. In a few patients atrial pacing might have a diagnostic importance for the tachycardia. Some patients will present with tachycardia which might resemble ventricular tachycardia. In one case we recorded clearly a regular sequence of P-waves followed by QRS complexes, or QRS complexes followed by P-waves. We could not find on this tracing whether we had an atrial tachycardia with aberrant conduction. In order to find out what type of tachycardia it was, we inserted atrial and ventricular electrodes. We then recorded lead V-4, simultaneously with an intra-atrial lead.

Thereupon we stimulated the heart with the atrial electrode and with the ventricular electrode and recorded the ECG during atrial stimulation at a high rate and ventricular stimulation at a high rate. The morphology of the QRS complexes during atrial stimulation was identical to the original tracing. Both differed from the other tracing during ventricular stimulation. This procedure made it clear that we were dealing with a supraventricular tachycardia.

PROPHYLACTIC PREOPERATIVE PACING

F.A. Pirzada, K. Venkataraman, J.E. Madias
and W.B. Hood Jr.

The threat of stress during anesthesia and surgery in patients with bifascicular block, precipitating complete heart block, raises the consideration of prophylactic temporary pacing. Guidelines for specific indications to pace in this high risk group are not as yet clear. Certainly the classification of the conduction pathway into a three fascicle system below the His bundle has made electrocardiographic recognition easy, but the involvement of the third fascicle making a patient more vulnerable to complete heart block cannot be reliably diagnosed. In right bundle branch block (RBBB) and left anterior hemiblock (LAH), one of the common varieties of bifascicular blocks confronted clinically, the estimated incidence of developing complete heart block is between 6 and 21 percent over a five-year follow-up period (1, 2). This range of probability especially under the stress of anesthesia and surgery creates the need for temporary pacing when such patients are confronted. Similar management problems also arise with other forms of bifascicular blocks which are also known to be forerunners of complete heart block. Clinical symptoms of dizziness and syncope indicate prior transient complete heart block in these patients, if no neurological reason exists, and thus are of help in the decision making. Increased PR interval on the suface electrocardiogram was thought to indicate tri-fascicular disease but has not proved to be of much significance as shown by Levites and Haft (3). Thus, with lack of guidelines in the decision making of to pace or not to pace in this clinical setting it may be argued that the insertion of a temporary pacemaker may be a relatively benign procedure as compared to the occurrence of complete heart block. However, the risk of infection, ventricular ectopy and occasional myocardial perforation warrants caution to such a statement.

To determine the need for prophylactic temporary pacing in bifascicular block, a retrospective analysis (Table 1) in 38 patients undergoing 74 surgical and other procedures was carried out (1). RBBB was diagnosed on the basis of a QRS $\geq$ 0.12 seconds, wide S in leads I and V_6 and wide R' in AVR and V_1. Left anterior hemiblock was diagnosed on the basis of the QRS axis more negative than –30 degrees, in the absence of inferior myocardial infarction and emphysema. Patients were divided into four groups. Group 1 consisted of 28 patients in sinus rhythm with a normal PR interval. Group 2 included 6 patients with a prolonged PR interval. Group 3 included 3 patients, two in atrial fibrillation and one in stable junctional rhythm. Group 4 consisted of one patient in sinus tachycardia with 2:1 AV block of the Mobitz 2 variety.

Table 1. The 4 patient groups of the study with RBBB + LAH. The total of 38 patients underwent 74 surgical procedures. (SR = sinus rhythm, AF = atrial fibrillation, JR = junctional rhythm, ST = sinus tachycardia). See text.

Prophylactic Preoperative Pacing		
Group 1	SR (PR $\leq$ 0.20 sec)	28
Group 2	SR (PR $>$ 0.20 sec)	6
Group 3	AF	2
	JR	1
Group 4	ST with 2:1 AV block	1
		38

Clinical and electrocardiographic features. In Group I, sixteen of the 28 patients had a diagnosis of organic heart disease, in the remainder the only manifestation of heart disease was the conduction disorder. Two patients had one or more syncopal episodes. In 20 patients, bifascicular block was noted for the first time during their hospitalization for surgery. The remaining eight patients were known to have conduction defects from 2 to 120 months prior to surgery (mean 42.1 months). Seven patients were receiving digoxin before operation, one was taking diuretics in addition and three were also receiving procaineamide. In Group 2, three of the six patients had no evidence of cardiac disease except for the conduction defect noted on the ECG. None had a history of syncopal spells in the past. The diagnosis of bifascicular block was made for the first time in two patients during hospitalization for surgery. The remaining four were known to have the conduction defect 6, 12, 69 and 74 months prior to surgery. Two patients were on maintenance digoxin and diuretics, and one patient was taking quinidine pre-operatively. In Group 3, one patient had hypertensive heart disease, another atherosclerotic heart disease and the third had no cardiac disease except the conduction abnormality. In two patients, the conduction disorder was noted for the first time pre-operatively and in the other, 34 months prior to surgery. All three were taking digoxin and one was on diuretics and procaineamide as well. In Group 4, the patient had sinus tachycardia with a 2:1 AV block of the Mobitz 2 variety. The bifascicular block had been present for 5 years. He was receiving digoxin and furosemide.

Anesthesia and pre-operative procedures. In Group 1 (Table 2) seventeen were major, and 34 were minor procedures. Fifteen were done under general and 15 under spinal anesthesia. Eighteen received regional or local anesthesia, and 3

Table 2. Surgical procedures and types of anesthesia for the 4 patient groups. (Maj = major, Min = minor, Gen = general, SP = spinal,Reg = regional). See text.

Prophylactic Preoperative Pacing	Procedures		Anesthesia			
	Maj	Min	Gen	Sp	Reg	None
Group 1	17	34	15	15	18	3
Group 2	5	11	3	5	7	1
Group 3	2	4	1	1	4	0
Group 4	1	0	0	1	0	0

were endoscopy procedures requiring no anesthesia. In Group 2, five major and 11 minor procedures were done. Three under general, 5 under spinal, 7 under regional anesthesia, one procedure did not require any anesthesia. In Group 3, 6 procedures were done, one under general, one spinal and 4 under regional anesthesia. The one patient in Group 4 had major surgery under spinal anesthesia.

Table 3. Preoperative measures and complications during the surgical procedures for the 4 patient groups. (BP = blood pressure, VPC = ventricular premature contraction, SB = sinus bradycardia, IVR = Idioventricular rhythm). See text.

	Prophylactic Preoperative Pacing			Complications		
	Atropine	Pacemakers	None	BP	VPC	SB
Group 1	23	8	46	3	1	1
Group 2	2	4	15	0	0	1
Group 3	2	2	6	0	0	0
Group 4	0	1	IVR requiring pacing			

Pre-operative procedures and complications encountered during the surgical procedures. As Table 3 indicates in Group 1, consisting of RBBB + LAH and normal PR, 23 patients had received atropine and 8 patients had received prophylactic temporary transvenous pacemakers. Forty-six procedures had no complications. During three operations, hypotension developed responding to volume expansion and pressors. One patient developed sinus bradycardia with hypotension responding promptly to atropine. No patients showed deterioration of AV conduction and the standby pacemakers were not utilized. In Group 2, consisting of patients with RBBB + LAH and 1st degree AV block, 2 patients got atropine and 4 patients received standby transvenous pacemakers. Out of the 16 procedures in this group only one episode of sinus bradycardia developed which responded to atropine promptly. No patient was observed to develop further impairment in AV conduction, and temporary pacemakers were not utilized. In Group 3, consisting of 2 patients in atrial fibrillation and one in junctional rhythm (2 of which received atropine) no further deterioration in conduction was seen and in 2 patients standby transvenous pacemakers that were inserted pre-operatively were not utilized. The single patient in Group 4 who had Mobitz type 2 block was observed to go into idioventricular rhythm at the time of recovery from anesthesia and required pacing to maintain normal blood pressure.

Discussion

A number of series have been reported in the literature similar to ours, providing more patient observation. Berg and Kotler (4) reported a retrospective analysis in 30 patients undergoing 36 surgical procedures. Twenty-six patients, forming the major part of the series, had RBBB and left axis deviation, and 4 had left bundle branch block (LBBB) with first-degree heart block. Eighty-three percent of patients had evidence of underlying cardiac disease, 2 patients gave prior history of syncope and dizziness. None of the patients intraoperatively or in the immediate post-operative period showed further deterioration in conduction. Similar conclusions can also be drawn from a series consisting of patients with RBBB and left anterior hemiblock reported by Kunstadt and his associates (5). A more recent observation has been made by Pastore* and associates as seen in Table 4. As shown, the majority of the procedures in that series were either

Table 4. Survey of the various ECG patterns and the type of anesthesia used in the 52 patients in the group of Dr. Pastore (St. Elizabeth Hospital, Boston). Courtesy of Dr. Pastore.

	Prophylactic Preoperative Pacing			
Rhythm	*Anesthesia*			*Total Operations*
	General	*Spinal*	*Local*	
Sinus (normal PR)	18	6	12	36
Sinus (prolonged PR)	4	4	4	12*
Atrial Fibrillation	1		1	2
Atrial Tachycardia with block	1			1
Atrial Flutter		1		1
Total Operations	24	11	17	52

* 2 pacemakers.

performed under general or spinal anesthesia, indicating major operations. None of their patients showed increase in the conduction abnormality in the

* Personal Communication.

intra- and immediate post-operative phase, except one patient in the first group who during induction of anesthesia went into high grade AV block which spontaneously abated. Pacemaker was not required in any of the patients.

Thus, it seems that patients with conduction abnormality in the right bundle and the left anterior fascicle seem not to progress to higher grades of AV block under the stress of surgery and anesthesia. In regard to the other forms of bifascicular blocks, namely left bundle branch block and right bundle branch block

Table 5. Summary of articles in support of prolonged H-V interval in predicting complete heart block. BBB = bundle branch block.

	QRS	Prophylactic Preoperative Pacing *PR(nor)*	*HV(nor)*	*HV(↑)*	Conclusions
Gupta (Amer J Card 73) Normal HV 35-55 msec; n = 16	RBBB + LAH (n = 10)	3	0	10	
	RBBB (n = 3)	2	1	2	Prolonged HV associated with CHB.
	Alternating BBB (n = 2)	2	0	2	
	RBBB + LPH (n = 1)	1	0	1	
Scheinman (Circ Abstr 75) n = 132 Normal HV 35-60 msec.	BBB	Unknown	53	79	Risk of sudden death high if HV > 75 msec.
Narula (His Bundle Electrocardiography FA Davis 75) n = 83 Normal HV 35-45 msec.	RBBB + LAH	30	25	48	Increased mortality in patients with HV↑
Vera (Circ 76) n = 50 Normal HQ 35-55 msec.	RBBB + LAH (n = 19)	6	0	19	Patients with CHB and Mobitz 2. had ↑ HQ
	RBBB (n = 5)	3	0	5	
	RBBB + LPH (n = 3)	0	1	5	
	Alternating BBB (n = 2)	0	0	2	
	LBBB (n = 18)	11	0	18	

with left posterior hemiblock (RBBB + LPH) very little is known as to how these patients do under stressful situations. Some valuable information could be drawn from His bundle electrocardiography in these patients by the measurement of the H-V interval. This, if prolonged, indicates an involvement of the third fascicle and thus could represent a parameter of identifying the high risk group for developing complete heart block prior to stress of anesthesia or surgery. However, some studies have failed to demonstrate this relationship, thus generating considerable controversy. Table 5 summarizes the articles in support of prolonged HV interval in predicting complete heart block.

Gupta (6) and associates in evaluating sixteen patients with second-degree or complete heart block and intraventricular conduction defect, showed that 15 patients had prolonged HV intervals. Scheinman (7) and associates in a preliminary report of 132 patients with bundle branch block, showed that there is an increased risk for either sudden death or development of higher degree of AV block if HV interval is prolonged beyond 75 msecs. Narula (8) and associates have also suggested an increased incidence of sudden death and higher degrees of AV block in patients with prolonged HV intervals. Vera (9) and associates have recently published a series consisting of 50 patients with bifascicular block and intermittent complete heart block or Mobitz 2 block. HQ intervals measured in all patients except one were prolonged. They also indicated that beyond three years of development of bifascicular block patients should be considered for diagnosis of trifascicular disease by His bundle study. Even though the evidence accumulated in these series is convincing due to the large group of patients studied, it is hard to accept totally in view of the evidence reported to the contrary by other investigators, summarized in Table 6.

Haft (10) noted normal HV intervals in four patients that subsequently developed complete heart block. Dinghra (11) and associates have recently published their experience in 18 patients with intraventricular conduction defect. Patients had prolonged HV intervals of 80 msecs and beyond and were prospectively followed for 711 ± 118 days. All those with symptoms did poorly having high morbidity and mortality while 5 asymptomatic patients had a benign course. Recently McAnulty et al (12) reporting on a larger group of patients with HV intervals followed for 10.5 months have shown a poor correlation with the onset of complete heart block. Thus, at the present moment as to how reliable His-bundle electrocardiography will be in predicting impending complete heart block in the asymptomatic patient, especially if stress of surgery or anesthesia is anticipated, has yet to be resolved.

Table 6. Summary of articles objecting prolonged H-V interval predicting complete heart block. AD = abnormal right or left axis deviation.

		Prophylactic Preoperative Pacing			
	QRS	*PR(nor)*	*HV(nor)*	*HV(↑)*	Conclusions
Haft (Chest 73) n = 5 Normal HV 35-45 msec.	RBBB + LAH (n = 3)	2 1*	2	1	CHB developed in 4 patients with normal HV intervals
	RBBB (n = 1)	1*	1	0	
	LBBB (n = 1)	1	1	0	
Dinghra (Circ 76) n = 18 Normal HV = 31-55 msec.	RBBB + LAD (n = 5)	1	0	5**	5 asymptomatic patients had benign course for 711 ± 118 days.
	RBBB + RAD (n = 2)	0	0	2**	
	LBBB (n = 11)	1	0	11**	
McAnulty (Circ Abstr. 76) n = 214 Normal HV 35-55 msec.	RBBB + AD (n = 109)			110	↑HV interval not particularly related to syncope and sudden death at an average follow-up of 10.5 months.
	LBBB (n = 90)				
	Unknown (n = 15)				

* Mobitz 2.
** HV ≥ 80 msec.

Conclusions

Based on our experience and evidence in the literature presented, we are using the approach as outlined in Table 7, when patients with bifascicular blocks are undergoing surgical procedures.

1) Patients with right bundle branch block and left anterior hemiblock of less than three years duration and normal PR interval and no symptoms of syncope seem to do quite well and do not require prophylactic pacemakers.

2) Patients with right bundle branch block plus left anterior hemiblock greater than three years duration with prolonged PR interval and no symptoms may have trifascicular involvement. As experience is limited at the present moment,

Table 7. Measure to be taken preoperatively in patients with various types of conduction defects.

	Prophylactic Preoperative Pacing			
EKG	*Duration*	*PR*	*Symptoms*	*Pacing*
RBBB + LAH	< 3 yrs	nor	–	–
RBBB + LAH	> 3 yrs	↑	–	?, His study
RBBB + LPH			–	?, His study
LBBB			–	?, His study
Bifascicular Block			+	+
Bifascicular Block with Mobitz 2				+

these patients should probably receive temporary pacemakers and at the same time His-study performed, if facilities are available, for prognostication. However, the small group of patients in our series and those reported in the literature, did quite well during surgery and perhaps may not require prophylactic pacemakers.

3) Patients with right bundle branch block plus left posterior hemiblock and left bundle branch block indicate greater involvement of the conduction system and perhaps should also be considered for temporary pacing, depending upon the procedure until more experience is accumulated.

4) All types of bifascicular blocks with symptoms of syncope should receive temporary pacemakers prior to the procedure.

5) Bifascicular block with Mobitz 2 AV block should also be considered for prophylactic temporary pacemakers.

References

1. Venkataraman, K, Madias, J.E., Hood, W.B. Jr., Indications for prophylactic preoperative insertion of pacemakers in patients with right bundle branch block and left anterior hemiblock. Chest 68: 501-506: 1975.
2. Kulbertus, H.E., Qualifié du, C., The magnitude of risk of developing complete heart block in patients with LAD-RBBB. Am Heart J. 86: 278-279, 1973.
3. Levites, R., Haft, J.I., Significance of first degree heart block (prolonged P-R interval) in bifascicular block. Am. J. Card. 34: 259-264, 1974.
4. Berg, R., Kotler, M.N., The significance of bilateral bundle branch block in the preoperative patient. Chest 59: 62-67, 1971.
5. Kunstadt, D., Punja, M., Cagin, N. et al., Bifascicular block: a clinical and electrophysiological study. Am. Heart J. 86: 173-181, 1973.
6. Gupta, P.K., Lichstein, E., Chadda, K.D., Intraventricular conduction time (H-V interval) during antegrade conduction in patients with heart block. Am. J. Card. 32: 27-31, 1973.

7. Scheinman, M.M., Brennan, M., Modin, G. et al., Comparative prospective study of bundle branch block. Circulation 51-(II): 113, 1975.
8. Narula, O.S., Gann, D., Samet, P., Prognostic value of H-V intervals. In His Bundle Electrocardiography, edited by Narula, O.S. Philadelphia. F. A. Davis Company 1975, p. 437.
9. Vera, Z., Mason, D.T., Fletcher, R.D. et al.: Prolonged His-Q interval in chronic bifascicular block. Relation to impending complete heart block. Circulation 53: 46-55: 1976.
10. Haft, J.I., Kranz, P.D., Intraventricular conduction intervals during orthograde conduction in patients with complete heart block. Chest. 63: 751-756, 1973.
11. Dhingra, R.C., Denes, P., Wu, D. et al., Prospective observations in patients with chronic bundle branch block and marked H-V prolongation. Circulation 53: 600-604, 1976.
12. McAnulty, J., Murphy, E., DeMots, H. et al., Natural history of conduction system disease: A prospective study. Circulation 54 (Suppl. II): 51, 1976.

CARDIAC PACING IN OPEN HEART SURGERY

G. RÁBAGO, J. FRAILE, N.G. DE VEGA AND T. MORENO

In the last few years the great utility of cardiac pacing after open heart surgery has been proven. Therefore we, in our Department, are using cables for eventual pacing of the surgical patient almost routinely.

After cardio-pulmonary by-pass, electrode needles are left in the left or the right (Fig. 1a) ventricular myocardium and in the anterior rectus muscle. The cables are passed through the skin and away from the operative incision (Fig. 1b) and will be firmly fixed to the skin (Fig. 1c) at their external portion to avoid any displacement. They are covered within a sterile dressing.

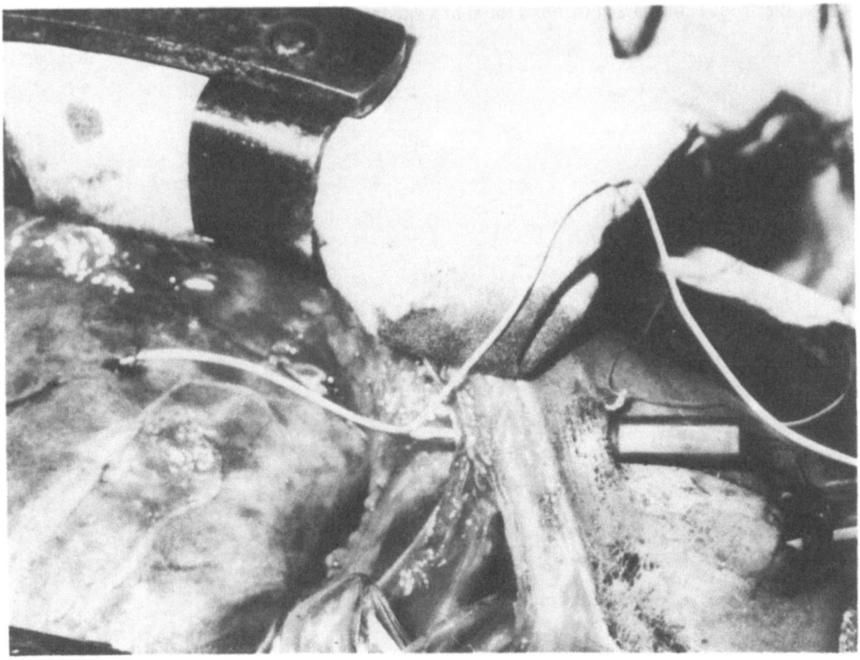

Figure 1. Needle electrode and cable for temporary post surgical pacing.
A) Needle electrode in the wall of the left ventricle.

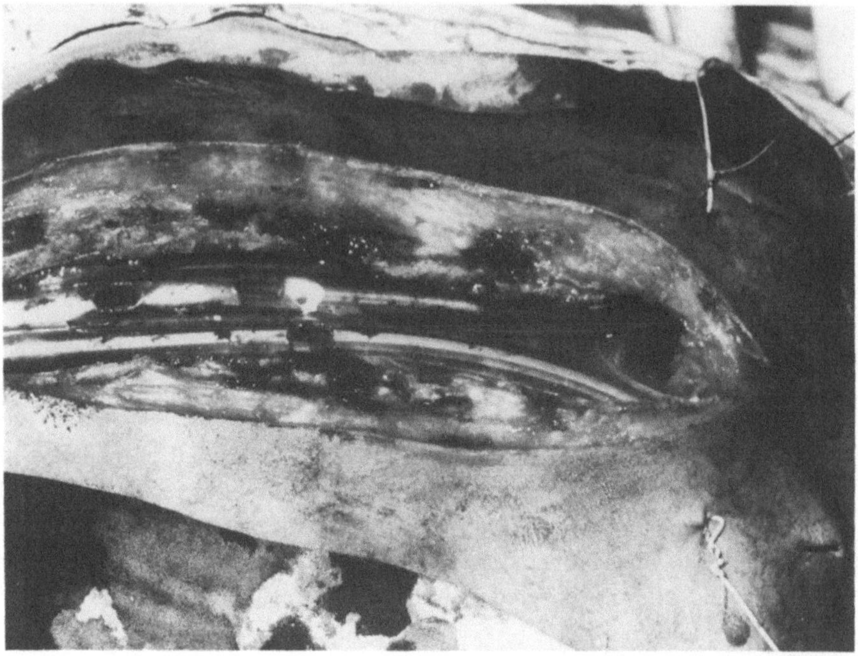

B) Electrode cable passed through the skin away from the operatory incision.

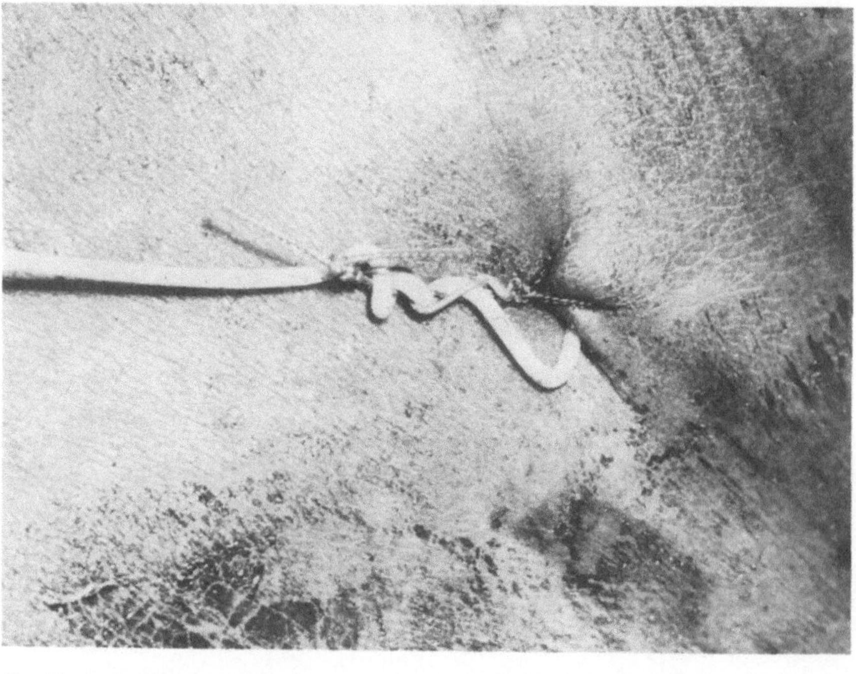

C) Electrode cable firmly fixed to the skin near the place of the skin perforation.

Cardiac pacing may be useful in the operating-room right after by-pass, whereas 10 to 20% of the patients might need a pacemaker in the immediate postoperative course during their stay in the Intensive Care Unit. It is very important for patients with coronary artery disease, who may develop a surgical myocardial infarction or disrhythmia.

It is also important for either mitral or aortic valve replacements or for patients in whom the tricuspid valve is corrected. In those patients, slow rhythms are frequent as well as extrasystoles or tachycardias.

After total correction of congenital diseases – specially Fallot's Tetralogy, Transposition of the Great Vessels, Atrioventricularis Communis, Ostium Primum – post surgical use of cardiac pacing would be worthwhile in cases of disrhythmias or auriculo-ventricular blocks, although these might be temporary. Pacing might be conditioned in bradycardias, A-V blocks, nodal or junctional rhythms. In those cases, a demand external pacemaker will increase the cardiac frequency and cardiac output, especially with aortic patients, as shown by the data of Ionescu. The fixed rhythm is useful to avoid extrasystoles which do not respond to medical therapy or to control with high frequency pacing tachyarrhythmias which affect cardiac haemodynamics.

However external pacing use does not rule out the necessity to identify the aetiology of the disrhythmia which has to be succesfully treated: blood transfusion for hypovolemia, potassium for hypokalemia, correction of digitalis overdosage, Xylocain for premature beats ... etc.

Generally, based on our own experience, transient pacing is only useful in the Intensive Care Unit period and cables should be removed on transfer from this Unit to the patient's room.

Only with some valvular patients or some cases of Fallot's Tetralogy with bradycardia or A-V block, pacing has been prolonged up to 30 days before the cables were removed. If the cause still persists by then, external pacing should be changed to a permanent pacemaker.

DISCUSSION II. TO PACE OR NOT TO PACE

Chairman: J. N. HOMAN VAN DER HEIDE *(Groningen, The Netherlands)*

G. FONTAINE *(Paris, France):* I would like to make some comments about the paper of Dr. Stopczyk about surface His bundle recording. There is no question that the main problem in this field arises as to whether the signal recorded is the depolarization of the A-V structure or an artifact produced by muscle potentials. The A-V conduction activation observed is not a brief deflection of the His bundle electrogram observed in the cath lab, but a wide deflection as the depolarization of the His bundle lasts tenths of milliseconds. We have found by experience that the most reliable criterion is the reproducibility of the phenomena recorded.

M. STOPCZYK *(Warsaw, Poland):* We found that the most difficult problem in achieving good results in external His bundle recordings is appropriate triggering from the QRS. There are many possibilities. You can for instance first record on tape and then play the tape back and trigger on the QRS complex and locate from there the His bundle deflection. In our studies, we put the first memory on digital registers into which the data were continuously fed. The memory was post-triggered and was stopped by QRS. In this way the capacity of the memory was read in a few milliseconds. The data were put into an averager to produce what we consider to be the real H-V time. I should also like to make some remarks about our trials with sinus node recording. From this work in cooperation with Drs. Wajszczuk and Palko already reported in Tokyo I show you a figure with recordings in a dog. (fig. 1) The first curve is recorded with an external surface lead and the last curve is an epicardial SA node recording from an electrode sutured directly over the sinus node. The middle curve gives the data recorded externally with our computer averaging technique. You can see that there is a good relationship between the direct recording from the sino-atrial node and the external recording. Fig. 2 shows the same, but now recorded in man. Of course there is no direct recording here from the sinus node, but the lower tracing shows the reference lead. We cannot say for sure in this case that the first deflection is the sinus node activity, as it could also be the muscular ring around the superior vena cava – the point of juncture with the atrial muscle – which is activated at the beginning of atrial activation. By now we are doing the

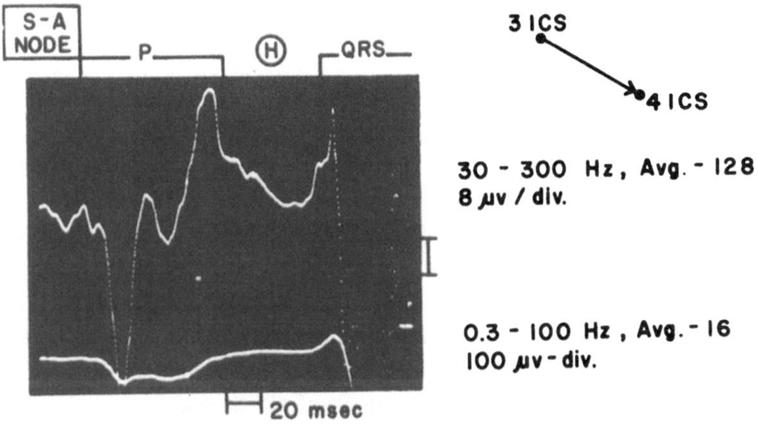

Figure 1. External recording of pre-P (S-A Node) activity. (Averaged QRS post-triggered.)

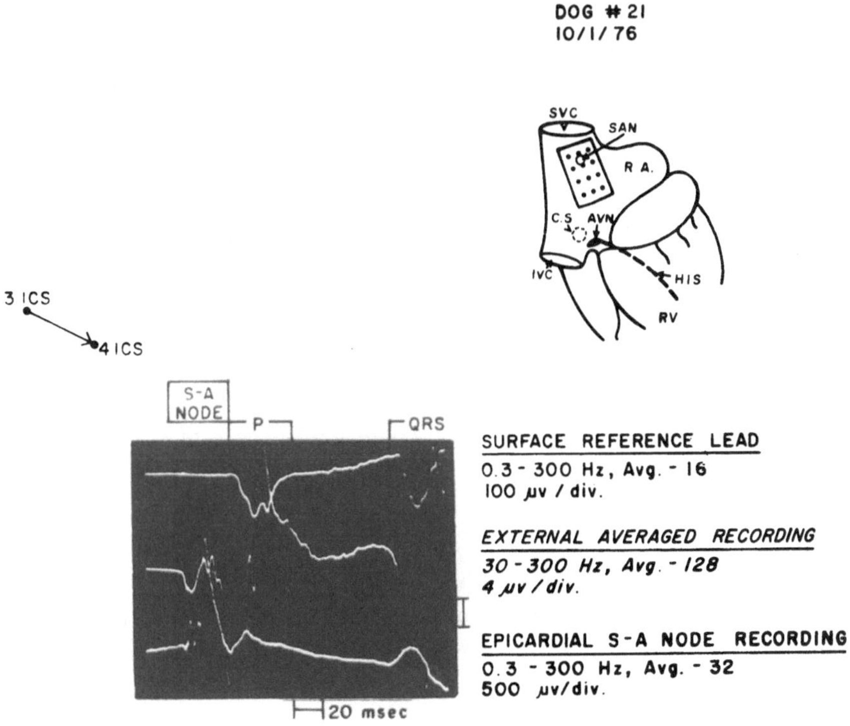

Figure 2. External recording of S-A Node activity. (Averaged P post-triggered.)

direct registration during open-heart surgery in man and I think this could confirm that we really recorded in this case externally the human sino-atrial activity. Perhaps we will discuss in future meetings also externally recorded sino-atrial conduction time.

S. SEQUERRA AMRAM *(Lisbon, Portugal):* It takes a lot of clinical judgement to pace or not to pace in acute myocardial infarction. I fully agree with Dr. Van Durme. But once you have made the decision to insert a stimulation catheter, for instance in a case of right bundle branch block, with or without left axis deviation, I believe one should also take the opportunity to make His bundle recordings both during introduction and, once you want to take out the wire, during withdrawal. These recordings have obvious prognostic significance for the immediate phase and may help us also with the decision for the implantation of a permanent pacemaker.

A second point that I would like to make regards pacing in bradyarrhythmias. Since the tendency nowadays in the treatment of acute myocardial infarction is to protect the ischemic myocardium, I wonder if by pacing, with the subsequent increase in oxygen consumption of the myocardium, we are not getting an opposite effect. It is my feeling that in bradyarrhythmias pacing should not be based only on the electrical instability but also on hemodynamic measurements. I would not do it without simultaneously introducing a second catheter for measuring wedge pressures and possibly also cardiac outputs by thermodilution. In most cases I would not be inclined – unless there is associated hypotension – to pace routinely bradyarrhythmias.

J.P. VAN DURME *(Gent, Belgium):* I fully agree with your first remark, that patients presenting bilateral bundle branch block during the acute phase should be investigated as well as possible in order to define their long-term prognosis and that a His bundle recording should therefore be performed in those patients in whom the bilateral bundle branch block persists after the acute phase. Whether it is useful – for other purposes than clinical research – to perform it in the acute stage, is not evident to me. As to your second remark, I would come back to what I said at the beginning of my paper i.e. that electrical stimulation is not an all-or-none decision. I again fully agree with you that bradycardia in itself is from a theoretical point of view often an indication for pacing in the acute phase, but one has to look at the clinical situation.

Let us be more specific: bradycardia, which is a-symptomatic from a hemodynamic point of view and which is not associated with serious ventricular dysrhythmias, we do not pace.

P.M. ZOLL *(Boston, USA):* I would like to direct a question to Dr. Pirzarda. If I understood your paper correctly, the only groups you examined who needed temporary pacing were those who had some degree of A-V block and who had symptoms. This constitutes a definition of Stokes-Adams disease and I would think that these patients needed more than temporary pacing during surgery and anesthesia and that they needed long-term pacemakers. I would think that, if possible, these people should have had long-term pacemakers put in before your procedures, so that you had secure, reliable stimulation going on, or, if that were not possible, you would have put in long-term pacemakers afterwards.

F. PIRZARDA *(Boston, U.S.A.)*: This paper was a retrospective analysis, Dr. Zoll. Some of these patients did get permanent pacemakers later on. I certainly agree with you that it has to be taken seriously when somebody comes in with syncope and has evidence of bifascicular disease.

S. DALLA VOLTA *(Padova, Italy)*: I would first like to make some comments on the beautiful presentation of Dr. Rabago about the problem of pacing after major open-heart surgery. While I agree with him on the major part of the indications, I would like to make some remarks. In the majority of cases, the problem is not bradycardia or reduced heart rate but irregular heart rate like atrial flutter or fibrillation. Three conditions prevail: repair of type II atrial septum defect without any previous cardiac rhythm disturbance; patients with mitral and aortic valvular defects with or without prolonged PR conduction before operation, who develop atrial fibrillation after heart surgery and the third group are young children or newborns, as you mentioned. In these cases, the problem is not the very high heart rate in itself, which can be controlled by digitalis, but the irregular ventricular contraction. This can be very well protected by cardiac pacing, where in our experience stimulation at 100-110 beats per minute has given the best results. Cardiac output which has been routinely studied before and after such cardiac pacing, has shown an increase of about 28-32% only by changing the irregular rhythm to regular rhythm by ventricular pacing. In our experience, the hypothermia we are employing in the last three years – our overall experience with open-heart surgery is about 4.000 cases operated in the last 12 years – is a good protection against the origin of arrhythmia. We do not find that coronary heart patients are very prone to this kind of problems.

I also would stress the importance of later cardiac disturbances during the sixth, seventh or eighth day after operation, when the patients are nor longer in an intensive care unit. We believe that in patients who had cardiac troubles or are high-risk patients for cardiac troubles, the possibility of stimulation by leaving the wires for eight or ten days is the best policy. Sudden death after ten days is so rare that we can safely remove the wires after ten days. So, cardiac pacing is a good indication, more for regularizing the ventricular contraction than for the control of the cardiac frequency after a major operation for a cardiac defect.

G. Rabago *(Madrid, Spain):* I agree completely with the points Dr. Dalla Volta made. I would like to mention experiences in cardiac surgery on valvular patients. Where we have trouble is with patients we operated on for mitral and aortic valvular disease. We are utilizing now the Hancock and the Björk-Shily valve for mitral valve replacement. We are using the technique described by our associate, Dr. de Vega, for mitral annuloplasty. Lately, we have done 250 cases. It means we operated on very high-risk patients, patients treated for a long time with medical therapy. In reality, most of our problems with this kind of patient is his low rhythm with very low output and I agree with you that it is a very good thing to have a regular rhythm instead of an irregular rhythm. I think it is very important in these cases particularly in those with low cardiac output because of very low rhythm.

M. Pieniak *(Warsaw, Poland):* I have some questions for Dr. Van Durme, regarding the ventricular overdrive pacing during myocardial infarction that seems to me a rather dangerous method from the metabolic point of view, as expressed in terms of oxygen supply and demand.

The first question is: How many patients with ventricular tachycardia in the course of acute myocardial infarction have been treated by ventricular overdrive pacing? The second is: How long did this ventricular overpacing last in your patients? The third is: Have you observed ventricular fibrillation induced by over-drive pacing of the ventricle in such situations?

J.P. Van Durme *(Gent, Belgium):* I will answer your last question first. So far we have had no incidence of ventricular fibrillation during overriding the heart for ventricular dysrhythmias. Coming back to the first two remarks, I would very strongly point out, that I am not trying to push overdrive pacing as the treatment of choice for ventricular dysrhythmias. It must be clearly understood that the patients with ventricular dysrhythmias for whom we would advise overriding by atrial or ventricular pacing in the acute phase of myocardial infarction are patients for whom we, with decent clinical judgement, feel that we have exhausted the possibilities of medical anti-dysrhythmic treatment. I agree that it is not advisable to increase the heart rate in patients with acute myocardial infarction and I am fully aware that it might increase oxygen consumption and infarct size. This is not the problem. As to the duration of cardiac overdrive pacing, it should last as long as it is needed. The need for pacing should be evaluated twice daily. The longest period of temporary pacing we have performed in a patient with acute myocardial infarction was 21 days; at this moment it was decided to implant a permanent pacemaker.

O.S. Narula *(Chicago U.S.A.);* Dr. Rabago's presentation reminded me of a comment I failed to make. What I wanted to indicate is: that especially in patients with stenotic aortic valve disease where you have an obvious cause for syncope, you should not forget the A-V conduction system. I think these patients also need to have their conduction system studied especially if the aortic valve is heavily calcified. They may not need a valve, they may need a pacemaker or both. In one of the patients we have seen for a number of years, we diagnosed aortic stenosis. During five years, we have done about three hemodynamic studies. Nothing did change. The sixth year, he comes back to us with syncope and dizziness. The hemodynamic study we did showed no change in cardiac output and the pressure gradient was again about 55-60 millimeters of mercury. Nothing had changed. We were puzzled: Why is this patient suddenly symptomatic? We had done a conduction study on this patient and we found that the A-V conduction system was normal and without any evidence or obvious evidence of sinus bradycardia. We had done the sinus node recovery time, which was extremely long. In view of that fact, we gave him a permanent pacemaker and did not elect to give him a prosthetic aortic valve. We have had a follow-up of approximately four years by now, and the man is totally asymptomatic with a pacemaker only.

So we have to keep in mind that in patients with severe aortic stenosis the heavily calcified ring may encroach on the main His bundle and these patients may need a pacemaker, either alone or with a prosthetic aortic valve.

M.E.M. Macedo *(Lisbon, Portugal):* I would like to ask Dr. Rabago and also our Chairman because he is a surgeon one question about pacing after surgery. We have not used it yet, because we are waiting for the unit, the sequential atrioventricular pacer. But I think this pacing is one of the things that has been a great benefit for the patients, because it increases really the cardiac output. I would like to ask you both if you have any experience with sequential pacing in post-operative patients. And secondly a short note regarding the remarks of Dr. Dalla Volta: we do not remove the pacing wires before we remove the stitches from the skin.

P. Rabago *(Madrid, Spain):* We have not used sequential pacing in patients after surgery. We use ventricular wires. We found that when we take the patient out of the intensive-care unit, the patient is not monitored anymore. It means that you take the pulse and you see if there is some extrasystole or some bradycardia. We found that sometimes you can have problems with infection of the wires. This is one thing that bothered us. So we have the stimulation wires routinely only 48 hours, in the intensive care. When the patient is sent back to the ward, we remove most of them except in patients who needed them during their stay in intensive care. Only in a few cases do the wires remain for 30 days, like in some cases of Fallot's tetralogy with A-V block. We have found that this A-V block can return to sinus rhythm up to 30 days. And we wait that time before we decide to put a permanent pacemaker in a small child with Fallot's tetralogy. But again we never use sequential pacing although it probably is a very good thing to use in some cases but not in all.

CHAIRMAN: To answer your question, we do not use pacemaker wires in all cases. We only use them on indication. Rarely we needed them afterwards, but most of the time we do not need them at all.

When you are talking about prophylactic use of pacemaker wires, you should also talk about the risk of introducing pacemaker wires and the risk of infection. I remember very well a patient from whom we removed the pacemaker wires, who died afterwards. Unnecessary use of external pacemaker wires introduces an extra risk and we do not want to introduce extra risks in open-heart surgery. So we do not use pacemaker wires as a prophylaxis.

J.G.SLOMAN *(Melbourne, Australia):* May I return to the paper on "Cardiac Pacing in Acute Myocardial Infarction," and in particular to the remarks Dr. Amram made in allusion to the value of the serial measurements of the H-V interval post-infarction. We have recently completed a prospective study on about 50 patients with major conduction abnormalities occurring during the course of acute myocardial infarction and carried out serial measurements of the H-V interval after their survival, with a follow-up for one year. We have found absolutely no relationship between the length of the H-V interval and the patient's long-term prognosis, that is, up to one year. We have found that the prognosis is related to the risk factors, if you like, that were originally described by Dr. Peel, Dr. Norris and others. We have now decided to abandon the use of routine electro-physiological studies on these people with acute infarction, unless they develop a clinical arrhythmia which, in itself, may be an indication for permanent pacing.

J.P. VAN DURME *(Gent, Belgium):* The problem of conduction abnormalities in acute myocardial infarction is a controversial subject. I do not think, that there are enough data in the literature to settle the problem of prognostic significance of electro-physiological findings and more about to decide whether some patients would benefit from long-term prophylactic permanent pacing. Therefore I believe that it is worth investigating these patients and, in this regard, if you want to validate the follow-up data, I think you need electro-physiological data.

S. DALLA VOLTA *(Padova, Italy):* Coming back to aortic stenosis and calcified aortic stenosis, while I agree with Dr. Narula's conclusion about the importance of His bundles, I would stress one more point. The importance of block, in our experience, has been more related not to the presence of calcification of the aortic valve, but to the pre-operative coronary angiogram. We routinely do coronary angiograms in cases of mitral and aortic disease. We have seen that one-third or more of the cases with a lesion of about 50% of the right coronary artery or in some cases the left circumflex artery, will need permanent transvenous or epicardial pacing. While in patients who do not have any kind of important lesion – not critical, 10% or less – usually, the heart block is temporary.

L. Giec *(Katowice, Poland):* I have some comments about Dr. van Durme's lecture on "Cardiac Pacing in Acute Myocardial Infarction." I think we all agree with you that in cases of bradycardias in myocardial infarction cardiac pacing is a matter of choice in coronary care unit. But I think that in some cases of tachycardias it is enough for proper diagnosis and treatment, to use esophageal leads ECG and trans-esophageal pacing, to obtain the same effect as by endocardial electrodes.

J.P. Van Durme *(Gent, Belgium):* I would not agree with the statement that esophageal leads allow you to get as close to the diagnosis of dysrhythmias. Between an esophageal lead and a small wire inserted in the atrium through puncture of the subclavian vein, I still prefer the subclavian puncture. As to trans-esophageal pacing I think that it is not reliable enough to have a real place in the treatment of tachycardias.

Chairman; Thank you Dr. Van Durme. This had to be the last comment. I thank all of you for your interesting comments and close this morning session.

Section III

ENERGY SOURCES AND ELECTRONIC CIRCUIT

PACEMAKER ENERGY SOURCES, OLD AND NEW

WILSON GREATBATCH

Introduction

Implantable cardiac pacemakers have used many of the power sources known to man, from Parsonnet's watch escapement mechanisms and piezo electric generators through primary power sources of most of the alkali anode metals against most of the halogen cathodes. Primary batteries, rechargeable batteries and isotope nuclear decay have all been used. Biological energy in biogalvanic cells, biofuel cells, and hybrids of both, have been investigated.

The most used was the Mallory Rubin zinc-mercury battery which dominated the field from 1960 through 1975. It made practical pacemaking possible and we owe much to it. However, by 1970, 50% of all implanted pacemakers were being removed in under two years, usually because of battery failure. The battery operated at some 300 pounds per square inch (PSI) of hydrogen pressure and it slowly (and innocuously) exuded hydrogen gas and sodium hydroxide electrolyte to its environment. Thus the battery could not be hermetically sealed. Pacemakers containing this battery could be hermetically sealed but only by going to engineering extremes. They generally were not.

It was obvious in 1970 that better pacemakers would require better batteries. In 1970 Moser and Schneider (1) reported a new lithium battery system with an iodine cathode. We successfully hermetically sealed batteries of this type in stainless steel cases (2) and they were introduced first into clinical service in Italian pacemaker clinical implantations in March of 1972. The first lithium powered demand pacemaker using this battery system was implanted in France in 1973.

The lithium iodine battery does not use a fabricated separator, as does the mercury system and some other lithium systems. The electrolyte itself serves as a nondestructible, self-healing separator which grows in thickness as the battery is used. Thus two primary battery failure modes (moisture infiltration and separator penetration) are eliminated in the lithium iodine system.

The lithium iodine system was the first lithium system to enter clinical service and it is the most used today. There are now, however, at least five other lithium systems, all of which have shown commendable clinical performance. The following table describes them.

Other Lithium Pacemaker Battery Systems

		Fabricated Separator?	*Volts /Cell*	*Hermetic Seal?*
Lithium Lead Iodide	Mallory (USA)	No	1.9	Yes
Lithium Silver Chromate	Saft (FRANCE)	Yes	3.5	No
Lithium Thionyl Chloride	GTE/Arco (USA)	Yes	3.6	Yes
Lithium Copper Sulfide	Dupont/Cordis (USA)	Yes	1.9	No
Lithium Bromide	WGLtd. (USA)	No	3.5	Yes

It is our practice to identify each lithium iodine battery by a serial number and to practice strict traceability of each process and each component, back to original sources. Each battery is "burned-in" for two months with six computer readings of loaded voltage and 1 Kilohertz (KHz) impedance during this period. Production samples are withheld for long-term test. Our test racks include three batteries which are still operative after seven years test, at body temperature and body load.

Rundown characteristics

Lithium batteries run down in three distinct phases. During the first phase, which is about 75% of battery life, electrolyte resistance gradually increases in a nearly linear fashion as the lithium iodine layer increases. After this point, in phase II, a shoulder is seen after which loaded voltage drops more rapidly due to iodine depletion of the cathode complex. However, anytime during phases I or II the open circuit voltage will return to 2.8 Volts (V) $\pm$ 10 millivolts (mv) anytime that the load is removed and the battery is allowed to rest without load for a day or two.

During the third phase, the open-circuit voltage falls about 100 mv to the end-of-life point. This drop is due to the fact that the available iodine concentration is under 2% and the classic Nerst equation predicts such a drop.

The open circuit voltage thus is a very useful indicator of approaching end-of-life. At the 1.8 V end-of-life point, several months warning is available before actual battery failure becomes imminent, allowing convenient scheduling of procedures on a truly elective basis.

Other halogens

We have built lithium batteries with cathodes of other halides. Bromine has proven successful in our hands and has seen some clinical service. We have also constructed batteries with chlorine and with flourine cathodes although we have not yet achieved practical designs with these systems. The lithium bromine battery has an open-circuit voltage of 3.45 V and an energy density of twice that of our best lithium iodine batteries. We hope to see considerable clinical use of the lithium bromine system in the 1979-1980 period.

Microcalorimeter battery evaluation

A recent most useful innovation has been the use of microcalorimetry for early evaluation of internal self-discharge in batteries and pacemakers. This concept was suggested to us in 1975 by Haaken Elmqvist and the Swedish Siemans Elema group in Stockholm and again two days later in Holland by Mr. Eikmans of Vitatron. The former group recently reported preliminary measurements on small batteries with a small commercial microcalorimeter.

We recently reported a large aperture microcalorimeter of our own design which is capable of seeing as little as 3 microwatts (μW) of generated heat. This is one-fifth of the energy generated by germinating a grain of rice! With this instrument we are able to nondestructively identify abnormal leakage paths in batteries and even in completed pacemakers. The time required for evaluation of internal self-discharge in batteries has been reduced from years to hours. We consider this instrument to be one of the major contributions of this decade to battery technology.

Nuclear pacemakers

Early problems with pacemaker batteries encouraged the development of atomic batteries operating on the nuclear decay of radioactive isotopes. Two isotopes were introduced to clinical practice: plutonium 238 with an excessive half-life of 87 years and promethium 147 with an inadequate half-life of 2.5 years. Tritium, with an ideal half-life of 13 years was considered but the problem of coping with its low energy level was not solved.

By 1973 no less than five manufacturers offered nuclear batteries for clinical use. If chemical batteries had not improved, probably all pacemakers today would be powered by nuclear batteries. However, lithium batteries did improve to the point where primary chemical batteries more than met the reliability objectives originally set for nuclear batteries.

Nuclear batteries themselves far surpassed their own objectives. However, the mandatory documentary requirements imposed by government regulatory authorities were such a deterrent to widespread use that nuclear powered pacemakers never did account for more than 1% of the pacemaker market. Few are implanted today.

Conclusion

Pacemakers and batteries are both becoming smaller and longer lived. We have predicted for some time that by 1980 the typical pulse generator will be under 10 millimeters thick, well under 50 grams in weight, will be rate-programmable and will have a ten year life. We also believe that halogens higher than iodine will come into use, providing still higher energy densities.

The reliability of sealed lithium powered pulse generators is already so high that nearly all surgical interventions today are for electrode related problems. When electrode problems too are eliminated, we will have arrived at the state where most pacemakers will outlive their host patients, without surgical intervention of any kind.

References

1. Schneider, A., Moser, J., Webb, T.H.E. and Desmond, J.E., A new high energy density cell with a lithium anode. Proc. Proc. U.S. Army Signal Corps. Power Sources Conf. Atlantic City (1970).
2. Greatbatch, W., Lee, J., Mathias, W., Eldridge, M., Moser, J. and Schneider, A., The solid-state lithium battery: a new improved chemical power source for implantable cardiac pacemakers IEEE BME Transactions 18-5: 317 (1971).

THE SAFT LITHIUM – SILVER CHROMATE BATTERY PERFORMANCES OF THE LI 210 TYPE

G. LEHMANN, M. BROUSSELY AND P. LENFANT

Introduction

After being involved in lithium power sources research since 1964, SAFT perfected in 1970 a new couple: lithium – silver chromate. In the light of the exceptional characteristics of this system, in particular its shelf life quality, a battery was specially designed and manufactured to power cardiac pacing devices. This battery is called Li 210. It was put on the market at the beginning of 1973, and immediately aroused the interest of pacemaker manufacturers so that a fairly large number of them are now using it in their apparatuses.

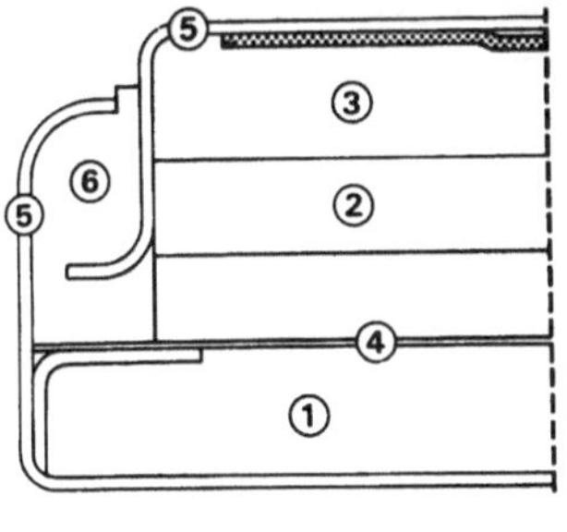

1. Silver chromate
2. Electrolyte impregnated in separators
3. Lithium anode
4. Barrier layer
5. Stainless steel container
6. Polypropylene gasket

Figure 1.

The technology of the cell is briefly described in Fig. 1, it is a button cell type, of 21 mm in diameter, 9 mm in height, weighing 9 gr. In this paper, we present the up-dated performances of the cell, extrapolating them in order to determine a projected life time. We indicate also our recent shelf life test results and, finally, we will give a figure of reliability for implanted pacemakers using this battery.

1. *Performances of the Li 210 SAFT batteries*

The realistic performances of the Li 210 battery at a pacemaker rate, have been estimated by two methods.

- By the first method, batteries are continuously discharged under a load equivalent to a pacemaker duty.

- By the second one, batteries are initially discharged under a rapid rate. When they reach a given cut-off voltage (2.4 V.), corresponding to a reaction efficiency of about 85% they are removed from the load and put on a higher one equivalent to the PM rate. In such a way, it is possible to obtain the realistic shape of the end of discharge of the cell. We choose a load of 300 K Ω as an equivalent PM duty; this load corresponds to a mean current of 10 μA; i.e. 20 μA for a pacemaker using two batteries in a parallel assembly. The two tests have been performed for more than two years by sampling each manufacturing day:
  - 2 batteries which are discharged on 300 K Ω (10 μ A)
  - 2 batteries which are discharged on 15 K Ω (200 μA) at a cut-off voltage of 2.4 Volts and afterwards put under 300 K Ω.

At present, we have accumulated a sufficient quantity of data to be able to determine with good accuracy the projected performances of the cell. A mean discharge curve for a Li 210 cell under the PM rate has an initial voltage of 3.24 V. and decreases steadily to 3.15 V. after 2.2 years, with a slope of 3.4 mV. per month (Fig. 2). The mean discharge curve under the rapid rate – represented in Fig 3 – shows that the delivered capacity is of 515 mAh at 2.5 V. (end of the first discharge reaction) and of 575 mAh at 2.4 V. Fig. 4 shows the mean voltage recovery curve obtained when a battery initially discharged on the rapid rate is put on the PM rate. The voltage increases and the remaining capacity is re-

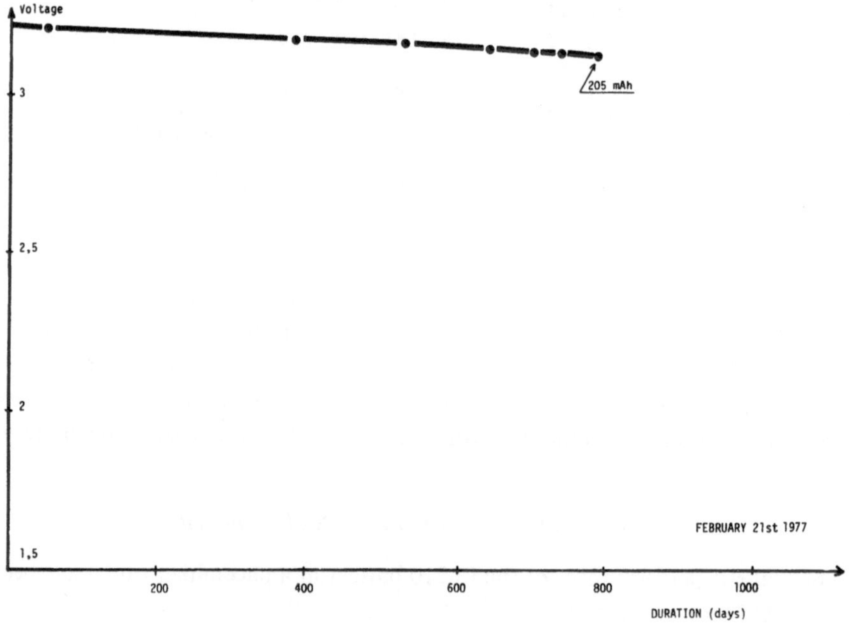

Figure 2. Mean discharge under 300 K Ω.

covered, i.e. 118 mAh; 59 mAh corresponding to the first reaction and 59 mAh to the second one. It should be noticed that this test is still in progress after 540 days, consequently the values given here are inferior to reality.

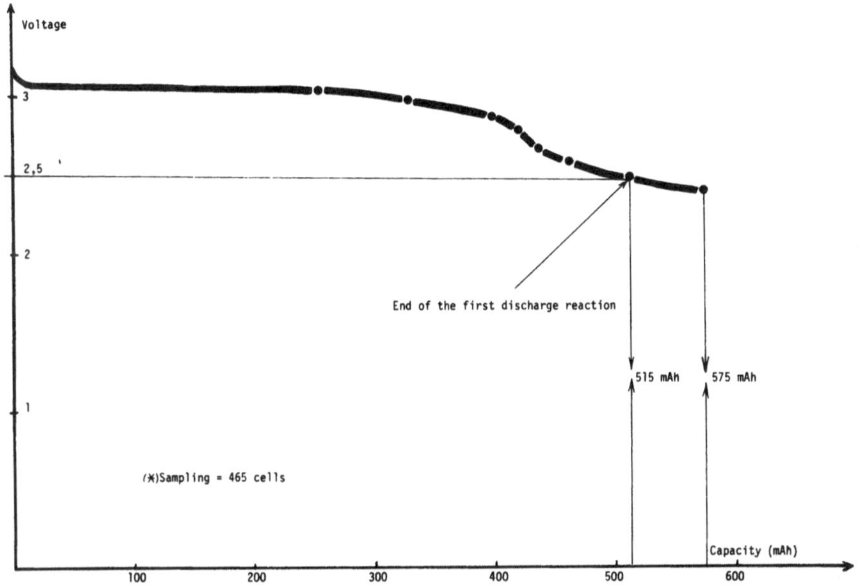

Figure 3. Mean discharge curve(*) under 200 μA (15 K Ω).

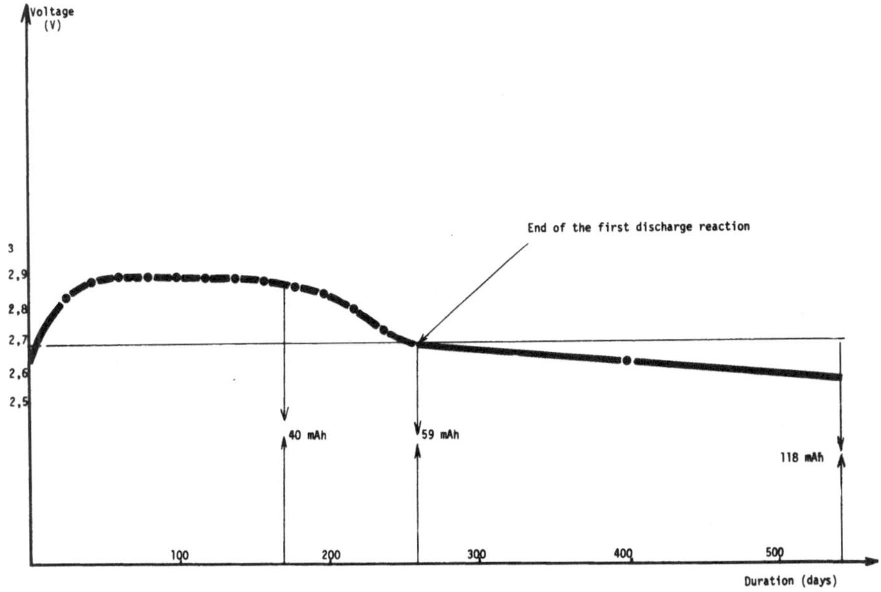

Figure 4. End of discharge under 300 K Ω (≃ 10 μA) for cells initially discharged under 15 K Ω (≃ 200 μA) at a cut off voltage of 2.4 volts. Mean value for 25 samples.

By association of the preceding results, we have determined the projected performances of the cell (Fig. 5). From this curve, it can be concluded that the useful life-time of the Li 210 cell will be of 6¼ years at 2.9 V., and of 7½ years at a cut-off voltage of 2.6 V. for a pacemaker having a current consumption of 20 μA and using two batteries in a parallel assembly. Fig. 6 represents on a larger scale

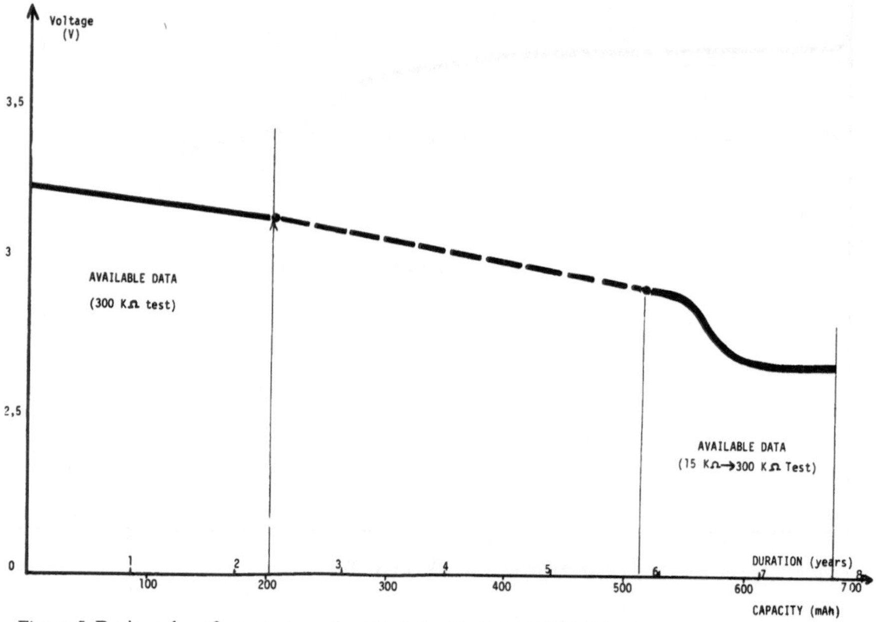

Figure 5. Projected performances under 10μA for the Li 210 SAFT battery.

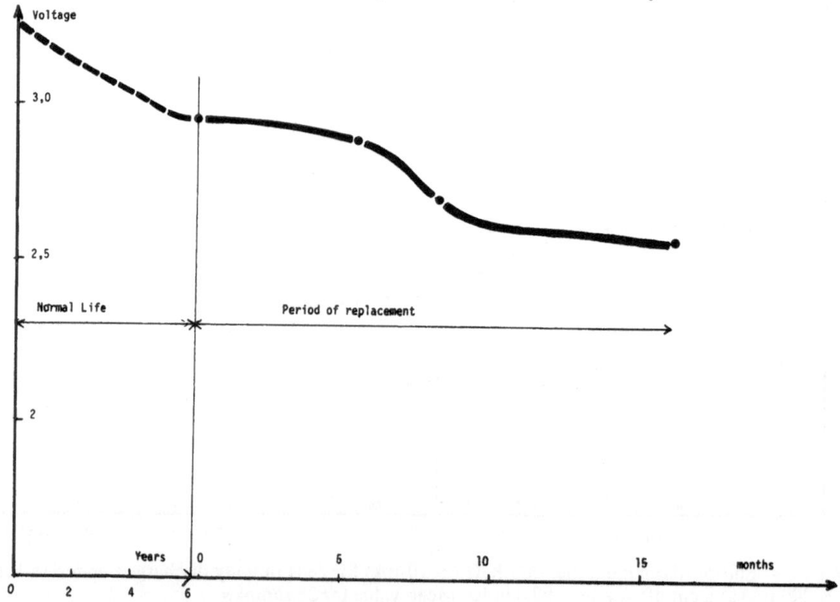

Figure 6. End of discharge under 10 μA (300 K Ω).

the realistic shape of the curve from the first plateau to the second one; it shows that the minimum prophylactic replacement period will be of 15 months, after the 6¼ years normal run of life. To conclude, SAFT benefits from the experience of the first 2½ years and the last 15 months of discharge. The only reason for a performance inferior to the estimated one, would be a self-discharge of the system. This problem has been studied in different ways.

2. *Self-discharge*

The theoretical reaction of self-discharge is as follows:

1. Solubilization of the active material:

$$Ag_2\,CrO_4 + 2\,Li^+ \rightleftarrows 2\,Ag^+ + Li_2\,CrO_4$$

2. Reduction on the lithium anode:

$$2\,Ag^+ + 2\,Li \rightarrow 2\,Li^+ + 2\,Ag$$

The overall self-discharge reaction can therefore be described as follows:

$$Ag_2\,CrO_4 + 2\,Li \rightarrow Li_2\,CrO_4 + 2\,Ag$$

Such a reaction is easily detected by various methods.

1. A rise in the storage temperature increases the solubilization of the active material and consequently accelerates the self-discharge (accelerated storage test).

2. The suggested reaction would involve during storage:

- the deposit of silver metal on the lithium anode,
- a loss of lithium,
- a loss of silver – chromate,

and these parameters can be measured by chemical analysis.

By the first method (high temperature storage test) it was impossible to detect the slightest loss of capacity after 14 months of storage at + 45° C. By the second one, (chemical analysis) we measured a deposit of silver on the anode of 0.25 mg after 14 months at + 45° C. This value corresponds to a self-discharge of 0.01%. From these two tests, it can be concluded that the self-discharge phenomenon is practically nonexistent in the lithium – silver chromate system.

3. *Reliability of the Li 210 battery*

In a preceding paper (1), we gave the failure rate value for Li 210 cells, in tests in our laboratories and we showed how our quality – control system is the guarantee of the high reliability of the product. Here, our purpose is to establish a figure of reliability for cells having already been implanted. On a large quantity of batteries dispatched all around the world, it is practically impossible to establish the accurate number of these having been implanted and the implantation duration of each one. Consequently, the figure of reliability indicated hereafter has to be considered only as an approximation based on the following hypotheses:

- two cells are used per pacemaker,
- 10% of the cells shipped to our customers are sampled for quality – control and not used in pacemakers,
- there is a 6 months delay between the delivery date of the cell and the implantation date of the corresponding pacemaker. With these hypotheses, and knowing the number of cells dispatched each month, we can calculate the number of "implanted pacemaker-month" using our battery. This calculation was made on the 1st of March 1977 and gives the following result:
- implanted pacemaker-month with Li 210 cells: 119 300. Our customers have never informed us of a failure due to the battery and so we conclude in a fourth hypothesis that no pacemaker failure has arisen from the battery. In such a case, the statistical calculation gives the following failure rate for the pacemakers.

Table 1.

	Failure Rate (λ) per hour	*Failure Rate (λ) % per month*
Confidence level 90%	$2{,}7 \times 10^{-8}$	0.0019
Confidence level 99.9%	$8{,}2 \times 10^{-8}$	0.0059

This is a rough idea of the failure rate due to the battery using the Li 210 cells; in particular, we have not considered that some of those pacemakers can be replaced for other reasons than for a battery failure (electrode or circuitry failure, unrelated death...). These replacements represent certainly a very small percentage of the total number of pacemakers, and this parameter is negligible in our calculation, taking into account the other approximations that we have been obliged to make.

A clinical evaluation based on a small number of implanted pacemakers followed with accuracy, was undertaken in collaboration with an Italian pacemaker manufacturer (LEM) and a cardiologist from the Hospital of Ferrara (Professor Antonioli) (2). This study is supported by a follow-up of 540 pacemakers using Li 210 batteries; the first having been implanted in June 1974. The results obtained are summarized in Table 2.

Table 2.

Number of cells per pacemaker	*Pacemaker Type*		*Failure*			
	Fixed Rate	*Demand Rate*	*Cell*	*Circuitry*	*Rejection*	*Death*
3 Li 210		48	0	1	1	
2 Li 210	7	492	0	2	1	1
Total	7	540	0	3	2	1
Percent			0	0.54	0.36	0.18

By the 31st of August 1976, 2678 pacemaker-months had been accumulated with no battery failure, the death being not related to the pacemaker functioning but to pulmonary cancer.

Conclusion

The Lithium – Silver Chromate cells, as power sources for pacemakers, confirm our previous expectations.

The present discharge data has already allowed us to cover a lot of ground and the chemical tests carried out, lead us to believe that the remainder will conform to our expectations, i.e. the realization of a small generator having an excellent reliability and capable of powering a pacemaker for seven years.

Finally, in view of the general aim for a "pacemaker for life," SAFT will produce from July onwards a higher capacity cell. This new Lithium – Silver chromate battery, model Li 355, which has been clinically and chemically tested for three years now, will offer a volumetric energy of 0.82 Wh/cm^3, giving to the pacemaker a projected life time of more than 15 years.

References

1. Gerbier, G., Lehman, G., Lenfant, P., Rivault, J.P., "Reliability of Lithium Silver Chromate cells" 10th International Power Sources Symposium – Brighton – Sept. 1976.
2. Antonioli, G.E., Baggioni, G., Grassi, G., Lehmann, G., "Lithium powered pacemakers – Our own experience since 1972" To be published.

THE LITHIUM-IODINE CELL

A.A. SCHNEIDER AND F. TEPPER

Introduction

In 1967 Catalyst Research Corporation (CRC) became involved in the invention and development of a new electrochemical system, the lithium-iodine cell. Since that time, over 100,000 cells have been produced by both lithium-iodine cell manufacturers, and to this time there has not been a single premature failure documented for any clinical cell.

This outstanding record is the result of two factors. The first is the quality designed into the cell and the extensive testing of each individual cell; at CRC each cell is subjected to a simulated pacemaker load for two months before it is accepted. Each cell design undergoes extensive environmental testing such as shock, vibration and thermal cycling. The second factor contributing to the outstanding record is the chemistry itself.

Cell chemistry – self-discharge

The cell is composed of three layers: lithium, lithium-iodide and an iodine-containing depolarizer abbreviated P2VP · nI_2.* When the cell is first formed, the lithium-iodide layer is very thin. This layer grows as iodine from the P2VP · nI_2 diffuses through to the lithium anode and reacts to form more lithium iodide according to the equation

$$2Li + I_2 = 2LiI. \tag{1}$$

This self-limiting reaction is the primary self-discharge process.

The layer formed is both electrolyte and separator. Unlike conventional cells, the electrolyte is not added during the construction process but is formed *in situ*. The layer is also self-healing. (A crack would result in more lithium iodide being formed at the crack site, sealing the flaw.)

* P2VP · nI_2 is poly (2-vinylpyridine) combined with n moles of iodine.

For any cell the self-discharge reactions are important since they play a significant role in determining how long that cell will run under pacemaker conditions. Only with very low self-discharge rates can one expect a pacemaker cell to run for more than five years. Measurements using the CRC Model 802/23 cell confirm that this cell does show such a low rate. Microcalorimetric data at 37°C are presented in Table 1 showing a decrease in heat output with cell age and with time under load. Cells A and B were run at 100 Kohm load for 10 and 2 months, respectively, then stored for one month under no load before measurement. Cell C was never subjected to loading and was measured at 1 and 2 months after manufacture.

Table 1. Heat Output from 802/23 Cells

Cell	*Months at 100 Kohm Load*	*Months Off Load*	*Heat Output*
A	10	1	5.0 microwatts
B	2	1	5.6 microwatts
C	0	1	23.8 microwatts
		2	8.8 microwatts

Cell A was also subjected to microcalorimetry measurements under load. With the cell in the calorimeter, current was increased in steps from zero to 200 microamperes. At the 5 microampere level, heat output decreased from 5.0 to 3.7 microwatts, suggesting that some iodine atoms, which would have contributed to self-discharge under no load were instead delivering useful electrical energy to the external load. At higher currents, internal i^2R losses obscured the measurement of any further decreases in self-discharge.

A self-discharge rate of 5.0 microwatts for cell A is equivalent to 0.7%/year capacity loss and a 3.7 microwatt rate to a 0.5%/year loss. Measurement of cell resistance increase under no load, a technique which can also be used to follow self-discharge, shows that cell capacity losses rise linearly with the square root of time; that is, equal amounts of capacity should be lost to self-discharge in 1, 4 and 9 years. This is a confirmation of the decrease seen in Table 1. In short, over a 10 year period, as little as 2% of cell capacity will probably be lost to self-discharge and, at worst, this number might be as high as 7% if the cell is not loaded.

Other investigators have reported considerably high microwatt outputs from lithium-iodine cells and have attributed these losses to reactions other than the prime reaction shown in equation (1). This points out the importance of experimental design when trying to measure the rate of this reaction. Very simple cells should be constructed which contain no cements or other materials whose heat of curing or reaction with iodine might obscure the basic rate. These side reactions may or may not be taking their toll in available cell energy, but in a worst case analysis, one must assume that they are.

Cell chemistry – electrochemical discharge

As one draws current from the cell, the following reactions occur:

$$\text{Anode:} \quad 2Li = 2Li^+ + 2e^- \tag{2}$$
$$\text{Cathode:} \quad P2VP \cdot nI_2 + 2e^- = P2VP \cdot (n\text{-}1)I_2 + 2I^- \tag{3}$$
$$\text{Overall:} \quad 2Li + P2VP \cdot nI_2 = 2LiI + P2VP \cdot (n\text{-}1)I_2 \tag{4}$$

At constant current, the lithium-iodide layer builds up linearly, resulting in a linear decline in voltage as is shown in Figure 1. The curves in this figure are

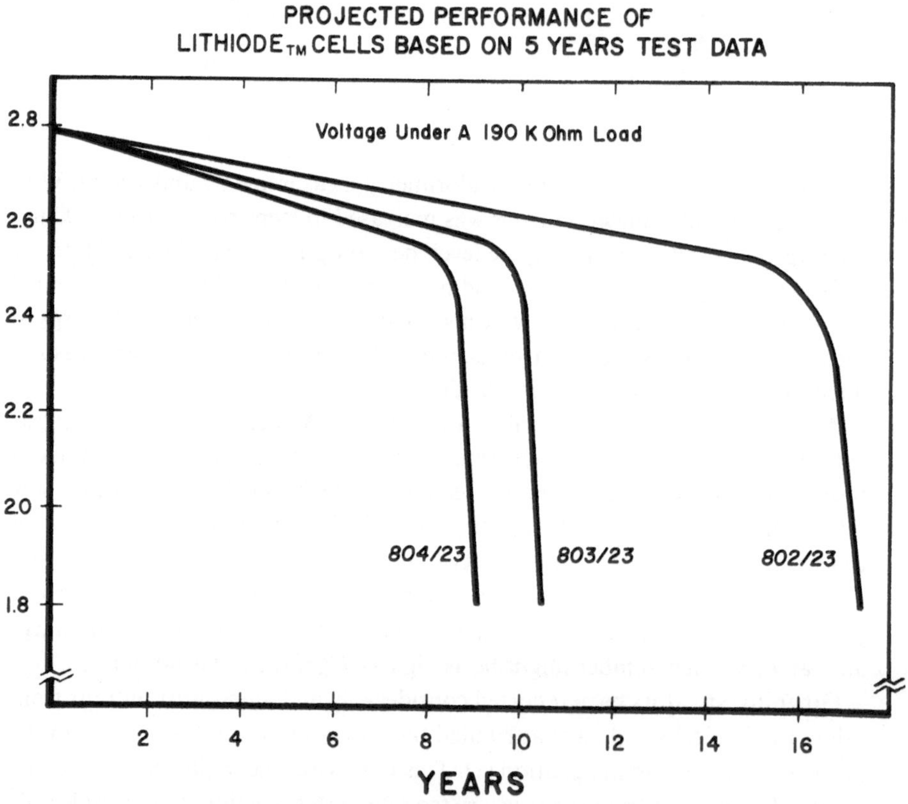

Figure 1. Sample discharge curves for 800 series cells.

based on six years hard data with lithium-iodine cells. Extrapolation from six to ten years appear justified, we feel, on the basis of experience with the cell design and the known properties of the metal and plastic cell encapsulants; beyond ten years, the extrapolation is tenuous.

The linear decline continues until the depolarizer is depleted of iodine and a "knee" in the curve is seen. This knee can be explained using the data in Figure 2

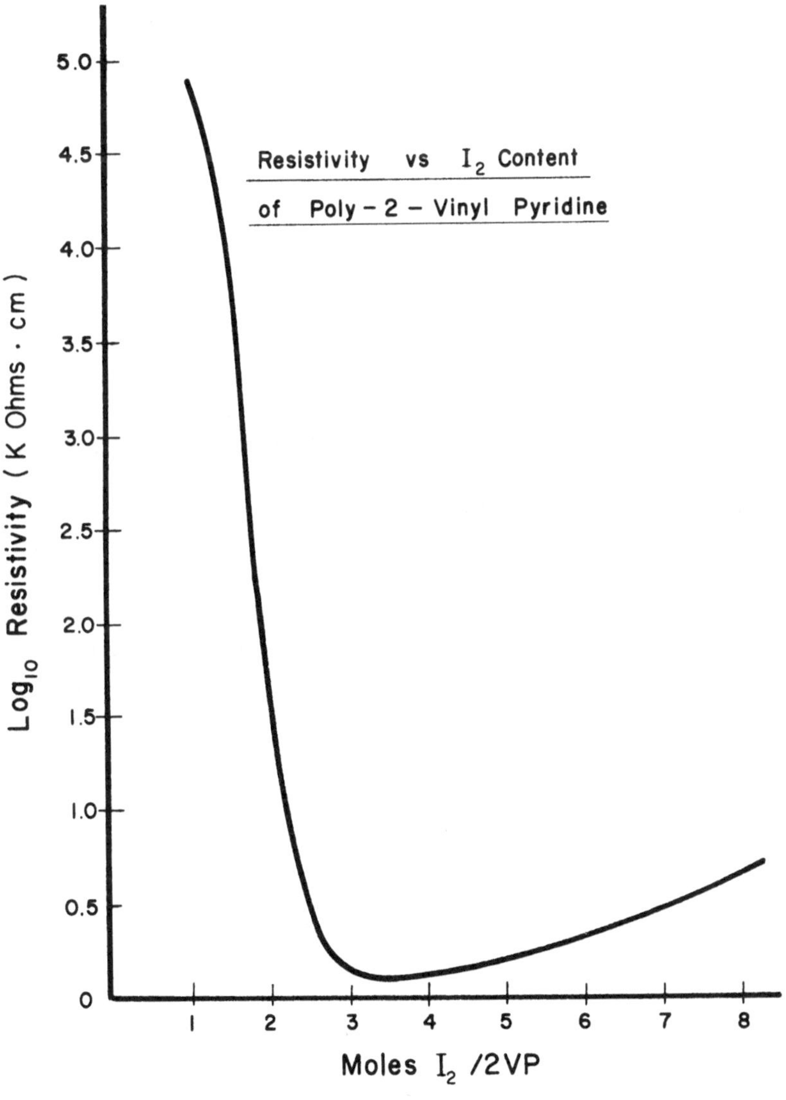

Figure 2. Depolarizer resistivity as a function of iodine content.

which shows the resistance of depolarizer as a function of iodine content. A fresh cell has 6.2 molecules of iodine per P2VP monomer unit (n = 6.2). As this number decreases to below 2, the resistance of the depolarizer rises, creating the "knee" in the curve.

Cell construction

The curves in Figure 1 illustrate the performance of CRC 800 series cells, which use triple encasement of the corrosive depolarizer material. The first encasement is the outer hermetic stainless steel case itself. Inside this is a fluoropolymer plastic envelope which is highly resistive to iodine attack. The third encasement is the lithium envelope itself which completely contains both the P2VP • nI_2 depolarizer and any iodine vapor.

The cell is constructed in a dry room where the relative humidity is 1%. After cleaning the lithium metal, it is formed into a cup and the depolarizer poured in. Following solidification of the depolarizer, the lithium cup is cold-welded shut and then the plastic envelope is added. The final stages of manufacture include welding, leak testing and two months of electrical testing of each individual cell.

Photomicrographs of partially discharged lithium-iodine cells reveal yet another encasement of the depolarizer material, the lithium-iodide electrolyte itself. This salt forms a hard layer between the lithium and depolarizer and when sufficient discharge has taken place, becomes an efficient barrier to depolarizer migration.

An interesting phenomenon seen in the photomicrographs is the apparent orientation of the lithium-iodide crystallites in columnar fashion, the axes of which are parallel to the direction of current flow. This arrangement might provide "highways" for the migration of lithium ions along the crystallite grain boundaries. Such a scheme could explain the high ionic conductivity of the electrolyte layer in the cell which is an order of magnitude larger than the conductivity of bulk lithium iodide.

Summary

The new self-discharge data presented in this paper show a maximum capacity loss of 2 to 7% in ten years for the lithium-iodine cell. These data support our former worst-case estimates of 10% maximum self-discharge loss in ten years. Predictions of the end-of-life characteristics of the cell have been calculated based on depolarizer resistivity data. These predictions can give circuit designers the necessary information to design an end-of-life indicator for lithium-iodine powered pacemakers which allows ample time for elective replacement.

Over the last two years, the lithium-iodine system has become the choice of the pacemaker industry. By 1978, more than one-half of all pacemakers manufactured will be lithium-iodine powered. With a reliable long-life power source such as this in hand, the industry has turned its focus to other areas which could not be investigated in years past when the mercury cell was the only choice available. Areas such as electronics reliability and efficiency, package miniaturization, lead reliability and long-term corrosion are now the main areas of concern for the pacemaker designer rather than the battery.

THE LITHIUM PACEMAKER, A FOUR-YEAR CLINICAL EXPERIENCE

J. KREUZER, O. ELERT AND P. SATTER

The main reason for unsatisfactory results in long-time stimulation of mercury-zinc batteries is a relatively high self-discharge and a small capacity. The reduction of energy for the single impulse will prolong durability but certainly not to the predicted time of 70 months. From March 7th 1973 to March 31st 1977 we implanted in Frankfurt 398 different Lithium-powered pacemakers as outlined in Figure 1.

STIMULITH	137	WG 702P/E
MINILITH	68	WG 752
MAXILITH	51	WG 702E
VITALITH S6	44	SAFT
ELEMA 207	40	CATALYST RES. 801
ELEMA 187/188	20	WG 702 E
ARCO L2	11	ARCO
CORATOMIC	6	MALLORY
BIOTRONIK	6	SAFT
LEM V12	6	SAFT
XYREL	5	WG 742
TELECTRONICS	2	SAFT
EDWARDS	1	SAFT
AMTECH	1	CATALYST RES. 801

Figure 1. Number of various types for 398 pacemakers implanted between March 1973 and March 1977 with on the right side the type of lithium battery.

1. We ourself implanted 59 pacemakers with the Saft Lithium cell 210.

2. Two such cells are placed in one pacemaker with a total capacity of 1,2Ah.

3. In 320 cases we have used pacemakers with Wilson Greatbatch and Catalyst Research Lithium cells.

4. The first implanted lithium pacemakers in 1973 had the Wilson Greatbatch 702P cells with only one anode. The inner resistance rose much quicker than expected and today 40 months after implantation 7 of those pacemakers are due for replacement. By introducing a second anode in the 702E cell, the increase of inner resistance could be reduced to 100 Ohm/month so that a durability of 72 months can be expected.

Today the development of Lithium batteries has reached a technical standard which gives us hope for the future and a possibility to choose the best pacemaker for a patient, according to his age and his expectation of life. Figure 2 shows the distribution of age of our patients.

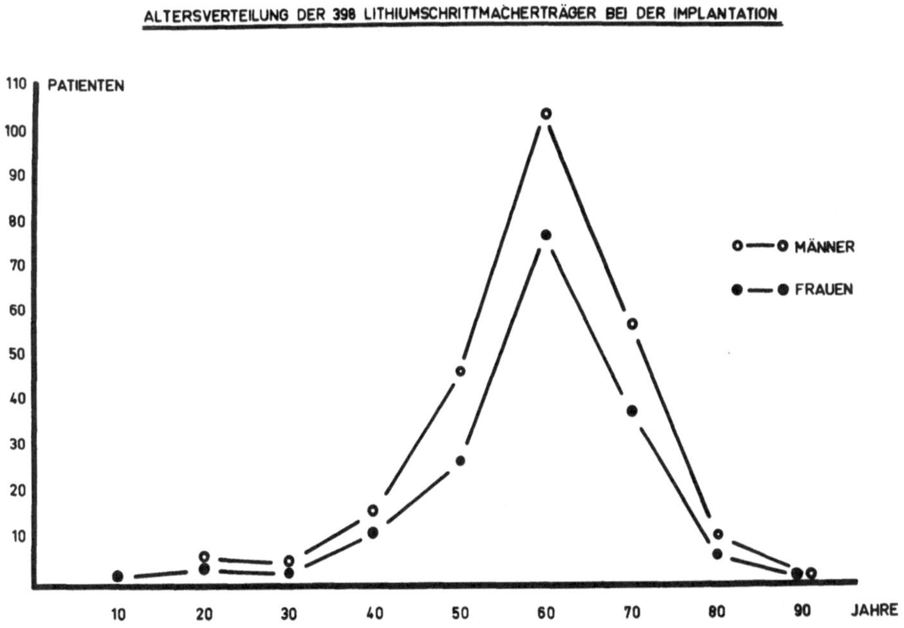

Figure 2. Age and sex distribution of the 398 patients at the first implantation of a lithium-powered pacemaker.

INDIKATIONEN ZUR LITHIUM-SCHRITTMACHER-IMPLANTATION		
MAS-ANFÄLLE	138	PATIENTEN
A.V. BLOCK 3°	106	"
BRADYARRHYTHMIE	39	"
A.V. BLOCK 2°	27	"
CAROTISSINUS SYNDROM	23	"
SINUSBRADYCARDIE	18	"
S.A.BLOCK	13	"
SONSTIGE	11	"
SICK-SINUS-SYNDROM	10	"
TACHY - BRADYCARDIE	9	"
BIFASC. BLOCK	4	"
GESAMTZAHL	398	PATIENTEN

Figure. 3. Indications for the implantation of a lithium-powered pacemaker.

Results

Electrically all 208 Elema 187-188 Maxilith and Stimulith pacemakers are functioning well. Nevertheless we had to replace 5 Stimulith pacemakers because of double stimulation and additional spikes.

Three pacemakers Vitalith S6 were defective on implantation due to an interruption within one of the circuits. A damage during transport could not be excluded. Pacemakers with discrete circuits proved equally reliable as those with integrated circuits. Pacemakers with MOS technique did not show any special advantages in power demand or reliability, compared with the others. The real advantage of all new developments is weight and size. Weight and size of the Elema Stimulith and Maxilith 187-188 were the reasons for stopping their implantation. But most other models are also far away from what would be possible to achieve. In our opinion the new Coratomic pacemaker comes quite close to the possible optimum. For many reasons – in particular resterilisation and lack of pyrogenicity – hermetically sealed all-metal bodies are preferred.

Unfortunately it is impossible to convince the companies to make a standard interchangeable connection between electrodes and batteries. An interchange is however possible between Cordis and Medtronic. Bulky connectors like the Biotronik could never really be satisfying.

Muscle twitching in particular with the Minilith pacemakers is a minor problem, but in some cases very annoying to the patient. This may be due to the fact that we still prefer the subpectoral implantation of the batteries because we did not have a single perforation in over 2.500 operations. Covering the pacemaker with a silicone boot could not prevent this twitching in every case. Other groups using subcutaneous implantation do not have this type of problem.

Problems still to be solved are in particular in the field of electrodes. The race for the smallest tip will soon be over just as the implantation of pacemakers with a stimulation time of less than 0,5 msec. The ideal electrode with no material fatigue and lifelong function when implanted in children, is still far away.

Conclusion

Today it is not possible to give a final opinion on the new Lithium-powered pacemakers. 4 years is a short time and experience has taught us to be cautious in prediction and in particular, in believing the prediction made by the industry. Industry has so often failed and the last two years have shown pacemakers with large series of recalls, but the progress is rapid. The Lithium-powered new generation of pacemakers with integrated circuits has already made the hazardous radionuclear pacemaker obsolete and will probably in a short time do the same to the mercury battery.

NEW PACEMAKER DEVICES FROM A TECHNICAL POINT OF VIEW

DAVID L. BOWERS

New pacemaker devices commercially available today have evolved from a simple functional device having limited life to a sophisticated system designed to operate for an extended period, hopefully the life of the pacemaker patient. The basic pacemaker function, demand pacing, remains the preferred choice for pacing but the technology used to generate this demand function has drastically changed. There are three major technical improvements in pulse generator design which help to extend pacemaker longevity and improve system performance. They are: (1) development of the lithium power source; (2) housing the electronics and power source in a hermetic package; and (3) utilization of thick-film hybrid circuitry.

The introduction of new technology to the pacemaker field has created a unique terminology vocabulary for describing new pacemaker devices. The descriptive terms are not medical terms but technical expressions describing significant improvements in pulse generator design. Therefore, today's pacemaker could be described using the following terms: *A hermetically sealed lithium pulse generator containing thick-film hybrid CMOS electronics.* To help associate each term as it relates to a pulse generator device, the terms are listed on the system interaction diagram shown in Figure 1.

The term *hermetically sealed* is associated with the pulse generator package and its primary function is to seal the electronics and power source in a controlled environment. The term *lithium* relates to the power source and is the new long-term battery source used to power the electronics and supply stimulus energy to the heart. The composite set of terms, THICK-FILM HYBRID CMOS, describes the type of electronic devices and circuit construction selected to improve pacemaker performance and provide additional features such as programmability.

The purpose of the hermetically sealed package is to provide a gas-tight as well as a fluid-tight housing preventing the controlled environment inside the housing from being altered by the presence of a gas or fluid outside environment. Placing the electronics and power source in a hermetic or controlled environment offers many advantages not possible with an epoxy (non-hermetic) pacemaker. The advantages can be related to improved pulse generator reliability and better

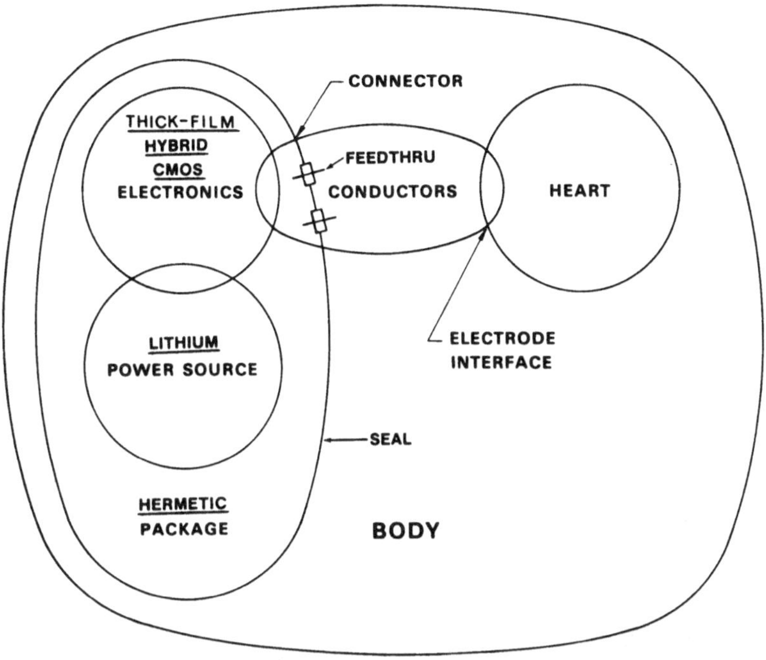

Figure 1. Technical terms are underlined within a pacemaker system interaction diagram.

prediction of system performance for long-term application. This does not mean epoxy pulse generators are less reliable than hermetically sealed devices, but it is more difficult to control and predict their long-term performance, beyond the 3 to 5 year longevity range associated with present epoxy devices.

Therefore, a hermetically sealed pulse generator has the best chance to reliably achieve its projected longevity and in terms of today's longevity predictions, this means an anticipated life of 5 to 10 years, with future devices projected to last 10 to 20 years. Another significant advantage for a controlled environment, is that it makes possible the use of advanced electronic circuits and special semiconductor devices which were impossible to use in an epoxy encapsulated device.

For the package to be hermetic and retain its hermetic properties over a 10 to 20 years period, requires the package housing to be carefully designed using proper materials and sealing techniques. The common materials used for the housing are stainless steel or pure titanium. There are various welding methods such as electron beam, plasma, TIG, etc., used to seal the metallic housing but the selection of the welding method will depend on the housing material and overall package design.

After sealing the package it is necessary to determine the level of hermeticity or simply stated, the degree of environment isolation between inside and outside of the package. One method to determine hermeticity is to monitor the leak-rate of a gas passing through the housing and quantitatively measure the amount of gas leaking out of a package. A practical method is to fill the pulse generator package with a gas such as helium at the time it is sealed and then measure the rate of helium escaping from the package after sealing. A practical guideline for a helium test is to have a leak-rate less than 1×10^{-8} standard cubic centimeters of helium per second per atmosphere escaping through the package. This is a very low leak-rate value but essential if the pulse generator is to operate reliably in a stable and controlled environment for 10 years with a design goal for 20 years.

The *lithium* battery has proven to be a reliable and predictable power source for pacemaker application. The combination of the lithium battery with advanced electronic circuitry, sealed in a hermetic package, has made it possible to achieve realistically the 5 to 10 year life pacemaker. Details regarding the lithium battery will not be presented in this paper but the author directs persons who are interested in this unique battery to refer to papers presented on power sources at the Pacemaker Colloquium.

The next subject relates to the pulse generator electronics and new circuit technology. The term *thick-film hybrid* describes the type of construction used to build the circuit structure. A hybrid circuit can be defined as a circuit structure which combines various technologies to form a complete electronic circuit. For example, in hybrid construction thick-film technology is used to make or print circuit resistors on a substrate combined with semiconductor technology to form active devices like transistors. This combination of technologies to form a hybrid circuit is an effective and reliable technique to construct sophisticated and low current drain electronics especially for pacemaker application.

The term CMOS also relates to the electronics and is the most difficult term to find a simple but descriptive technical definition. CMOS is a special type of semiconductor transistor used for low current and battery powered applications. Therefore it is well suited for pacemaker application where low current drain and battery operation is essential. What do the letters C-M-O-S represent? The letters CMOS are derived from the first letter of each word in the following statement: Complementary Metal Oxide Semiconductor. The CMOS principle is based on a complementary two transistor design with the transistors connected in series, always having one transistor in the off- or non-conducting state. Figure 2a shows a simple schematic comparing a CMOS circuit (2 transistors) with a standard circuit (1 transistor) which represents a standard, bipolar transistor. The CMOS circuit has two series connected switches, A & B, representing 2 transistors. The waveform patterns in Figure 2b illustrate the opening and closing sequences for switches A and B. Note, when switch A is closed switch B is open; the reverse condition is also true.

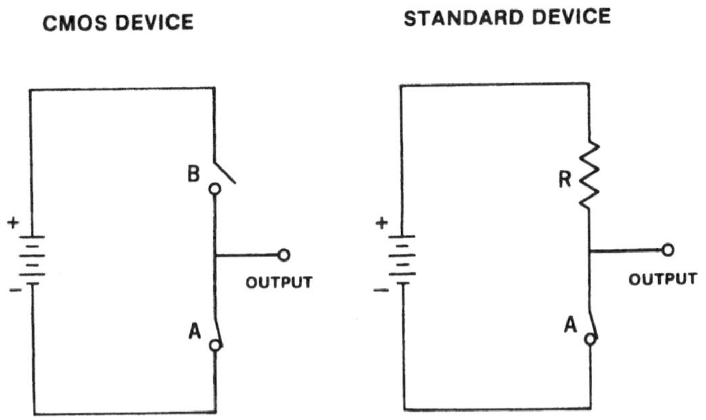

Figure 2a. A simple schematic diagram comparing a CMOS circuit to a standard circuit.

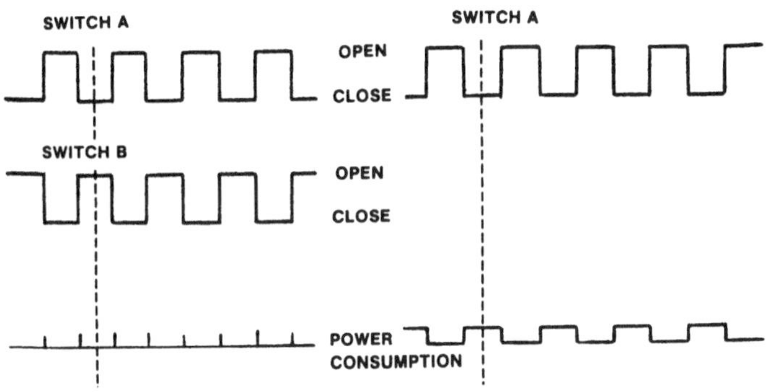

Figure 2b. Switching and power consumption waveforms associated with the respective CMOS and standard circuits.

The standard circuit contains only one switch or transistor in series with a limiting resistor R. The opening and closing sequence for switch A is shown in the appropriate waveform pattern in Figure 2b. The important comparison between the CMOS and standard circuits is in the power consumption area. Refer to the power waveforms in Figure 2b and note that the CMOS circuit only consumes power when switches A and B change or switch state (open to close or close to open) but the standard circuit consumes power on a continuous level when switch A is closed. Therefore, if the switching rate is slow or remains static (inhibited), like for pacemaker operation, the CMOS circuit will consume little or no power when compared with the standard circuit.

The pacemaker has technically evolved since the early 1960's from a very simple electronic device for generating fixed rate pulses to a sophisticated system operating in conjunction with heart demand. To illustrate this evolution trend,

Figure 3 displays a 17-year trend pattern and a 3-year growth projection for circuit complexity and changes in total source current drain.

The evolution chart in Figure 3 was initially presented at the 1975 Pacemaker Colloquium in Arnhem, Holland. In 1975 circuit complexity was established to be approximately 100 components and total source current drain (100% pacing) at 15 microamps. In a short two-year period, 1975 to 1977, there was a threefold increase in component count to 300, attributed to new circuit design techniques while the total source current was reduced to approximately 12 microamps. One would expect source current drain to increase with increased levels of circuit complexity. Instead, circuit design improvements along with technological

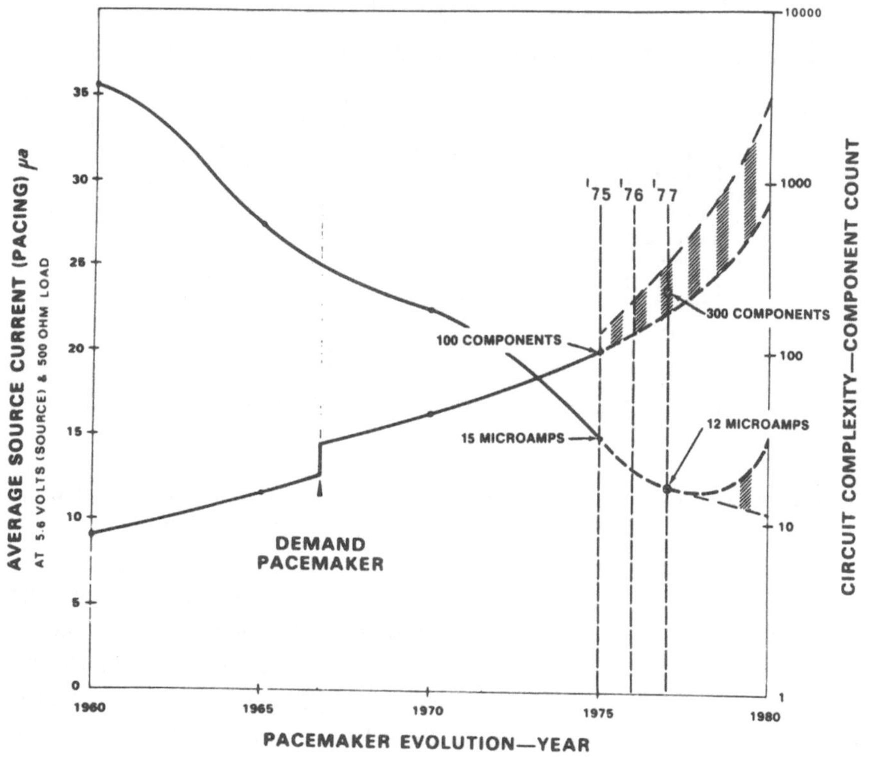

Figure 3. A pacemaker evolution chart showing pulse generator power source current and circuit complexity trends over a 20-year period, 1960 to 1980.

breakthroughs have increased circuit efficiency and therefore contributed to reducing current drain from the power source. If future growth projections are correct, between 1977 to 1980, current drain will continue to decrease, but the most dramatic change will occur in circuit complexity with component count exceeding 1000 by 1980.

NEW PACEMAKER CIRCUITRY FROM A CLINICAL POINT OF VIEW

G.E. Freud

Pacemaker therapy is one of the most successful procedures in the medical field. Without a pacemaker only about 45% of the patients with total block are surviving after one year. With a pacemaker 50% of the patients are still alive after 12.1 years (Furman). This means that life expectancy of a pacemaker patient who survives the implantation procedure and its complications is restored to 92% of the normal. Death rate in the first four weeks after implantation is very variable from clinic to clinic, from 1-2% to 14-15%. About half of the later deaths are caused by the condition of the heart of the patient, the other half by problems resulting from re-implantation procedures and technical pacer-related problems. The overall result is that of each year-class about 5% of all patients are lost because of surgery related complications and about 3% because of system failures (wire and pacemaker).

Pacemaker lifetime and costs of pacing

Smaller, longer living and more dependable pacers will decrease those numbers by causing less need for repeated surgical interventions, fewer sudden breakdowns and fewer late complications. Moreover such pacemakers will cause a sharp reduction in the total number of interventions by reducing the need for reimplantation of fresh units (up to 25% of today's number). They will cause a 60% reduction in the overall costs of wearing a pacemaker and up to 75% reduction in pacemaker related hospital turnover. These data are calculated with help of our own hospital data, the assumption of a 12-year + pacemaker versus a three-year pacemaker, the assumption of a 12-year + electrode and a reduction of the policlinical control frequency from four times to once a year.

Hermetic encapsulation of the pacemaker, made possible by lithium batteries which do not produce gas and have no other factors causing volume expansion, is statistically significantly better than epoxy housing of batteries and components. By keeping the body fluids outside, leakage-currents are prevented which increases the percentage of the battery-contained energy that is available for stimulation of the heart. Moreover corrosion of the components is effectively prevented in this way.

The lithium batteries have a very high energy-content which increases the life expectancy of pacemakers by a factor of two to three, and this energy is packed in a minimal volume which enables the construction of small pacemakers.

Small surface electrodes (in the order of 4-6 mm^2) reduce the current drain of the pacemaker because they have a lower stimulation threshold allowing for a lower energy output of the pacemaker and they have a higher resistance so that the load of the pacemaker is higher, however this causes a higher energy-dissipation at the tip of the electrode reducing slightly the efficiency of the system. This is one of the reasons that the size of the electrode can not be reduced below the dimensions mentioned above. Reduction of the current drain prolongs pacemaker life because it is effective each day a hundred thousand times.

Circuit design

Modern electronic circuitry can be designed in such a way that it is optimally adapted to the battery, to the electrode as a stimulating tool and to the electrode as a part of the sensing system. The two first points are sufficiently solved in a number of pacemakers. The last one is not. This is caused by incomplete knowledge of the properties of the ECG signal derived from the wire. We did fast-Fourier-analysis on this ECG signal with help of a PDP 11 computer. The signal was derived with a high input impedance ECG amplifier (Elema, 10 Mohm input impedance) and put on tape (Ampex FR 1300 instrumentation recorder). The signal was sampled during 500 msec, with a sample frequency of 4000 samples a second in such a way that the sample started before the onset of QRS and ended after the T wave. The digitized signal was calculated in the frequency domain and displayed on an oscilloscope from which photographs (Polaroid) were taken. The frequencies between 2 and 35 Hz made out the bulk of the signal. They result from the repetition frequency of the signal, the Q-T interval, the Q-S interval and the Q-, R-, and S- wave. Between 35 and 70 Hz very little signal was found. Between 70 and 90 Hz in 10 patients considered normal about 15% of the energy-content of the signal was found. In 4 patients with a small-amplitude ECG from the wire this figure was even higher. The signal in this high frequency band is caused by the intrinsic deflections and the different notches in the QRS complex. As the combination of the two frequency bands in noise is extremely rare and they are present in all our studied cases (14), they might be used for a more certain QRS complex detection in sensing amplifiers.

Circuit quality control

Modern electronics can be divided in four groups: 1) consumer electronics, 2) industrial electronics, 3) military electronics, 4) space technology electronics. In each group there is a rather strong conformity in properties such as reliability, repairability, price, number of units produced, consequences of breakdown and requirements resulting from the environment. According to these criteria pacemakers are somewhere between 3) and 4). Also pacemaker technology has a strong resemblance to that used in space and military electronics. Based on the experience in these fields quality control criteria are defined by NASA and the US defence office (MILL-STD). Quality control is establishing according to a well-defined protocol, if a given product has or has not a number of also well-defined properties. If it has the result is positive, if it has not the product can not pass the control. In my opinion a pacemaker only can serve its purpose during the many years it is meant to, if it fulfills the mentioned quality criteria. Quality control on a number of pacemakers was performed with the help of the

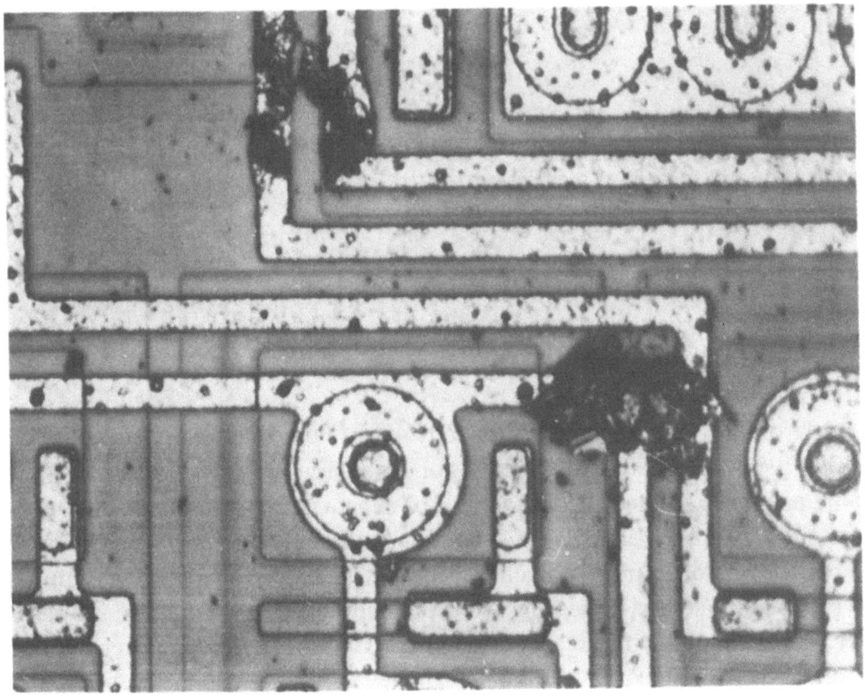

Figure 1. Extensive damage on the surface of a micro circuit leading to short-circuiting or a break in the circuit.

European Space Technology Research Centre (ESTEC) at Noordwijk. It appeared that none of these pacemakers could pass the control.

The number of problems found ranged between 8 and 13 in 22 circuits that were studied. Fig. 1 shows extensive damage on the surface of a microcircuit leading to short-circuiting or a break in the circuit. Fig. 2 shows again a scanning

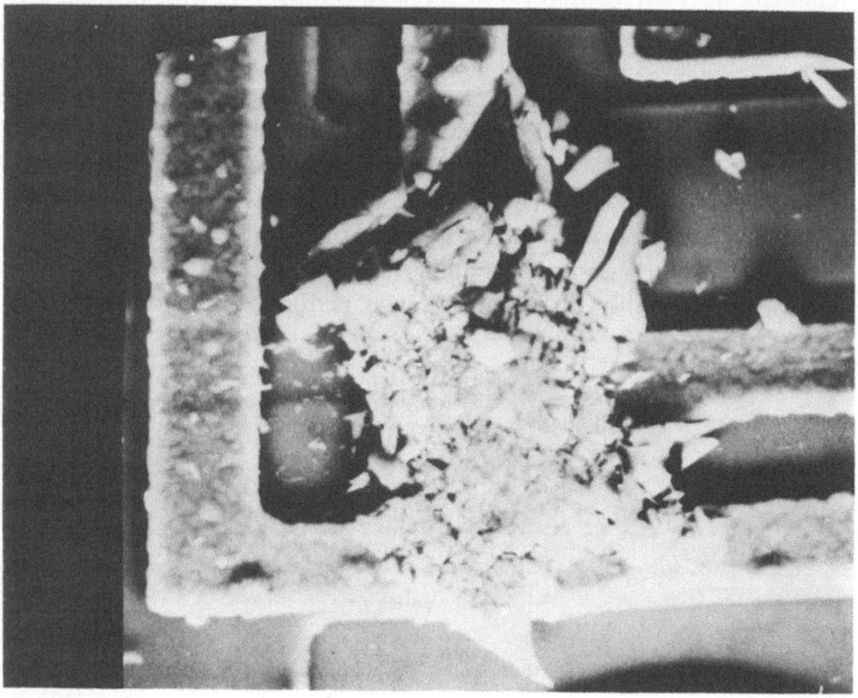

Figure 2. Detail of damage from fig. 1 (400 ×).

electron microscope picture (originally 400 ×) demonstrating a detail of such damage. Remnants of etching fluids or conducting epoxy or solder (fig. 3) were frequently found increasing the risk of short-circuiting or breaks more than desirable in pacemakers. Fig. 4 shows the mounting of a new wire on top of a broken one on a transistor chip. This has to be considered as an improper production method increasing the probability of metal migration, specially in case of an even slight increase of the humidity. The manufacturers were informed about these detected problems of which they were at that moment unaware. The conclusion has to be that quality control was insufficient at that time in all factories that were studied. The industry showed much cooperation to solve the demonstrated problems, resulting in most cases in an important improvement of

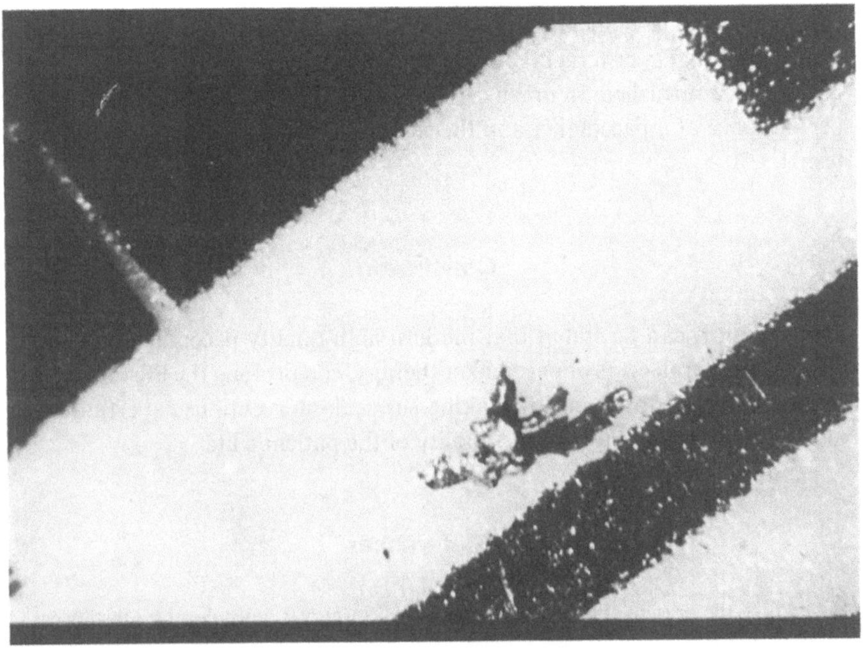

Figure 3. Remnants of solder on micro circuit.

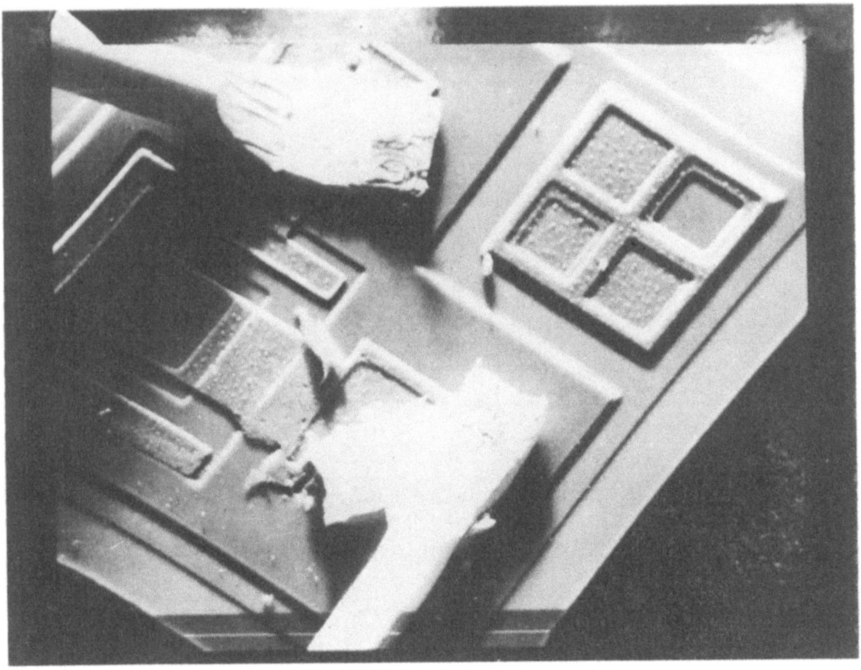

Figure 4. Mounting of a new wire on top of a broken one on a transistor chip.

the product. The conclusive proof that pacemakers have to fulfill space-technology quality criteria in order to function dependably over a range of years has not been furnished. In practice there seems to be a clear relation between the performance of a pacemaker and the standard according to which its quality is tested.

Conclusion

Concluding it can be stated that modern high-quality pacemaker circuits can reduce the overall costs of pacemaker therapy, can prolong the life of the patient by not breaking down and by making surgical interventions superfluous. This last factor also will improve the quality of the patient's life.

References

Furman, S. the present status of cardiac pacing. Surgery, Gynecology & Obstetrics; 143, 645-659, 1976.

END-OF-LIFE INDICATIONS FOR LITHIUM PACEMAKERS

A.C.M. RENIRIE

Introduction

The increasing use of lithium instead of mercury-zinc power sources in cardiac pacemakers has resulted in a change of end-of-life characteristics. In this paper we will describe the methods used to make an accurate assessment of end-of-life of the lithium batteries used by Vitatron. These are the lithium-silver chromate cell (S.A.F.T.) and the lithium-iodine cell (Catalyst Research Corp.), which are used in the Vitatron S 6000 and C 2000 series of pacemakers.

The lithium-silver chromate cell (S.A.F.T., Poitiers, France)

This cell has a low internal resistance and an initial voltage of 3.2 V. The discharge of the cell is coupled to a number of chemical reactions. At the anode there is oxidation of Li to Li^+, whilst at the cathode there is initially a reduction of Ag^+ to Ag, followed by a reduction of Cr^{6+} to Cr^{5+}. According to figures supplied by the battery manufacturer there is sufficient lithium available for 800 mAh, and silver for 600 mAh of energy (chemical capacity). The total capacity of the cell is determined by the amount of lithium taking part in the reaction.

During the initial discharge of the battery the voltage, and therefore the pulse rate, remains almost constant for a long period. During this period a voltage plateau exists that corresponds with the reduction of Ag^+. This is followed by a voltage drop to a lower plateau as a result of Cr^{6+} reduction. The existence of this second plateau is a unique characteristic that makes the S.A.F.T. cell highly suitable for use in the pacemaker industry.

In a Vitatron pacemaker the load on the battery is 10 μA, which results in a 90% efficiency of the chemical reaction. This means that for the first plateau more than 550 mAh of energy are available, which is equivalent to a lifetime of at least 7 years.

Figure 1 shows the projected pulse generator lifetime and the rate change during this period. At the beginning of life the pulse generator has a typical rate of 71 ppm and the mean rate of 70 ppm is reached at 3.1 V per battery. This

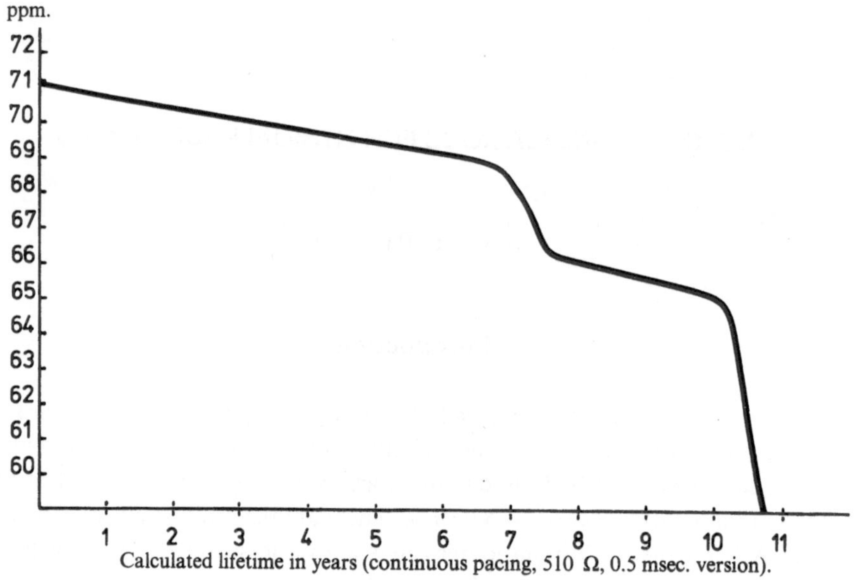

Figure 1. Projected Performance of Vitalith pacemaker equipped with two Saft Li 210 batteries.

occurs at approximately half-life, half-way through the first plateau. The second plateau is not taken into account when calculating pulse generator life, as it is only used to provide a safety margin. Therefore we advise replacement of the pulse generator as soon as a voltage drop to the second plateau is established. In this way a lengthy safety margin is guaranteed.

The clear indication of the voltage drop and this safety margin, coupled to the fact that the lithium-silver chromate cell has safe, reliable characteristics and low weight and dimensions, make this cell very suitable for pacemakers.

The lithium-iodine cell (Catalyst Research Corp., Baltimore, U.S.A.)

The lithium-iodine cell is by comparison a completely different power source. In contrast to the lithium-silver chromate cell and the mercury-zinc cell, there is no change in the open circuit voltage of the lithium-iodine cell during its discharge. There is, however, a change in its internal resistance. To explain this, we first need to understand the chemical characteristics of the cell.

The batteries have a lithium anode and a cathode of iodine and poly-2-vinylpyridine. Between the two is the electrolyte of solid lithium iodide.

When current is drawn from the cell a chemical reaction takes place, resulting in the formation of more crystalline lithium iodide – which gradually accumulates within the hermetically sealed battery. The result of this is an increase in the cell's internal resistance (R_i) which is made up of two main factors: the continually increasing resistance of the lithium iodide and the resistance of the charge-transfer complex, which remains constant until just before the end of battery life.

Initially there is a linear increase in internal battery resistance. However, when the cathode has released most of its iodine there is a sharp increase in cathode resistance and the curves of both battery voltage and internal resistance show a sudden, sharper change. This is a sure sign of impending battery depletion. (See Fig. 2).

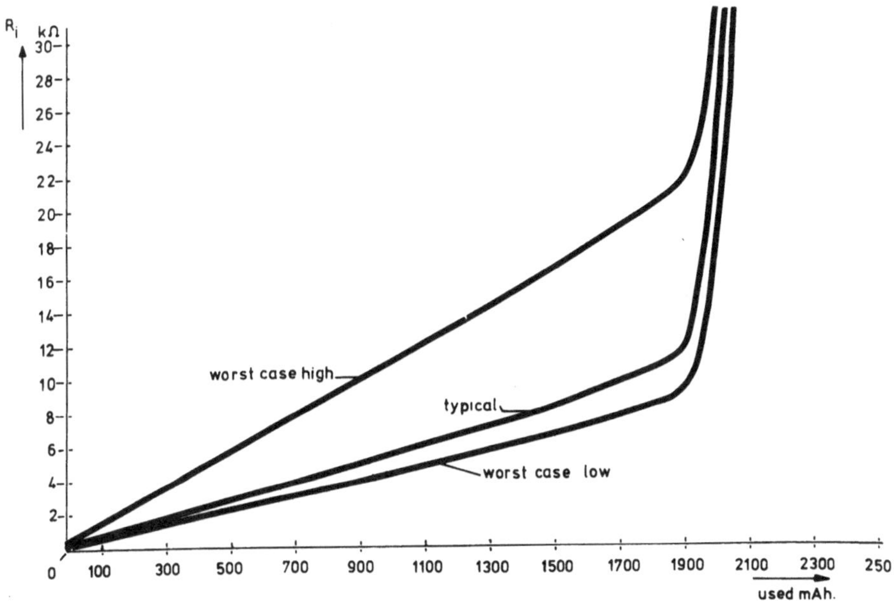

Figure 2. Internal resistance CRC type 802/23 Li-I battery at 15 μA current.

In principle the remaining battery capacity can be determined on the basis of either battery voltage or internal resistance. These can both be calculated from the measured pulse rate. The relation between these parameters can be expressed as follows:

$$V_{bat} = V_{oc} - I\,R_i$$

in which V_{oc} is the constant open circuit voltage of the battery, V_{bat} is the battery voltage, R_i is the internal resistance and I is the current drain.

The decrease in battery voltage δV_{bat} is in fact caused by a voltage drop across R_i as a result of current drain by the electronic circuitry and the output circuit.

Although the current consumption of the electronic circuitry is known to be of a constant value, the output current is load dependent. This is because the output impedance can vary between 400 Ω depending among other things on both the type of electrode used and on physiological circumstances. The total current drain, therefore, varies according to the load. This becomes apparent when studying the following example: At a battery voltage of 2.8 V, the Vitalith C 2130 circuitry consumes 5 μA. If the output impedance is 1 k Ω, the current drain for a pulse width of 1.0 ms is 10 μA, whilst the current drain at an output impedance of 400 Ω is 20 μA. The total current drain therefore varies between 15 and 25 μA.

If the electronic circuitry and the output circuit are both connected to the battery (Fig. 3), the total current drain is variable – as the above example shows.

Calculated lifetime in years (continuous pacing, 510 Ω, 0.5 msec. version).

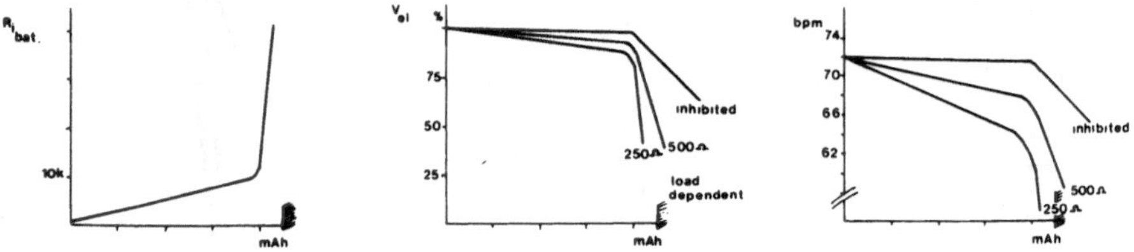

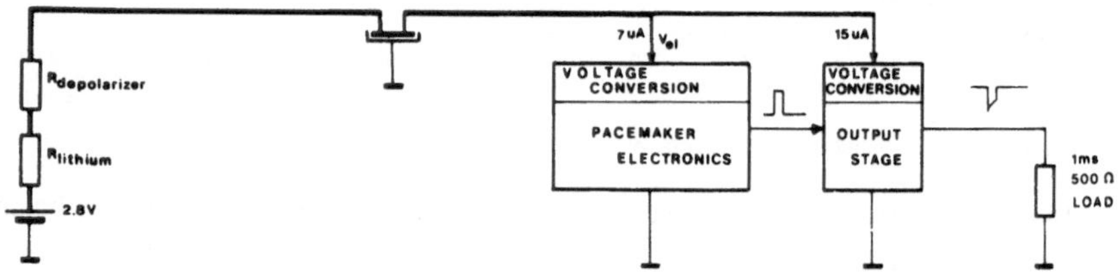

Figure 3. System: rate & E.O.L. indication are voltage dependent (also load dependent).

A direct result of this is that the voltage over the circuit and therefore the rate varies with the load. This makes it extremely difficult to make an accurate and reliable determination of end-of-life of the pacemaker. Apart from this the stability of the electronic circuitry is also very difficult to check.

This problem can be solved by keeping the oscillator frequency stable for a long period and then switching to a lower, equally stable frequency.

The disadvantage of this approach, however, is that the voltage is influenced by a number of variable factors, making it difficult to give an accurate indication of end-of-life. As a rule 2.2 V is given as E.R.T. (Elective Replacement Time) for this type of battery, whilst E.O.L. (End-Of-Life) is given as 1.8 V. The period between E.R.T. and E.O.L. is very short and the risk of a too early, or worse still, a too late indication of E.O.L. is a real possibility.

Therefore, to determine the remaining battery capacity we use another method, i.e. the internal resistance which, as we mentioned earlier, correlates with the discharge of the battery. A simple graph showing R_i against load is, however, impossible to give because resistance at a certain output voltage is dependent on the current drain from the cell – which varies between patients and depends on the regularity with which the pulse generator is inhibited.

We have developed a circuit which enables us to measure the remaining battery capacity on the basis of R_i only, thereby eliminating the influence of the output stage. To achieve this the Vitalith C 2000 series of pacemakers has been equipped with a special converter, that not only acts as a voltage doubler, but also as an electronic switch. This switch connects the electronic circuitry and the output circuit to the battery alternately, so that these components take turns in drawing current from the cell. (Fig. 4)

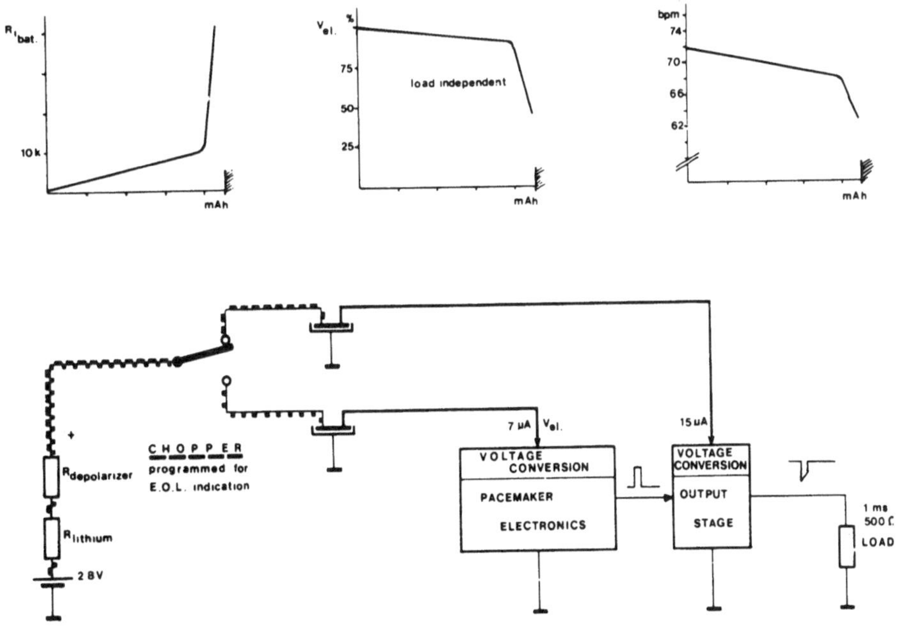

Figure 4. System: rate only dependent on battery resistance.

The ratio between the period during which the electronic circuitry withdraws current, and the period during which the output circuit withdraws current, can be factory set. Using this ratio the dynamic R_i can be coupled to the interval duration, so that internal resistance can be calculated on the basis of interval duration.

The R_i can be accurately determined by measuring the interval duration and by checking the result against the pacemaker Final Test Card, which shows specific characteristics of the pulse generator in question. In this situation the pulse duration can be used to check the interval duration measurements.

As long as the absolute value of R_i remains under 10 kΩ the condition of the battery is good and 6 to 12 month checks are sufficient. If the R_i exceeds 10 kΩ, a regular 6 monthly check is necessary.

At this stage the △ interval duration, i.e. the rate at which the interval duration varies, becomes important. If the change exceeds 10 ms a year, it is advisable to replace the pulse generator.

If the △ interval duration remains fairly stable, however, explantation is not necessary unless R_i exceeds 20 kΩ.

If the internal resistance rises above 20 kΩ the pulse generator must always be replaced, even though it will continue to function correctly until resistance reaches 30 k Ω. This method of converter in combination with the Final Test Card offers excellent possibilities of making an accurate assessment of end-of-life for the lithium-iodine cell.

References

1. Gerbier, G., Lehmann, G., Lenfant, P., Rivault, J.P., Reliability of lithium-silver chromate batteries for cardiac pacing and the related quality control systems; S.A.F.T. – Dry battery division, Poitiers, France.
2. Broussely, M., Lehmann, G., Lenfant, P., The S.A.F.T. lithium-silver chromate battery – Performances of the Li 210 type; S.A.F.T. – Dry battery division, Poitiers, France. DC.3.04.77.10016.2.
3. Catalyst Research Corporation: Lithiode, Lithium-iodine batteries.
4. A.C.M. Renirie: United States Patent 3,031,899; June 28, 1977.

DISCUSSION III. ENERGY SOURCES AND ELECTRONIC CIRCUIT

Chairman: W. IRNICH *(Aachen, F.R. Germany)*

W. IRNICH *(Aachen, F.R. Germany):* It is an unusual opportunity to have all the lithium manufacturers – or the major ones – in one colloquium. One of the problems about which I would like to hear their comments is the issue of cost effectiveness. There has been some discussion now that lithium is universally available, that the increased costs may not be justified when you select a patient who has a very short life expectancy and that there is still a place for the use of mercury batteries in certain patients. The question is: will the cost of the lithium batteries come down as the use becomes more widespread and thus we will not have to worry about making a choice between mercury and lithium.

W.G. GREATBATCH *(Clarence, U.S.A.):* I think there is no question about the fact that the cost of lithium will come down. Actually, the difference in the cost of a lithium battery, as contrasted with the cost of a mercury battery is less than $ 100. Why it is that the pacemaker manufacturers charge about $ 500 more, I do not really know. A lithium battery is fundamentally simpler than a four-cell mercury battery and, therefore, as time goes on and systems become automated and as the capital investment becomes paid off, I believe that the cost of the lithium battery will be considerably less than that of the mercury. But we must observe too that the hospitalization costs for a patient having a pacemaker replacement are much, much greater than the differential between the price of a lithium battery and a mercury battery. I was talking to a doctor from Wales, this morning, who made this point very strongly: that if we are to go to the point where there are 1.000 pacemaker patients per million population – we are going to have to worry about availability of beds for these people. And also a doctor may have to consider very carefully: Is he sure that this patient will not live five years before he puts in a shorter life unit?

A.A. SCHNEIDER *(Baltimore, U.S.A.):* I think that the cost of a lithium battery could well be the same as that of a mercury cell, but I think the reason for the additional cost is simply the quality that is put into the lithium battery. It is definitely the major cost of the battery and I think it is well worth the trade: the improved lifetime, the kinds of records we have been talking about today, for not too many more dollars.

A.C.M. Renirie *(Dieren, The Netherlands):* One remark on the Vitratron side. We thought last year that we would have, at this moment, a lithium pacemaker and that the mercury powered pacemaker would almost drop out. Now, I must admit that we are almost in trouble, because the demand for mercury pacemakers is extremely high, higher even than last year. It is my opinion that the price really makes a difference. The price of the lithium pacemaker is not higher because of the price- difference of the lithium battery compared to the mercury-zinc battery only, but it is also more expensive because we are trying to develop systems with a life expectancy of ten years or more and a confidence level of, let us say, more than 95%. The costs of developing and testing of these electronic circuits are high and also contribute to the higher prices. It is not only the battery that causes the higher price of the lithium pacemakers.

F. Tepper *(Baltimore, U.S.A.):* I would like to comment on Mr. Greatbatch's remarks about the energy density of batteries. I think it is appropriate to indicate that there are finite thermodynamic limits to how much energy one can get in a chemical battery. I know Mr. Greatbatch is aware of it, but perhaps the medical industry might not necessarily be. Engineering limits with respect to voltage also are generally in the order of 4 volts per cell whereas the energy consumption is limited by the fact that we have already chosen the most energetic anode that one can find on the periodic table. In effect, we have a sort of genies-in-a-bottle; we crack the bottle just a bit and let him out a bit at a time rather than try to open the whole bottle.

P.M. Zoll *(Boston, U.S.A.):* I am a little confused between the projections of 15-year life spans of lithium powered pacemakers and the relatively short time that they have been in use clinically. So I direct this question primarily to Dr. Elert, the first speaker, who presented experiences with a series of 300 pacemakers. Now his pacemakers have been in for only a maximum of three years, I would like to know how many patients have had lithium-powered pacemakers in for two years or three years. When we get a three-year total experience in a total number of months experience, this does not tell me how many pacemakers have been in for a long period of time. I presume that of these last 300 pacemakers, 250 may have been put in during the last six months. That is less of a clinical experience than if we would have had a much larger number of an earlier period of time.

Chairman: Dr. Elert, do you want to answer this question?

O. Elert *(Frankfurt, F.R. Germany):* Mr. Greatbatch, are you familiar with the data of C.P.I.? The first lithium pacemaker has been produced by them and implanted in November 1972, four-and-a-half-year ago. Is there any exhaustion?

W. Greatbatch *(Clarence, U.S.A.):* Of a thousand pacemakers which I showed on a slide in my paper, five are now over four years old and I believe close to a hundred are three years old. I agree, I do not like to see 15-year projections on 3-year data. I am willing to double my experience in projections. We now have three lithium batteries which have run since October of 1970. So we have about five- and-a-half years of bench testing and 53 months of clinical implants, some of which are still working. On that basis, I would think we can perhaps start talking in the realm of ten-year pacemakers. But even that is stretching things a little bit. Dr. Chardack said to me one time: when you talk about pacemaker longevity, you had better talk in the past tense. So it is better if we do that and certainly not advance our projections more than twice our actual test time.

W. Vulto *(Dordrecht, The Netherlands):* A question for Mr. Greatbatch. Do you think different makes of lithium batteries have the same reliability? In the same field a question for Mr. Renirie perhaps. Is this why Vitatron is using two different types of lithium batteries in their pacemakers?

W. Greatbatch *(Clarence, U.S.A.):* Once again, I think we must base reliability on past experience. I would rather state positively that, to the best of my knowledge, most of the lithium systems which we showed, have shown no clinical failures of any kind. The oldest system, of course, is the lithium-iodine system with over four years of clinical implant. So we have to qualify our statements on which is the most reliable as which has seen the most service. I do not think there is enough data around now to clearly state that one is greatly superior to another. We like to think that we get the longest service, but yet we must realize that Mr. Lehmann's battery also has seen no clinical failures. So I think we can say in general that most of the lithium systems that we have seen have demonstrated their reliability as superior to the older battery systems. But the specifics as to which of the lithium systems is better and just how much better they are than mercury, I think we will just have to let time tell.

A.C.M. Renirie *(Dieren, The Netherlands):* Part of the question was addressed to me. I think that at this moment it is still good that we have two lithium battery systems, because, in our case, the lithium battery of SAFT has a very simple and stable character and has a lot of safety built in, as I showed. It has a lower internal resistance and the price is lower. I think that the price is also an important point, as pointed out earlier.

Mr. Schöttelndreier *(Haarlem, The Netherlands):* This question is not from me but from my son. As a 15-year old boy, he is involved in recycling problems at his school, losses of energy and so on. He saw in a room all these pacemakers which contain a lot of energy and he asked me: what can you do with them? I asked around and nobody knew. Could the panel say what can be done with pacemakers with a lot of energy in them, but which have been used in patients?

CHAIRMAN: Anybody wants to answer this question?

W. GREATBATCH *(Clarence, U.S.A.):* There is really not that much energy there, when you think that we are talking about three ampère-hours being too much for clinical use. I could suggest to your son that if you take perhaps three hundred thousand old pacemakers, maybe he could run his automobile with them.

R. GOLD *(Consett Durham, England):* I have a similar question, actually. Our crematorium medical officers are getting very worried, in parts of Britain, following one or two problems with the mercury pacemakers in patients. Now we have reassured them that with these lithium pacemakers, hydrogen is not involved and, therefore, the risk of explosion is much less. However, I wonder if the panel could reassure us as to whether there is any danger, at temperatures reached either in a crematorium or in the refuse collector's incinerator, of the lithium element's itself exploding?

A.A. SCHNEIDER *(Baltimore, U.S.A.):* Just like any hermetically sealed container, the hermetically sealed lithium batteries will explode if burned. I think you should expect nothing different from a lithium battery than you experience is from a mercury battery. I am not sure about the SAFT system, perhaps Mr. Lehmann could comment.

G. LEHMANN *(Poitiers, France):* I agree with you. It is the same. We have a hermetic system, so if you heat it, it blows up. But it is the only danger.

A.A. SCHNEIDER *(Baltimore, U.S.A.):* One more comment. We do suggest that all pacemakers should be disposed of as solid waste, rather than being cremated. I think we should state too that the hazard of a mercury battery in a crematorium is quite high, that the toxicity of the effluents is far higher than it would be with any of the lithium systems.

F. TEPPER *(Baltimore, U.S.A.):* There have been no known explosions in lithium batteries, in both systems that were discussed today. I think one should distinguish these from what history there exists of high-rate lithium batteries which can, upon shorting in fact explode even under ambient thermal conditions. With these particular pacemaker systems, with low rate discharge and high impedance batteries, it is just not possible. I think I also speak for SAFT.

G. Lehmann *(Poitiers, France):* I agree with you. There is absolutely no danger at normal temperatures. But if you heat the battery to 200 or 300 degrees centigrade, it is normal for all kinds of batteries to explode.

Chairman: We have to close this interesting discussion here. Time will tell us more about the lithium batteries. I sincerely hope that in the future we may find a possibility to extend this discussion between the lithium specialists and thank all of you for your contributions in this discussion.

Section IV

STIMULATION ELECTRODES

A. Atrial Electrodes

TRANSMEDIASTINAL AND TRANSTHORACIC ATRIAL ELECTRODES

STURE LARSSON

Atrial pacing, atrial synchronous ventricular pacing, and atrioventricular sequential pacing have obvious physiological advantages over conventional ventricular pacing. However, current methods of ventricular pacing give very good results in most cases of arrhythmia in which pacemaker treatment is indicated.

Indications and the necessary conditions for atrial synchronous ventricular pacing are present in roughly 10-15% of pacemaker patients. Atrial pacing may be used to abolish attacks of tachycardia and for treatment of supraventricular brady- and tachy-arrhythmias. Permanent atrial pacing is very rarely indicated probably in less than 1% of patients. Patients with sinus arrest, SA block, and the sick sinus syndrome should, with few exceptions, be given a conventional QRS-synchronous pacemaker. This is the safest method of treatment at present.

Transthoracic atrial sensing

There are only a few electrodes specially designed for detection of atrial activity. The first Atricor system consisted of the pacer and three epicardial leads. Nowadays Cordis has a separate electrode for detection of the atrial signals. We have used the flexible Elema electrode 588 or the Elema epicardial type of electrode. The techniques we have employed for fixation of electrodes for atrial sensing or atrial pacing are shown in Fig. 1. The 588 electrode has either been inserted in the atrial appendage through a hole in the atrial wall and been fixed to the inside by two or three interrupted sutures or U-sutures tied over teflon pledgets or applied to the surface of the atrial wall and fixed with a few interrupted sutures. The epicardial electrode has been fixed to the surface of the atrium by means of two sutures through the two holes in such a way as to avoid damaging the myocardium below the electrode.

An electrode for detection of the atrial activity has been implanted in 5 patients during open heart surgery. The results of atrial synchronous ventricular pacing in these patients are shown in Table 1. In one patient in whom the electrode was inserted into the atrium and merely fixed with a purse string suture, defective triggering occurred due to dislocation of the electrode. A re-

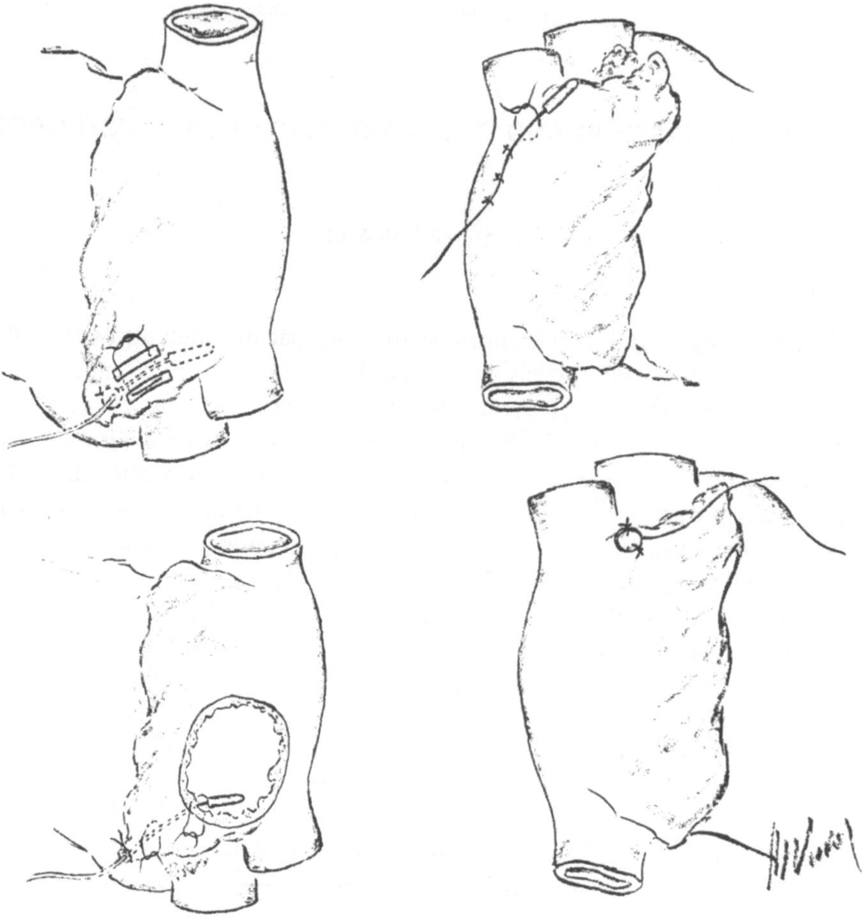

Fig. 1. Example of placement and fixation of the atrial electrode.

Table 1. Atrial synchronous pacing in 5 patients with an atrial detector electrode implanted during open heart surgery

Patient number	*Age of patient*	*P signal in mV*	*Duration of atrial synchronous pacing in months*
1	15	6	67
2	7	1.8	53
3	6	4	4
4	6	2.5	8*
5	63	1.5	39**

* Atrial synchronous pacing discontinued

sternotomy was performed and the electrode was successfully placed outside the right atrium. In three patients the pacemaker has functioned well – in one for more than 5 years. The atrial synchronous pacing was discontinued in two patients because of atrial arrhythmia and impending skin necrosis, respectively. Although our experience with transthoracic application of an atrial sensing electrode is limited we definitively prefer the transmediastinal approach.

Transmediastinal atrial sensing

There is no electrode specially designed for detection of the atrial signals transmediastinally. I have used the flexible Elema electrode 588 with a large surface area.

The first atrial-triggered pacemaker in Gothenburg was implanted in October 1966. The series comprises 130 patients. The results represent our experience of atrial synchronous pacing during a 10-year period. Sixty-two patients have had atrial synchronous pacing for more than 5 years and seven patients for more than 10 years.

There have been 29 deaths during the 10-year period. There were 8 sudden deaths at home, and two in hospital. The two patients who died in hospital had Adams-Stokes attacks early postoperatively. Ventricular fibrillation was recorded on the ECG. This method of stimulation should be used when the right conditions exist, and there should then be no problem of arrhythmias during treatment. Patients with abnormal atrial rhythm or ventricular tachyarrhythmias should not be given an atrial-triggered pacemaker. With the development of atrial synchronous ventricular demand pacemakers, however, ventricular arrhythmias would be no contraindication to atrial synchronous pacing.

Table 2. The causes of cessation of the atrial synchronous pacing in 30 patients

	No
Atrial arrhythmia	15
Ventricular arrhythmia	2
Dislocation of the electrode	4
Decrease in P-wave amplitude	5
Infection	1
No reason	3
Total	30

The atrial synchronous pacing was discontinued in 30 patients, i.e. 23%. Table 2 shows the causes of discontinuance. The cause was arrhythmia in more than half of the patients. Problems associated with the method of detection of the atrial signals caused discontinuance of the atrial synchronous pacing in 9 patients, i.e. 7%, including two cases of iatrogenic dislocation of the electrode in connection with replacement of the pacemaker.

Impaired detection of the atrial potentials occurred in 29 patients in all, including 4 iatrogenic dislocations of the electrode and one dislocation caused by the patient. The position of the electrode was adjusted or a new detector electrode was successfully inserted in 22 patients. Spontaneous dislocations of the electrode occurred in 13 patients, i.e. 10%. It was diagnosed within the first postoperative week in all cases. Two of those patients in whom the electrode was re-positioned later had a critical decrease in the P wave amplitude. A decrease in the P wave amplitude below the level for triggering a pacer with conventional sensitivity was observed in another 11 patients, making 10% in all.

Atrial pacing without thoracotomy

Atrial pacing without thoracotomy can be achieved by inserting a stimulation electrode in the right atrium, right atrial appendage or coronary sinus transvenously. At my request a special electrode for inserting in the right atrial appendage and a special P-triggered atrial pacemaker with an input sensitivity between 0.5 and 1 mV was produced. I implanted the first pacemaker system of this type in April 1968. Unstable pacing was observed two weeks later and the electrode was re-positioned. The patient died from cancer after 82 months of atrial pacing.

I tried this method in another two patients but the position of the electrode was unstable and pacing was defective. Both patients were subjected to thoracotomy for application of an atrial electrode.

Atrial pacing can also be achieved by insertion of a *transmediastinal stimulation electrode*. In 1967 I tried to stimulate the atrium in two patients with sinus rhythm. I applied an electrode behind the atria in connection with mediastinoscopy for pulmonary carcinoma. I used the Elema electrode 588 with a large surface area. The stimulation threshold was 3.5 V in one patient and 4 V in the other.

In July 1968 I tried this method of stimulation in a patient with bradycardia. I obtained satisfactory atrial pacing at an output of 1.5 V. I therefore applied a P-triggered atrial pacemaker. Two weeks after the implantation, however, defective pacing was observed and I changed to a high-output pacemaker. A few days later defective pacing was registered once again. I removed the pacemaker system and switched to ventricular demand pacing. If a better electrode can be developed it should be possible to achieve long-term atrial pacing with this method of stimulation. Recently transmediastinal retrocardial stimulation of the left atrium has been tried by other authors (Kleinert et al. 1976).

Table 3. Data on 5 patients with atrial pacing. Transthoracic application of the stimulation electrode

Patient number	*Diagnosis*	*Surgical procedure*	*Type of pacemakers used*
1	Sinus arrest	Sternotomy	Fixed-rate
2	SA block Atrial flutter	Anterior thoracotomy. Defibrillation	External fixed-rate
3	Sinus bradycardia Atrial arrhythmia	Sternotomy	P-triggered Fixed-rate
4	SA block	Sternotomy	P-triggered P-inhibited
5	SA block Sinus bradycardia	Sternotomy	Fixed-rate P-triggered P-inhibited

Atrial pacing with thoracotomy

In 5 cases I have done a thoracotomy in order to achieve atrial pacing (Table 3). I now consider that the indications and conditions for successful atrial pacing were present in only one patient, namely case 5. Two patients have had good atrial pacing for many years but they have both had episodes of atrial fibrillation, probably due to defective sensing owing to the use of pacemakers with too low input sensitivity (Table 4). The atrial pacing was discontinued in 3 patients because of exit block, atrial arrhythmia, and 2nd degree A.V. block, respectively. In my opinion, this method of pacemaker treatment should only be used upon strict indications.

Table 4. Atrial pacing. Transthoracic application of the electrode

Patient number	*Type of electrode*	*Electrode position*	*Stimulation threshold (V)*	*Duration of treatment in months*
1	EMT 588	Intraatrial	–	1.5*
2	EMT 567	Epicardial	1.5	1*
3	EMT 588	Intraatrial	2.0	48*
4	EMT 588	Intraatrial	–	88
5	EMT 588	Intraatrial	2.6	66

* Atrial pacing discontinued

Reference

1. Keinert, M., Beer, P., Taylessani, A., Möglichkeiten der Elektrostimulation des Herzens mittels transmediastinal retrokardial verlegter Elektroden. Thoraxchir. 24, 484-492, 1976.

THE USE OF CORONARY SINUS PACING

MYRVIN H. ELLESTAD, JOHN MESSENGER, PAUL GREENBERG AND MARK CASTELLANET

Introduction

Permanent atrial pacing from the coronary sinus has been used since 1958 (1-5) and has been shown to provide better cardiovascular function. (6-9). This is a report of our experience with this method of 66 consecutive patients. A special lead was used with a flexible tip extending beyond the distal electrode to prevent dislodgement from the coronary sinus during inspiration (Fig. 1).

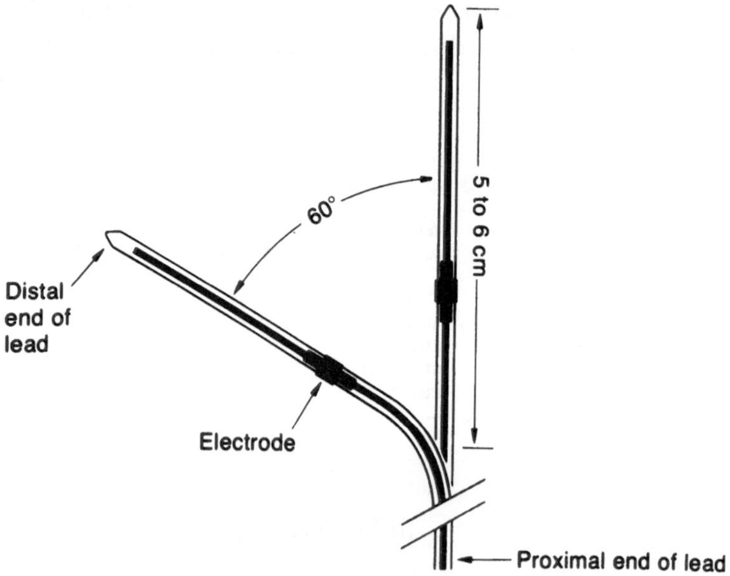

Figure 1. The tip of the unipolar coronary sinus pacing catheter is shown. The guide-wire extends almost to the tip (made by Cordis).

Methods

The lead is passed from the external jugular vein or the cephalic vein into the coronary sinus and the great cardiac vein which is then explored for pacing and sensing threshold (Fig. 2). A cavity electrogram is recorded (Fig. 3), and rapid

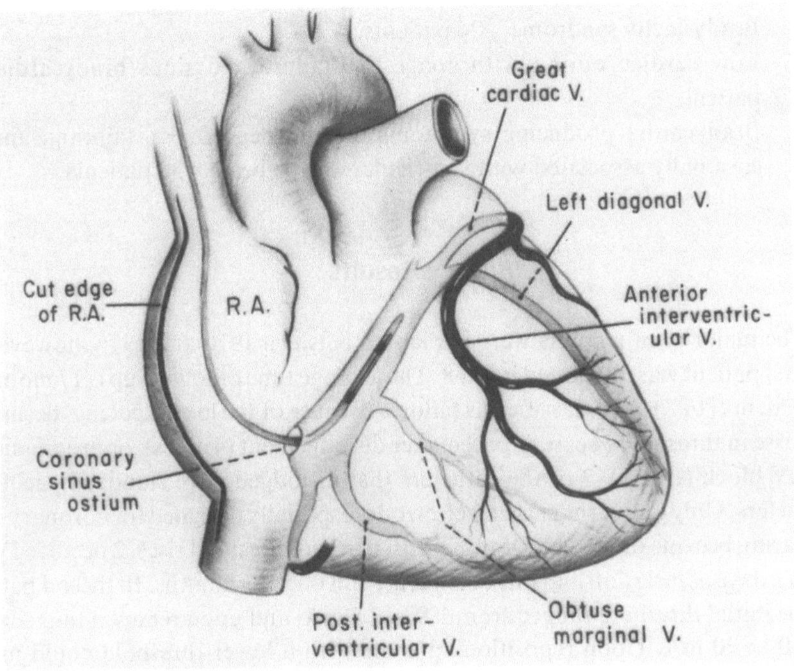

Figure 2. The bipolar pacing catheter (Medtronic) is positioned in the great cardiac vein at the site usually selected for optimum pacing.

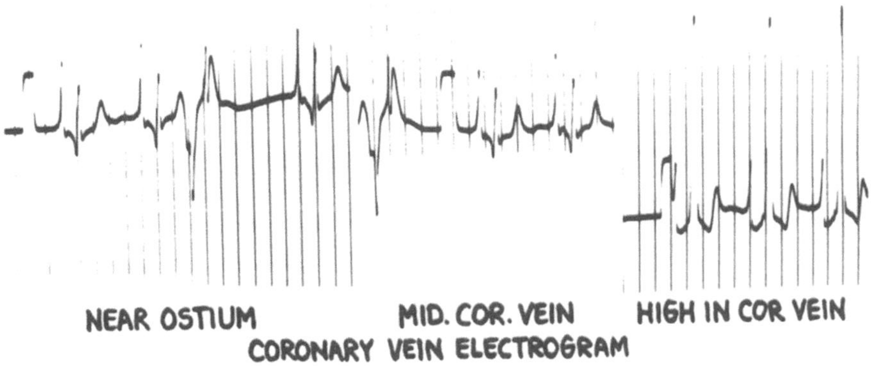

Figure 3. Coronary sinus electrogram. The P waves near the ostium and proximal part of the great coronary vein show very high voltage, but as the catheter is passed higher into the coronary vein, a taller R wave is recorded.

atrial pacing, up to rates of 130 or more is carried out to identify the tendency to develop AV block. Sudden termination of rapid atrial pacing then allows the measurement of the sinus node recovery time to evaluate for the presence of sick sinus syndrome.

The indications for atrial pacing include:

1. Uncontrolled ventricular tachycardia – 4 patients.
2. Brady-tachy syndrome – 24 patients.
3. Low cardiac output with congestive failure and sinus bradycardia – 8 patients.
4. Bradycardia producing symptoms of light-headedness, fainting, and occasionally associated with ventricular escape beats – 30 patients.

Results

The majority of patients were implanted between 1970 and 1976, however the first patient was implanted in 1968. The average time of follow-up is 17 months. 9 patients (14%) were classified as failures because of the loss of pacing, because of a rise in threshold (4 cases), pacemaker dislodgement (4 cases), or progression of AV block (1 case). 3 of the catheters that dislodged were standard pacing catheters. Only one of the catheter electrodes especially designed for coronary sinus pacing became displaced. Of those with marked threshold rises, 2 occurred within 3 days of insertion and one at 3 weeks, and one at 2 months. In these 4 patients the initial threshold ranged from 1.8 to 2.8 mA, and upon removal ranged from 9.0 to 20 mA. Upon repositioning a site with a lower threshold could not be located. The initial threshold did not indicate in any way that it would later be found to be too high for capture. The patient had developed complete AV block at an initial threshold of 1.9 mA.

Degree of A-V block

19 patients had either first degree A-V block at rest or developed second degree A-V block with atrial pacing.

P-R intervals

The pacer spike-R interval was measured on insertion and on follow-up visits and was of no predictive value in terms of eventual pacemaker failure. None of the 9 patients with intervals over 200 msec went on to complete A-V block.

Deaths

4 patients died during the follow-up and none were due to pacing complications. The autopsy on one woman who died of a cerebral hemorrhage 5 years after pacemaker implantation, revealed that the electrode in the coronary sinus was not associated with a thrombus and did not compromise the lumen in any way. Fibrous bands attached the catheter to the endocardium of the atrium and in the coronary sinus in 3 or 4 places.

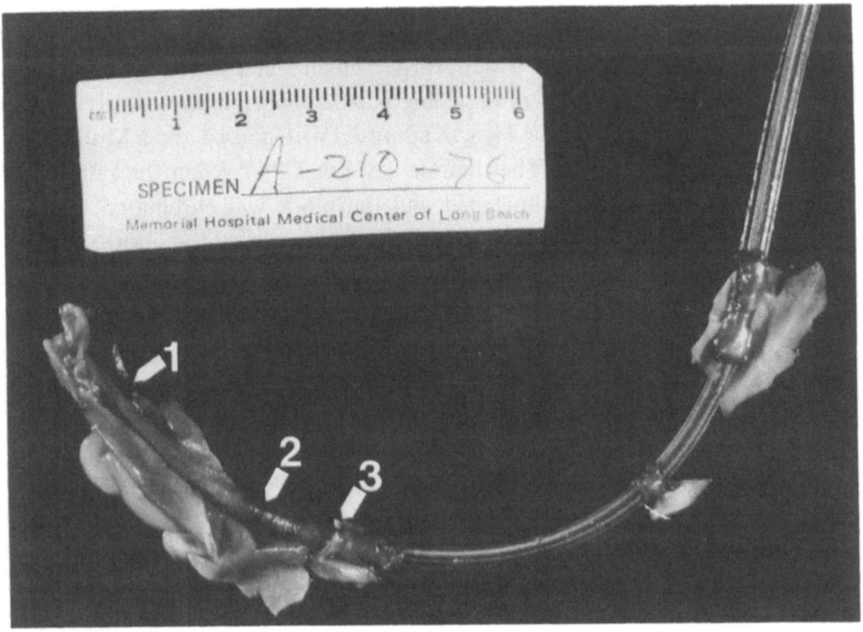

Figure 4. Coronary sinus catheter removed at autopsy. One is the tip of the catheter residing in the coronary sinus. Two electrode. Three coronary sinus ostium. Attachment to the endocardium occurred at 2 sites in the coronary sinus and 2 in the atrium. There was no evidence of obstruction or undue trauma.

Case reports

R. D., a 77-year old female with congestive heart failure and a low cardiac output associated with a slow sinus rhythm varying from 46 to 50, was selected for coronary sinus pacing. Satisfactory pacing at 3-4 mA was accomplished with the catheter in an area near the ostium of the coronary sinus. Pacing at various rapid rates was done to determine whether A-V block would occur. As pacing at a rate near 90 beats per minute did not develop block, although the P-R interval remained long, permanent pacing at 90 beats per minute was established which improved cardiac function so that congestive failure could be adequately controlled.

D.B., an 80-year old male physician with severe angina and a brady-tachy syndrome. Coronary sinus pacing at 80 beats per minute along with Propranolol 160 mg. per day, resulted in control of the tachycardia and the angina. Atrial pacing often is an aid in the control of angina when Propranolol is indicated, but ordinarily would reduce the heart rate to prohibitive levels.

G.G. is a 66-year old male with coronary heart disease, sick sinus syndrome and intermittent paroxysmal atrial tachycardia. The pacemaker was placed in an attempt to minimize the atrial tachycardia which seemed to come on more frequently when the rate was very slow. Digoxin 0.25 mg. per day was given to help prevent the atrial arrhythmia. He was admitted with nausea and a Mobitz type 1 second degree A-V block. The digitalis level was 2.6. When the rate was decreased, the P-R interval shortened and the block was eliminated. After the digitalis was eliminated the pacer could be reprogrammed to a more rapid rate. This pattern has been seen several times.

Discussion

Atrial pacing has been a special help in patients similar to those illustrated in the case reports above. Although an occasional failure occurs when a sudden, unexplained increase in threshold supervenes, the functional benefits seem worth the problems encountered. Catheter dislodgement, fairly common with standard leads have all but been eliminated with the new tailed electrode. Transient, remediable problems are fairly common, such as intermittent failure to sense, resetting on the R wave with the resultant reduction in heart rate and a number of others, can usually be managed with some experience. The dictum (Ref. 4) that a prolonged PR interval (over 0.26) and evidence of A-V block on rapid pacing are contraindications to permanent atrial pacing has not been borne out in our experience. Patients with both these findings have been successfully paced for long periods from the atrium and have not had an increased incidence of eventual complete heart block. We have also found that the high thresholds (average 3.5 mA) have not progressed significantly with time, so that we do not hesitate to use this modality unless the threshold is above 6 mA.

The importance of the atrial component of stroke output is well documented (Ref. 6-9). This has been a significant factor in the control of congestive failure. We also have found that the atrial pacer seems to prevent a return to atrial fibrillation in an occasional patient who otherwise can not be maintained in a sinus mechanism. This concept needs further exploration. If sensing is lost, and the patient's own sinus rate exceeds that of the pacer, atrial extrasystoles or atrial fibrillation may result. However the latter is quite rare. There seems to be no danger of causing stimulation of the ventricle during the vulnerable period in this situation, which is always a possibility with ventricular pacing.

When the advantages of atrial pacing are considered, it seems surprising that it has not gained greatly in application. In our hospital each year sees a greater percentage of pacemaker leads being implanted in the coronary sinus. We would estimate that only 30 or 40% of the pacers should be placed in the ventricle if optimum function is to be realized. This trend will continue as pacemaker circuits are designed primarily for atrial pacing. We would also expect that double catheter units for sequential and other more complex approaches would gain in use when an atrial lead system is well accepted. At this time the coronary sinus seems to be an excellent site to establish atrial pacing.

References

1. Moss, et al., Pervenous atrial pacing; JAMA, Vol 209 No. 4 , pg. 543-545, July 28, 1969.
2. Kramer, Moss., Permanent pervenous atrial pacing from the coronary vein; Circulation 42, pg. 427-436, Sept. 1970.
3. Moss, Rivers, Kramer, Permanent pervenous atrial pacing from the coronary vein – Long-term follow-up; Circ. 49, pg. 222-225, Feb. 1974.
4. Moss, A.J., Therapeutic uses of permanent pervenous atrial pacemakers: A review, Electrocardiology, 8 (4) 373-380, 1975.
5. Furman, S., Therapeutic uses of atrial pacing: American Heart Journal 86, No. 6 pg. 835-840, Dec. 1973.
6. Brokman, Stanley, Dynamic function of atrial contraction in evaluation of cardiac performance; American Journal of Clinical Physiology 204 (4) 597-603, 1963.
7. Martin, Richard, Cobb, Leonard, Observations on the effect of atrial systole in man; Journal of Laboratory and Clinical Medicine, Vol. 68, No. 2, Aug. 1966.
8. Benchimol, Alberto et al., Hemodynamic consequences of atrial with ventricular pacing in patients with normal and abnormal hearts; American Journal of Medicine 39, pg. 911-922, Dec. 1965.
9. Parker, John, Ledwich, Rodney et al., Reversible cardiac failure during angina; Circ. 39, pg. 745-757, June, 1969.

PERMANENT ATRIAL ELECTRODES WITH SPECIAL CONSIDERATION TO TRANSVENOUS ENDOCARDIAL FORMS

M. KLEINERT

Introduction

Atrial programmed permanent pacemaker therapy, using devices such as 1) atrial demand pacemakers (AAI or AAT, 1, 2) atrial sensing ventricular stimulating, commonly referred to as P-wave synchronous pacemakers (VAT, 1) and 3) A-V sequential or bifocal (DVI, 1) units offers the most physiologic form of bradycardia rhythm disturbance management (2, 3, 4, 5, 6, 7, 8, 9, 10, 11, 12, 13, 14) in properly selected cases. A key benefit of these modalities is the maintenance of the atrio-ventricular contraction sequence with the consequential homeostatic response (6). According to the investigations of Irnich (15), atrial programmed pacing should be considered in approximately 77% of all patients with symptomatic bradycardias. Evaluation of our patient population generally agrees with this figure. In 1976, 84 out of 98 (85%) were judged to be candidates for atrial programmed pacing. Of these, 54 actually received atrial devices. The disparity between the indication and utilization figures was due primarily to the absence of good, reliable, commercially available A-V sequential and P-wave synchronous pacemakers. Atrial electrode problems such as electrode instability and high thresholds, long considered to be the limiting factor to more widespread utilization of atrially programmed stimulation (16, 17), have been overcome to a large degree with new lead designs and techniques. The report which follows describes our experience with 147 atrial electrodes of 4 designs used over a period of 58 months.

Material and methods

From March 1972 to January 1977 we treated 145 patients (63 women and 82 men) with an average age of 65.39 $\pm$ 7.96 years, the youngest 21 and the oldest 86 years old, with a total of 147 atrial electrodes. During this time, the number of electrode insertions increased continuously from year to year. Hence, in 1976 the ratio of implanted atrial electrodes was 55% (54 out of 98).

The atrial electrodes used were:

a) EMT 588 (Elema)
b) Hooking (Biotronic)
c) Tined J-tip (Medtronic)
d) Endocardial Screw-in (Bisping)

Three lead emplacement methods were available for the positioning of atrial electrodes:

1. Transthoracic myocardial placement (12). This method has only historical significance in our opinion because of the increased stress placed upon the patient (e.g., general anesthesia, thoracotomy) and was not used in our described patients.
2. Transmediastinal, retrocardial electrode placement, and
3. Transvenous electrode placement.

We will concentrate on our experiences with the latter two techniques.

Transmediastinal retrocardial placement

We have placed 37 atrial electrodes by the transmediastinal retrocardial technique first described by Swedish investigators (18, 19, 20, 21, 22, 23, 24, 25). The lead used was the Elema EMT 588 with electrode surface area of 47 mm^2. The atrial electrograms sensed by these electrodes had an average value of 3.93 ± 1.38 mV (Table 1). The minimum signal detected was 1.5 mV; the maximum was

Table 1. Magnitudes of atrial signals measured by 147 atrial leads of different types and emplacement techniques.

	Transmed-iastinal	Transvenous		
Lead Model	EMT 588 (Elema)	Hooking (Biotronik)	Tined J-tip (Medtronic)	Screw-in (Bisping)
No. of Leads	37	19	86	5
Action Potentials (mV)				
Average Value	3.93	3.21	5.29	4.20 (5.30)
Maximum	10.00	7.00	10.00	6.00 (8.00)
Minimum	1.50	1.50	1.50	2.50 (3.50)

10 mV. These leads were used exclusively for sensing (detection) of the atrial electrogram in 36 cases (Table 2). In the case of one female patient, the lead was used to effect atrial pacing and sensing. The atrial electrode was removed in one

Table 2. Emplacement techniques and functioning of 147 atrial leads of different forms.

Emplacement Technique	n	Electrode Type	Mode of Operation	n
Transmediastinal Retrocardial	37	EMT 588 (Elema)	Sensing	36
			Sensing/Pacing	1
Transvenous Endocardial	110	Hooking (Biotronik)	Sensing	9
			Sensing/Pacing	10
		Tined J-tip (Medtronic)	Sensing	36
			Sensing/Pacing	50
		Screw-in (Bisping)	Sensing	1
			Sensing/Pacing	4

patient in spite of atrial electrogram amplitude of 4 mV due to A-V dissociation which appeared intraoperatively.

These atrial electrodes functioned trouble free in 26 of the 37 patients (70%) in whom they were implanted for follow-up periods of up to 58 months (average 38 months). In 7 cases, electrode related aberrant atrial signal detection occurred 4 to 37 months postimplantation. Electrode dislodgement occurred in 5 patients (14%) which is somewhat higher than the approximately 9 respectively 10% reported by the Swedish studies (19, 26). Our higher dislodgement rate may be ascribable to our lack of lateral X-ray equipment, thereby having to rely on posterior-anterior illumination only.

Because of the relatively high dislodgement rate experienced and the subsequent availability of alternative approaches, we have abandoned this lead placement technique.

Transvenous lead placement

The transvenous method of atrial lead placement, initiated by Rodewald and coworkers (27), obviates many of the difficulties encountered with previously mentioned atrial electrode placement techniques. Two broad types of transvenous atrial leads exist:

1. Conventional atrial leads, including
   a) coronary sinus leads (28, 29) and
   b) J-shaped leads for placement in the right atrial appendage (23, 30, 31, 32, 33, 34) and
2. Penetrating anchoring atrial leads such as
   a) hooking or barb electrodes (23, 35, 36, 37, 38, 39, 40),
   b) umbrella electrodes (41), and
   c) endocardial screw-in electrodes (42, 43)

Our experience is limited to the emplacement of the hooking type, modified J-shaped and endocardial screw-in leads. Because of difficulties encountered in locating and catheterizing the coronary sinus, we have had little experience with coronary sinus atrial leads.

Introduction of atrial electrodes via the transvenous route corresponds closely to the approaches and methods commonly used for endocardial ventricular lead placement. Table 3 shows the veins used and distribution for the three lead types to be described in greater detail.

Table 3. Routes of emplacement using 110 transvenous atrial leads of types hooking, tined J-tip and screw-in.

	Hooking		Tined J		Screw-in	
Rt. external jugular v.	15	79%	43	50%	1	20%
Rt. internal jugular v.	4	21%	28	33%		
Rt. cephalic v.			15	17%	4	80%
Total	19	100%	86	100%	5	100%

Hooking electrodes

We have inserted 18 electrodes described by Wende and Schaldach (39). These can be inserted only via a large diameter, stiff, pre-bent guide trochar. The acute angle of the metal barbs often makes myocardial positioning and anchoring of the electrode difficult. In addition to these leads, we have attempted to position 4 electrodes of the type developed by Irnich (35, 36) with an obtuse angle between barbs and electrode body. Only one of these could be brought into the right atrium and positioned successfully.

9 of the 19 hooking electrodes served as sensing electrodes; 10 were used as

pacing and sensing electrodes (Table 2). The atrial electrograms sensed on the inner wall of the right atrium by hooking electrodes averaged 3.21 ± 1.31 mV (Table 1). The minimum was 1.5 mV; the maximum was 7.0 mV. These values are below the atrial signals that were registered with other atrial leads studied. We suspect localized injury and scarring may have an attenuating effect on signal amplitudes.

The acute intra-atrial pacing voltage thresholds averaged 1.04 ± 0.40 (0.47 minimum to 2.00 maximum) V at a pulse width of 1.0 ms. At a pulse width of 0.5 ms, they were on the average 1.42 ± 0.75 (0.66 to 3.30) V, undergoing an additional increase up to mean values of 2.05 ± 0.89 (1.00 to 4.00) V at 0.25 ms. The 4 V output limit of our stimulation threshold device was exceeded in one case.

In spite of acute atrial threshold values which exceed intraventricular thresholds by a factor of 2-3 (33, 34), no pacemaker output blocking was observed, even when using pacemakers having pulse widths of only 0.5 ms (5 cases).

In 2 cases where the initial intraatrial action potentials were quite low at 2.0 and 1.5 mV, sensing problems occurred temporarily within the first 10 days following electrode insertion.

In the case of hooking electrodes, dislodgements were absent with the exception of one case. In this case, the atrial electrode dislodged 12 months after implantation because of fracture of the steel barbs at the apex of the electrode structure. Stimulation became ineffective.

If one now applies the same considerations for hooking electrodes as were used for determination of the long-term performance of atrial electrodes inserted retrocardially then we note that 17 out of 19 still functioned properly 16 to 30 (average 22.5) months following implantation. As was already mentioned, one atrial electrode had become ineffective because of broken barbs, another induced a painful sympathetic excitation of the right phrenic nerve shortly after implantation of the atrial generator. This forced our abandoning of this particular lead.

J-shaped electrodes

J-shaped atrial leads, intended for electrode positioning within the right atrial appendage have been offered previously by at least two manufacturers. These (30, 44, 45) have not enjoyed widespread application of implantation. A modified J-lead (Fig. 1) developed by Smyth and Citron (31), containing an arrangement of nine pliant silicone rubber fixation tines at the distal end represents a significant evolution from previous designs. We have implanted 86 of these leads. 36 of the leads were used for sensing purposes alone; 50 were used for sensing/pacing (Table 2). Atrial electrograms averaged 5.29 mV (1.5 mV minimum, 10.0 mV maximum, Table 1). To our knowledge, these represent the highest level of atrial signals to be reported for any permanent atrial electrode. In only 8 of the 86 cases (9%) was the acute action below 3.0 mV. Stimulation thresholds at 0,5 ms pulse width averaged 1.5 ± 0.46 V (0.69 V minimum, 2.16 V maximum). We have not observed any instance of "exit block" during patient follow-up.

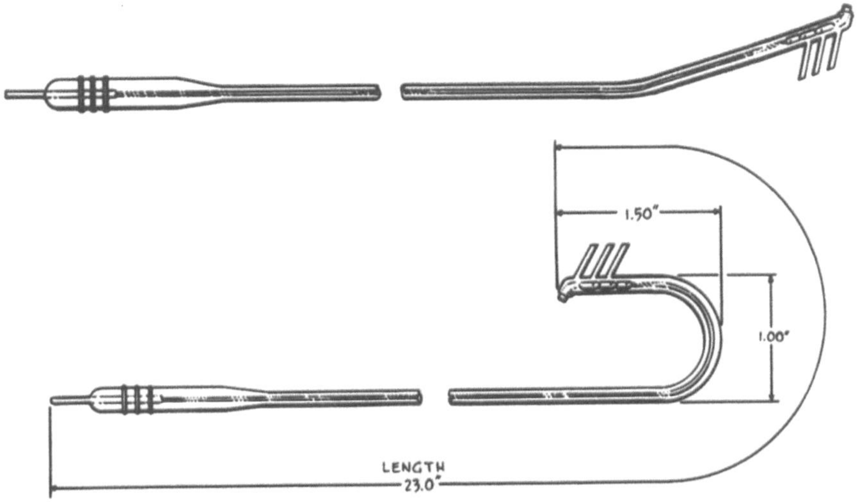

Figure 1. Schematic representation of the tined endocardial J-lead. Above, lead with guide stylet inserted. Below, lead with stylet removed.

In 5% of patients (4 out of 86), electrode microflotations led to sensing problems. However, with the exception of one case, they were only transitory in nature and occurred in the immediate postimplantation period. In the case of this one patient who was being treated with an atrial stimulating device because of a sick sinus syndrome, intermittently ineffective sensing which resulted in fixed rate pulse trains were still in evidence six weeks after implantation. Subsequently, however, this electrode also assumed a stable position.

Lead dislodgement occurred in 6 out of 86 cases (7%). In the majority of cases, the dislodged leads were replaced without any difficulty. In the case of 2 patients, however, we did not succeed in repositioning due to a strong degree of atrial dilatation which made the tines ineffective. The leads wêre easily removed in both cases. We consider the dislodgement rate to be quite low since at the beginning of our activity with this lead we had absolutely no experience in the catheterization of the right appendage. Further, the more recent implantations have been carried out by four young doctors who have not had any previous heart catheterization experience before using this lead. It appears that a short learning curve is necessary to master the positioning and secure placement of this electrode.

In this respect, it appears worthy to mention something about the localization of the right atrial appendage, since locating it initially may offer considerable difficulty to those unfamiliar with it. The exact location of the right atrial appendage can be seen from the following Fig. 2 and 3. It lies ventromedially at the level

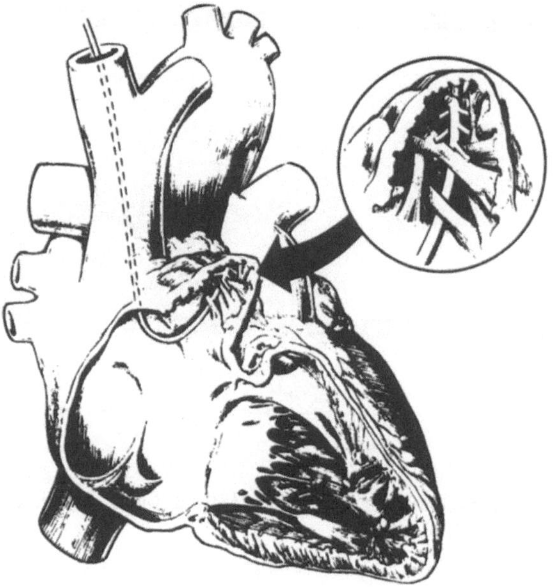

Figure 2. Diagrammatic representation of the tined endocardial J-lead in position in the right atrial appendage.

of the root of the pulmonary artery, immediately behind the sternum; however, it does not come quite as close to this latter as does the conus pulmonalis that lies cranially from it. The appendage proves to be of varying size and can encompass a relatively large portion of the atrium. In cases of high pressure on the right atrium with atrial dilatation, fluoroscopic visualization of the appendage may be obscured.

Allusions to the fact that the silicone tines may induce thromboembolisms have not been demonstrated clinically to the present time. Angiographic studies which we conducted in 10 patients one year after emplacement of the electrodes also lent no support for this concern (46). Furthermore, no thrombotic activity was noted in two post-mortem studies.

We have been using the tined J-lead for over 21 months (average 11 months for

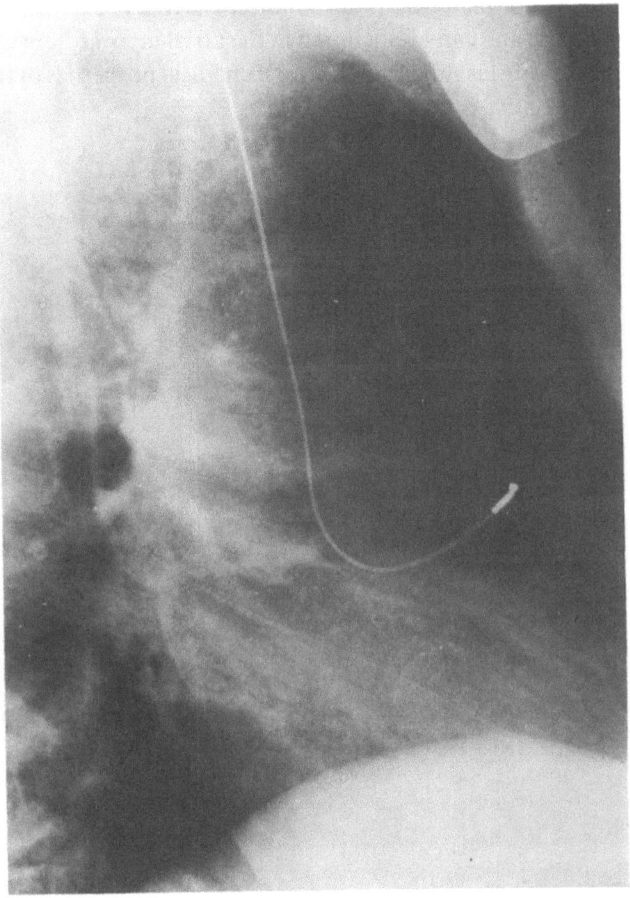

Figure 3. Transverse x-ray view of the tined endocardial J-lead in position in the right atrial appendage in a 74-years-old patient.

the population) and acknowledge the outstanding performance of this lead's design.

Atrial screw-in studies

We have recently used 5 endocardial screw-in electrodes developed by Bisping and Rupp (42) for atrial applications. Our preliminary results (43) with this lead design (Fig. 4) are encouraging. The active portion of the lead consists of two corkscrew-like turns of electrode material with an effective surface area of 5.3 mm^2. The electrode attains a penetration depth into the myocardium (Fig. 5) of 2 mm. For this small series, the average atrial electrogram potential was 4.2. mV

(Table 1). After approximately 15-30 minutes, this rose to 5.3 mV. The electrodes are easy to handle and can be anchored in the atrial myocardium quickly and in an anatomically safe fashion. The electromechanical properties of this design are encouraging.

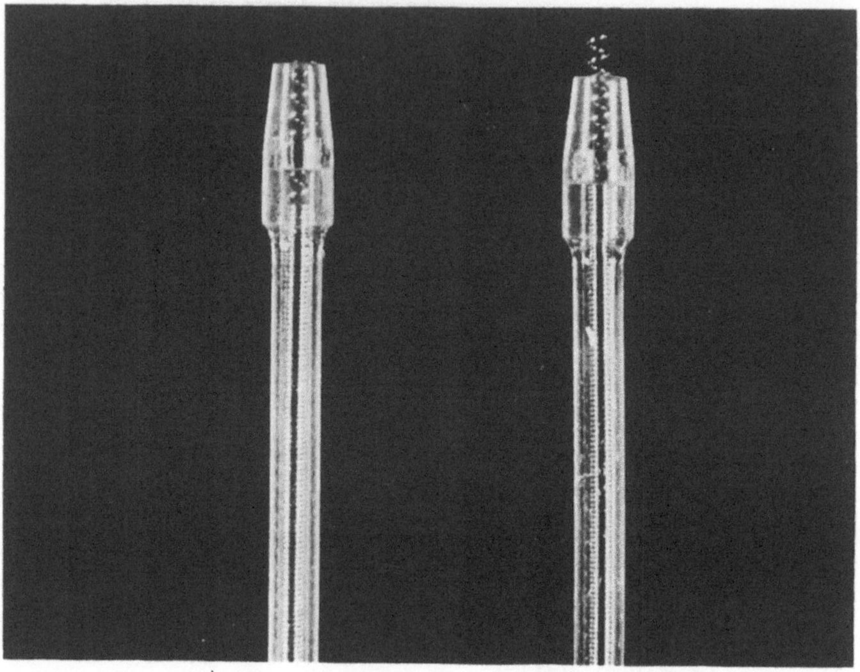

Figure 4. Screw-in electrode. On the left "corkscrew" within the silicone cover. On the right extended for penetration into the myocardium.

Discussion and summary

The necessity for implantation of atrial programmed pacemakers is undisputed. We constantly hear references to these modalities and their potential benefits in patient management. At the same time, it has been resignedly noted that there continues to be an absence of suitable atrial electrodes. Electrodes which are easily emplaced, achieve stable position, sense sufficiently large intraatrial electrograms and demonstrate reasonable stimulation threshold behavior are felt not to exist.

We feel these objections no longer apply. Our experience with the tined J lead

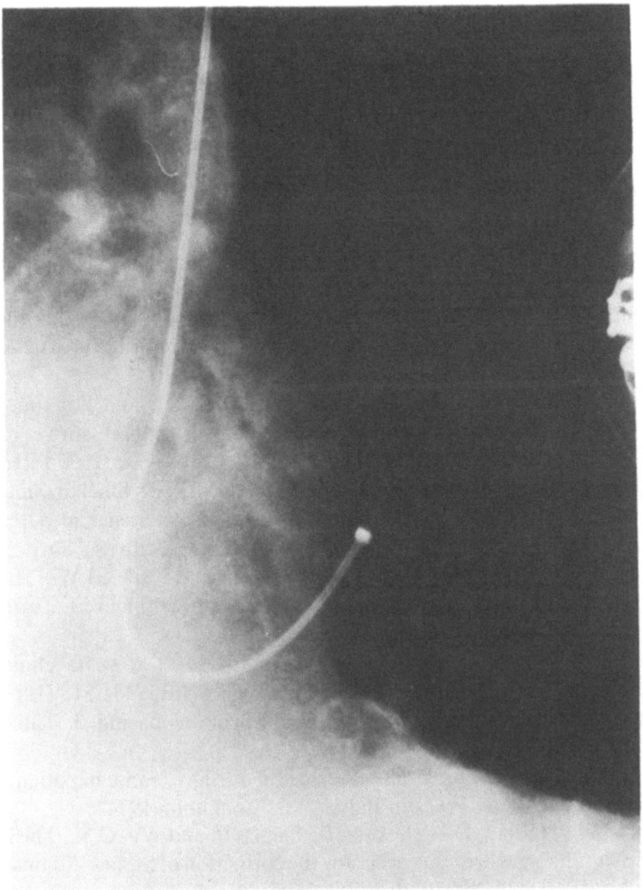

Figure 5. X-ray view (I. oblique diameter) of the screw-in electrode in position in the right atrial appendage in a 76-years-old patient.

in particular demonstrates that, for the first time, transvenous atrial electrodes are available which can be emplaced quickly and securely. Placed in perspective, the dislodgement rate of 7% for these leads corresponds quite well to the experience with standard transvenous ventricular leads. Stated another way, transvenous atrial electrodes can be emplaced with the same confidence as ventricular electrodes.

The high action potential of 5.29 ± 1.75 (1.5. to 10) mV measured from the right atrial appendage with the J lead is noteworthy. Consistently high atrial electrogram potentials have not, to our knowledge, been reported to the present time. Finally, in spite of the high initial stimulation threshold, in no case did exit block occur. I might also add that up until now, progression to AV-block has not as yet appeared with permanent atrial stimulation (47).

Our experience with atrial programmed pacing over the past 58 months leads us to believe that the problems with these modalities lie not with leads and electrodes, but with the development of state-of-the-art generators.

References

1. Parsonnet, V., Furman, S. and Smyth, N.P.D., Implantable cardiac pacemakers status report and resource guideline. Circulation 50, A-21 (1974).
2. Benchimol, A., Ellis, J.G. and Dimond, E.G., Hemodynamic consequences of atrial and ventricular pacing in patients with normal and abnormal hearts. Am. J. Med. 39 911, (1965).
3. Bevegard, S., Jonsson, B., Karlöf, J., Lagergren, H. and Sowton, C., Effect of changes in ventricular rate on cardiac output and central pressure at rest and during exercise in patients with artificial pacemakers. Cardiovasc. Res. 1 21, (1976).
4. Brockmann, S.K., Collins, H.A., Bloomfield, D.A., Sinclair-Smith, B.C. and Gobbel, W.G., Physiological studies and clinical experience in patients with synchronous and asynchronous pacemakers. J. Thor. Cardiovasc. Surg. 51 864, (1966).
5. Center, S., Nathan, D.A., Wu, C.Y., Samet, P. and Keller, J.W., The implantable synchronous pacer in the treatment of complete heart block. J. Thor. Cardiovasc. Surg. 46 744, (1963).
6. Center, S., Nathan, D.A., Wu, C.Y. and Duque, D., Two years' clinical experience with the synchronous pacer. J. Thor. Cardiovasc. Surg. 48 . 513 (1964).
7. Center, S. and Castillo, C., Pervenous synchronous pacing. J. Thor. Cardiovasc. Surg. 53, 508 (1967).
8. Karlöf, J., Hemodynamic studies at rest and during exercise in patients treated with artificial pacemakers. Trycken Balder AB, Stockholm 1974.
9. Keller, J.W., Nathan, D.A., Center, S., Samet, P. and Wu, C.Y., The application of an implantable synchronous pacer for the correction of Stokes-Adams attacks. Ann. N.Y. Acad. Sci. 111, 1093 (1964).
10. Martin, R.H., Cobb, L.A., Sun Ling Han and Samson, W.E., Reduction in cardiac output caused by asynchronous ventricular pacing in man. Circulation XXIX Suppl. III, 122 (1964).
11. Nager, F. und Kappenberger, L., Hämodynamik und Herzschrittmacher-implantation. Internist 18, 1 (1977).
12. Nathan, D.A., Center, S., Wu, C.Y. and Keller, W., An implantable synchronous pacer for the long-term correction of complete heart block. Am. J. Cardiol. 11, 362 (1963).
13. Samet, P., Castillo, C. and Bernstein, W.H., Hemodynamic consequences of atrial and ventricular pacing in subjects with normal hearts. Am. Heart J. 72, 725 (1966).
14. Westermann, K.W., Untersuchungen zur Hämodynamik bei Schrittmacherträgern. Habil.-Schrift. Hamburg 1971.
15. Irnich, W., Stand der Schrittmachertherapie: Bisherige Erfahrungen und Entwicklungstendenzen. Aus Donat, K., Kleinert, M. und Meißner, J., Herzschrittmacher mit nuklearen Batterien. Symposion im Forschungsinstitut Borstel, 2. November 1973, Verlag G. Witzstrock, Baden-Baden.
16. Parsonnet, V., Quoi de neuf dans les pacemakers en 1975. Stimucoer 2, 70 (1975).

17. Witzfeld, A. und Himmler, Ch., Technischer Entwicklungsstand künstlicher Herzschrittmacher. Internist 18, 1 (1977).
18. Carlens, E., Johansson, L., Karlöf, J. and Lagergren, H., New method for atrial-triggered pacemaker treatment without thoracotomy. J. Thor. Cardiovasc. Surg. 50, 229 (1965).
19. Lagergren, H., Johansson, L., Karlöf, J. and Thornander, H., Atrial-triggered pacemaking without thoracotomy: Apparatus and results in twenty cases. Acta Chir. Scand. 132, 678 (1966).
20. Larsson, St., Alestig, K., Bojs, G. and Bergh, N.P., Treatment by atrial-triggered pacemaker. Scand. J. Thor. Cardiovasc. Surg. 3, 186 (1969).
21. Larsson, St., Mediastinoscopy in pacemaker treatment. Mediastinoscopy. Proceedings of an International Symposium. Odense University, June 18-20 1970.
22. Kleinert, M. und Nahrstedt, J., Zur transmediastinalen Verlegung von Detektorsonden bei vorhofgesteuerten elektrischen Stimulationssystemen. Z. Kardiol. 63, 862 (1974).
23. Kleinert, M., Beer, P. and Taylessani, A., Comparative studies of transmediastinal retrocardial and transvenous endocardial placement of atrial electrodes. Vth International Symposium on Cardiac Pacing. Tokyo, March 14-18, 1976.
24. Kleinert, M., Beer, O. and Taylessani, A., Special pacemaker catheter techniques: The transmediastinal placement of sensing electrodes. J. Thorac. Cardiovasc. Surg. 71, 4 (1976).
25. Larsson, St., Carlens, E.Edhag, O., Karlöf, J., Lagergren, H., Levander-Lindgren, Pehrsson, K., Schüller, H. and Westerholm, K.-J.: Long-term follow-up of 254 patients treated with atrial-triggered cardiac pacing (ATPC) – a Swedish multicenter study. Vth International Symposium on Cardiac Pacing. Tokyo, March 14-18, 1976.
26. Larsson, St., Transmediastinal and transthoracic atrial electrodes. 2nd European Pacemaker Colloquium Brussels, April 21 and 22, 1977.
27. Rodewald, G., Giebel, O., Harms, H. und Scheppokat, K.D., Intravenös-intrakardiale Applikation von vorhofgesteuerten elektrischen Schrittmachern. Zschr. Kreisl.-Forsch. 53, 860 (1964).
28. Zimmermann, H.B. and Bergmann, M., Permanent coronary sinus pacing. 35th Annual Meeting, American College of Chest Physicians. Chicago, 111, Sept. 8, 1969.
29. Zucker, I.R., Parsonnet, V., Gilbert, L. and Newark, N.I., A method of transvenous implantation of an atrial electrode. Am. Heart J. 85, 3 (1973).
30. Smyth, N.P.D., Keshishian, J.M., Bacos, J.M., Massumi, R.A., Fletcher, R.D. and Boivin, M.R., Permanent pervenous atrial pacing. J. Electrocardiol. 4, 299 (1971).
31. Smyth, N.P.D. and Citron, P., Permanent pervenous atrial sensing and pacing. Vth International Symposium on Cardiac Pacing. Tokyo, March 14-18, (1976).
32. Smyth, N.P.D., Citron, O., Keshishian, J.M., Garcia, J.M. and Kelly, L.C., Permanent pervenous atrial sensing and pacing with a new J-shaped lead. J. Thorac. Cardiovasc. Surg. 72, 4 (1976).
33. Kleinert, M., Beer, P. and Taylessani, A., Erfahrungen mit 87 permanenten Vorhofelektroden verschiedener Ausführungen und Verlegungstechniken. Z. Kardiol. 65, 10 (1976).
34. Kleinert, M., Bock, M. und Wilhelmi, F., Einjährige Erfahrungen mit einer neuen Vorhofelektrode (J-Version) an 53 Patienten. Z. Kardiol. 66, 2 (1977).
35. Bleifeld, V., Irnich, W. and Effert, S., A new transvenous electrode with myocardial fixation for permanent pacing. Digest Ninth International Conference of Medical and Biological Engineering. Melbourne, Australia, 1971.

36. Irnich, W., Bleifeld, W. und Effert, S., Permanente transvenöse Elektrostimulation des Herzens mit einer myokardial-fixierten Elektrode. Thor. Chir. 20, 6 (1972).
37. Rosenkranz, K.A., Technik, Indikationen und Ergebnisse bei der Anwendung der "Widerhaken-Elektrode." Z. Kardiol. 62, 8 (1973).
38. Vogel, I., Dressler, L., Witte, J., Warnke, H., Porstmann, P. and Schaldach, M., Atrial synchronized pacing using a new transvenous technique. Ann. Cardiol. Angiol. 20, 381 (1971).
39. Wende, U. und Schaldach, M., Neue intrakardiale Schrittmacherelektrode zur Vermeidung von Dislokationen bei stark dilatiertem Ventrikel. Med. Wschr. 95, 40 (1970).
40. Witte, J., Dressler, L., Schröder, G. and von Knorre, G.H., Transvenous atrial synchronized pacing. Vth International Symposium on Cardiac Pacing. Tokyo, March 14-18, 1976.
41. Udall, J.A., Permanent pervenous transseptal atrial pacing. Am. J. Cardiol. 33, 6 (1974).
42. Bisping, H.J. and Rupp, M., A new permanent transvenous electrode for fixation in the atrium. Vth International Symposium on Cardiac Pacing. Tokyo, March 14-18, 1976.
43. Kleinert, M. und Bisping, H.J., Erste klinische Erfahrungen mit einer neuen transvenös endokardialen Schraubelektrode in Vorhof- und Kammerposition. 43. Jahrestagung der Deutschen Gesellschaft für Kreislaufforschung. 15-17 April 1977, Bad Nauheim.
44. Smyth, N.P.D., Vasarhelyi, L., Mc Namara, W. and Katascik, G.E., A permanent transvenous atrial electrode catheter. J. Thorac. Cardiovasc. Surg. 58, 6 (1969).
45. Smyth, N.P.D., Keshishian, J.M., Basu, A.P. Bacos, J.M., Massumi, R.A., Fletcher, R.D. and Baker, N.R., Permanent transvenous atrial pacing: An experimental and clinical study. Ann. Thorac. Surg. 11, 360 (1971).
46. Kleinert, M. and Wilhelmi, F., Angiographic findings in 10 patients with tined-J-leads positioned in the right atrial appendage. Paper in preparation.

Section IV

STIMULATION ELECTRODES

B. Ventricular Electrodes

RESULTS OF 57 CASES WITH MIP 2000 ENDOCARDIAL ELECTRODE, COMPARED WITH A SERIES OF 1200 ENDOCARDIAL ELECTRODES

G. Pioger, R. Dian and A. Bianchini

Introduction

Our clinical experience concerning the living patients who are at present followed up at our Cardiac Stimulation Center, comprehends 1200 endocardial leads of 14 different types.

We began to use the MIP 2000 Vitatron electrode in July 1973, i.e. 45 months ago, especially in order to stimulate the big hearts of elderly patients with deteriorated general state of health, who show a greater rate of electrode dislocations. Doing so, we succeeded in avoiding the hazard of general anesthesia for the direct suturing of the electrode on the myocardium. From July 1973 to November 1976, 165 MIP 2000 were implanted and 57 patients were followed up in our Center.

Features and implantation technique

The MIP electrode, developed by G. Schmitt, possesses a device which attaches the termination of the electrode to the endocardium. It consists of four nylon wires which are brought forward from the electrode tip into the myocardium. After appropriate intraventricular placement, thresholds are evaluated and the nylon wires are then gently forced into the myocardium by pressing forward adequately the stylet (fig. 1), after which the intracardiac ECG with this electrode shows during about 15 minutes an elevated St segment. (fig. 2 on pp. 180-182).

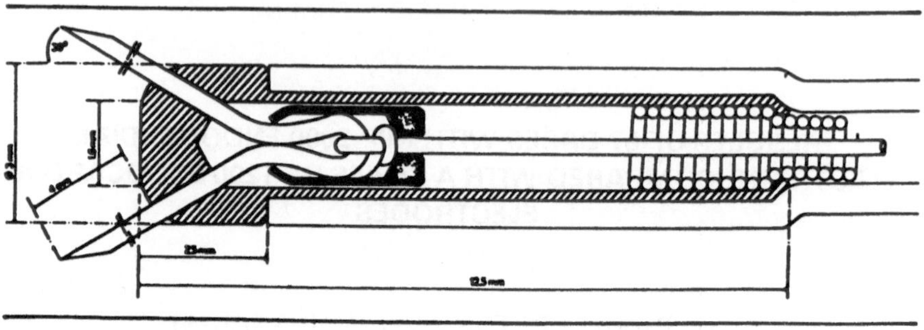

Figure 1. The MIP electrode, developed by G. Schmitt, possesses a device which attaches the termination of the electrode to the endocardium. It consists of four nylon wires which are brought forward from the electrode tip into the myocardium. After appropriate intra-ventricular placement, thresholds are evaluated and the nylon wires are then gently forced into the myocardium by pressing forward the stylet (fig. 1), after which the intracardiac ECG with this electrode shows during about 15 minutes an elevated ST segment (fig. 2).

Surveyed materials

Among the *57 patients* we are following up (out of the 165 into whom a MIP 2000 was implanted):

There was in 22 cases a first implantation and in 35 cases a replacement with a MIP 2000 after dislocation of another type of electrode.

All the patients showed megalocardia:
- 29% of type V2
- 25% of type V3
- 26% of type V4

Average age is 76.5 years.

12 patients died (3 females and 9 males); their average age at the implantation was 81.7 years:
in 3 cases it was recurring infarction
- in 1 case, complication of bradycardiatachycardia syndrome
- in 1 case, renal deficiency
- in 7 cases, terminal evolution of cardiac deficiency.

None of these patients showed any dislocation of the MIP 2000 electrode.

45 patients are living (21 females and 24 males) with an average age of 75.2 years namely:
- 18 as primary implantation with megalocardia (V2, 11.2%), (V3, 55.5% and V4, 33.3%); there was no dislocation of MIP 2000.
- 27 as replacement with MIP 2000 after 1 or 2 dislocations of another type of endocardial electrode; we had then 7 additional dislocations with MIP 2000 in large-size hearts: V2, 29%, V3 41%, and V4 30%.

Methods

The *early complications* (PDp) occurring up to one month and including mostly dislocations and the *late complications* (P average) after one month, of a greater variety, are summarized in the tables. The histogram of the cumulated late complications for monopolar leads shows a greater occurrence of complications between the first and the 8th month, whereas, later on, distribution is more or less uniform with a slight increase between 2 and 2½ years.

The *energy requirements* of the artificial stimulating systems are directly related to the following product: voltage multiplied by intensity and by the duration of stimulus. We studied the tendency of evolution of the chronic stimulation thresholds of the MIP 2000 as compared with the other electrodes, taking as a comparison parameter the voltage for an impulse duration of 2 ms (milliseconds). For that stimulus duration, the intensity values are practically in line with the potential difference, according to Keller.

The average value of the acute thresholds is .44 volt for the 14 types of 1200 electrodes; it is of .4 volt for the MIP 2000 one (table 1). Then, after 2½ to 3 years it is 1.2 V for the whole of them and 1.5 V for the MIP 2000. Thereafter, thresholds become steady for the MIP 2000 and, as for the whole of the 1200 endocardial electrodes, there is no increase of energy requirements with time, according to our 9 years experience (fig. 3).

Additional information and conclusions

– Among our series of 1200 endocardial electrodes on living patients, some cases were found where no satisfactory permanent pacing was feasible; many patients have a markedly enlarged right ventricle with thinned myocardium and smoothed out trabeculae.

– In the seven cases with dislocated MIP 2000 already referred to, all have shown an increased heart size: volume V3 or V4 on chest x-ray.

– From July 1973 up to date, for such peculiar difficult cases, we used MIP 2000 only and had 11.4% dislocations, which appeared just at the beginning of our MIP 2000 series, i.e. in 1973/74.

– That electrode permitted avoiding general anesthesia for direct myocardial stimulation in nine out of ten cases with critically ill and elderly patients.

– We introduced successfully the MIP 2000 electrode about four years ago in the panoply of various leads used in our Cardiac Stimulation Center.

– We introduced it, at the time, to treat dislocation of electrodes. Now, we usually use it, in addition, for primary implants on patients with an enlarged right ventricle.

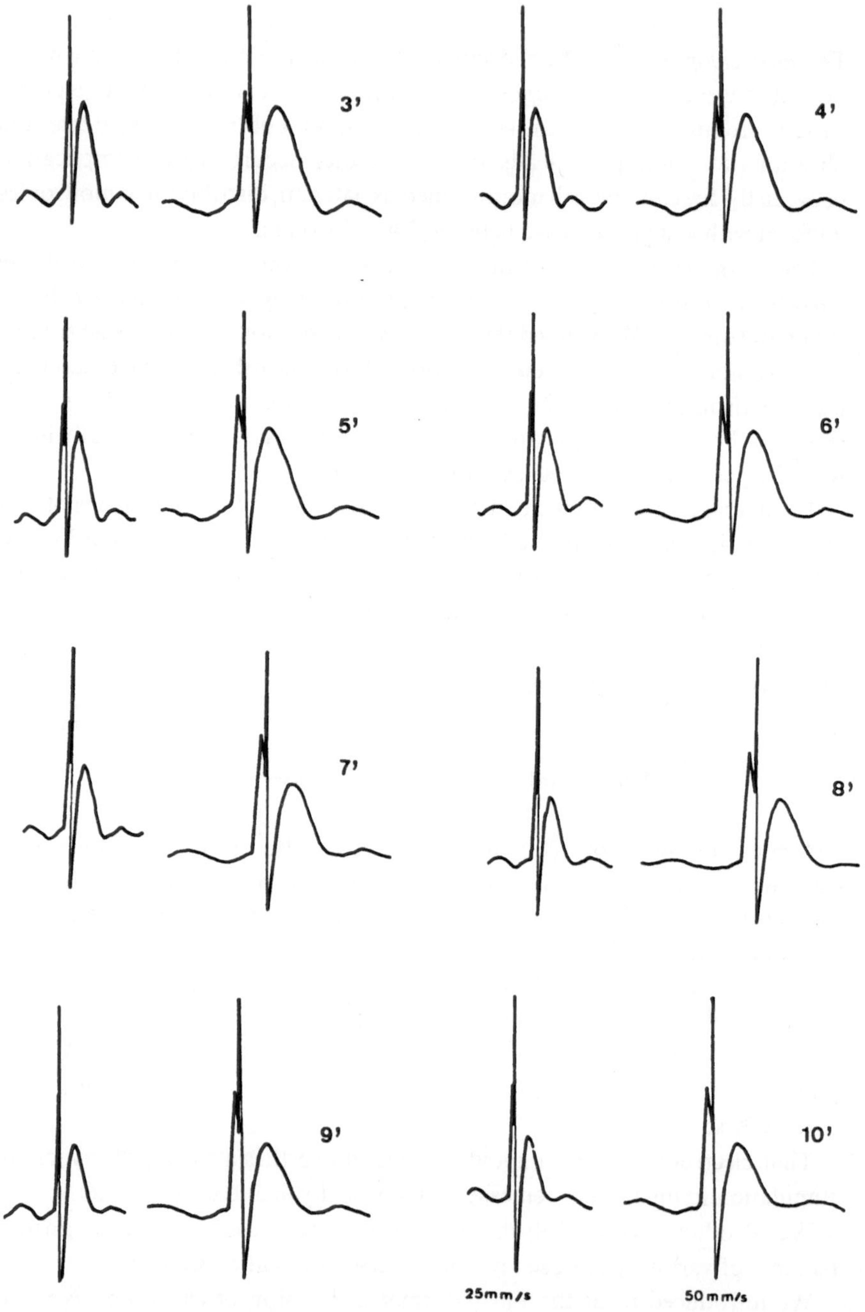

Figure 2. Intracardiac ECG by the MIP 2000 25' after implantation ST is almost normal. (ST segment elevation)

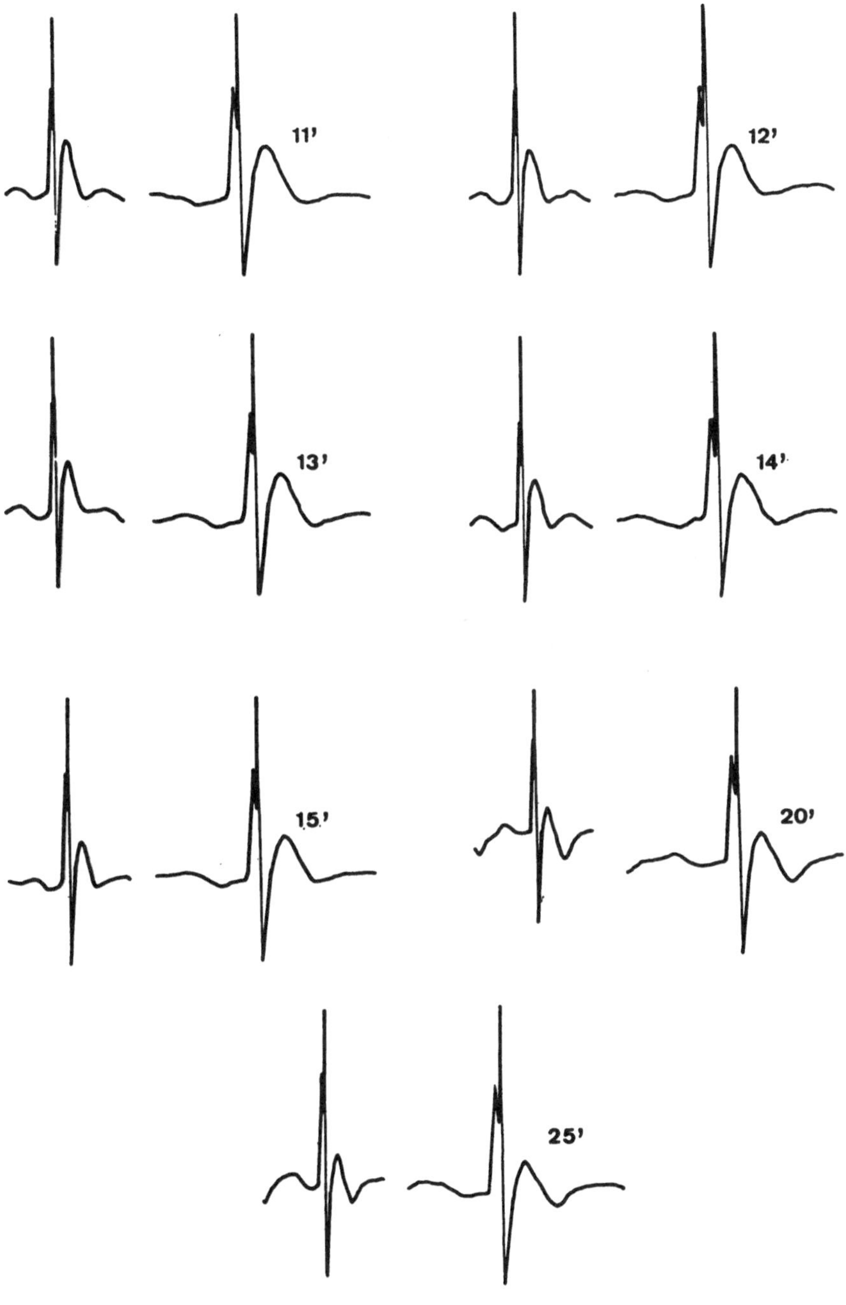
11'
12'
13'
14'
15'
20'
25'

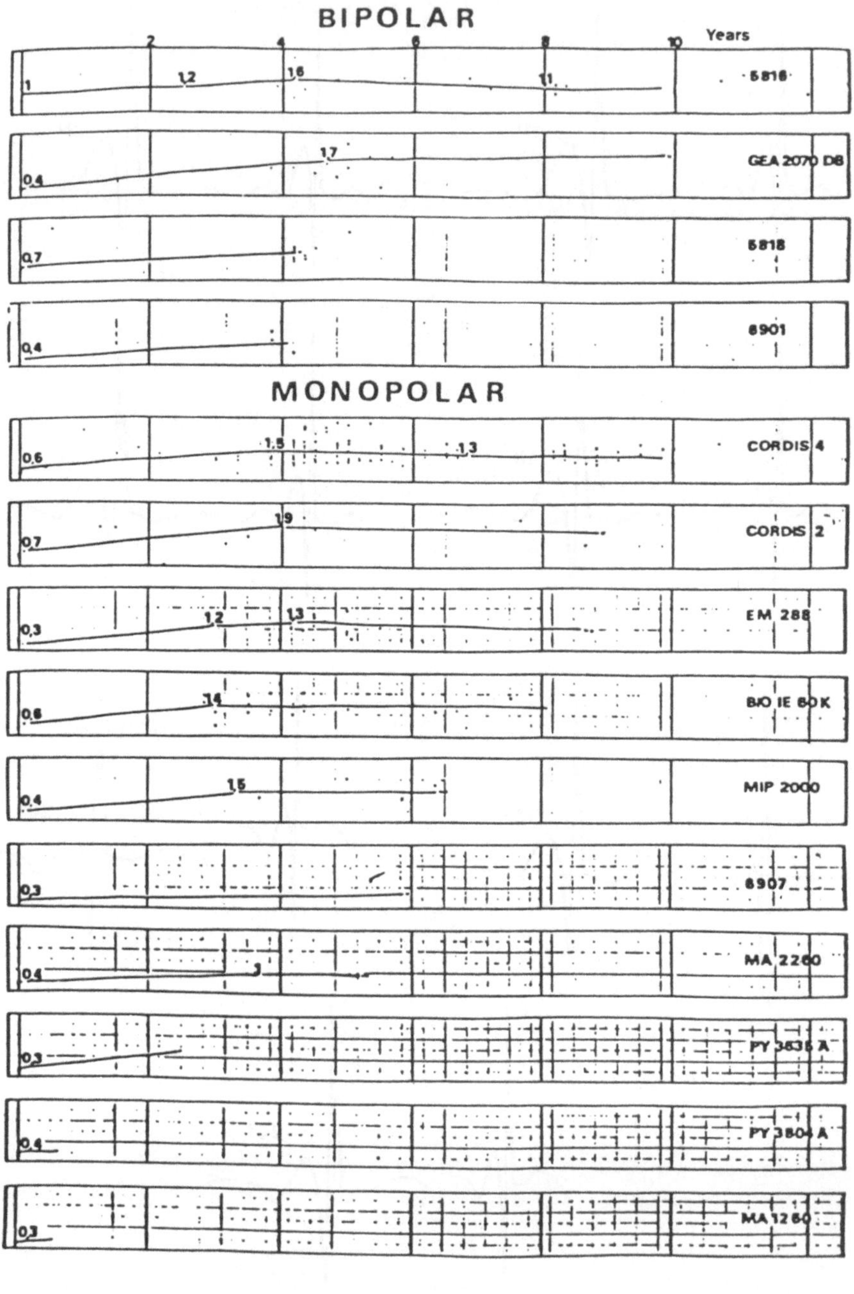

Figure 3. Evolution of chronic thresholds: 1024 cases.

Table 1. Survey of 1204 cases of 14 electrode types with the electrode identifications, acute threshold and acute (1 month) and late (1-7 months) failure rates (G. Pioger).

Model	*Mono/ Bipolar*	*area* mm^2	*Impedance Ohm*	*Section*	*Constitution conductor*	*TIP*	*N*	*Max. impl. time in months*	*Acute thresh.*	*Failure rate %* 1 month	*Failure rate %* 1-7 months
Biotronik 1E 60 K 10	M	10	100	Cylind.	ELGI	ELGI	82	89	0,60 V	1.23	0.11
Cordis											
2 mm.	M	12	80	Cylind.	ELGI	ELGI	67	59	0,7 V	6.34	4.98
4 mm.	M	28	65				310	112	0,6 V	3.7	1.24
E.L.A.											
MA 1260	M	12	85	Cylind.	A. INOX	PT + IRR	38	24	0,3 V	28.2	
MA 2260	M	22	85	Cylind.	A. INOX	PT + IRR	90	41	0,4 V	15.3	1
Elema											
EM 288	M	24	90	Cylind.	ELGI	ELGI	71	58	0,3 V	2.98	0.77
G.E.											
A20 70 DB	B	11	100	Cylind.	A + AG	PT + IRR	25	69	0,4 V	4.34	0.83
Medtronic											
6901	M	11	75	Cylind.	All NI	PT + IRR	28	52	0,4 V	3.85	0.56
6907	M	11	75	Cylind.	All NI	PT + IRR	22	41	0,3 V	4.76	2.85
5818	B	53	75	Cylind.	ALL NI	PT + IRR	60	101	0,7 V	1.92	1.34
5816	B	85	75	Cylind.	ALL NI	PT + IRR	74	100	1 V	3	1.17
Telectronics											
PY 3635 A	M	15	70	Hybrid	A. INOX	PT	76	30	0,3 V	5.5	2.02
PY 3804 A	M	15	70	Hybrid	A. INOX	PT	220	22	0,4 V	4.6	0.99
Vitatron											
MIP 2000	M	25	250	Hybrid	ELGI	PT + IRR	41	44	0,3 V	11.43	5.1

References

1. Bianchini, A., Intérêt de l'électrode de stimulation endocavitaire MIP 2000 – A propos de 140 observations – Thèse 1975 (Paris).
2. Braun, R. and Schmitt, G., Experimental and clinical studies with a new transvenous catheter-electrode. 4th international Symposium on cardiac pacing - Groningen, April 1973.
3. Keller, W., Les stimulateurs cardiaques – ANPVC.
4. Pellegrini, R.V., The Vitatron 2000 intracardiac electrode – Pacemaker Colloquium – Arnhem, The Netherlands, 1975.
5. Pioger, G. and Dian, R., A propos de 1204 electrodes de stimulation cardiaque endocavitaires implantées. Expérience sur près de 9 ans – Résultats – 6ème Entretien de langue française – Dakar, 7-12 février 77. 1e Congrès International de Cardiologie en Afrique noir.

CLINICAL RESULTS WITH INTRAMURAL AND ENDOCARDIAL ELECTRODES IMPLANTED FOR OVER 8 YEARS

M.F. Lefèbvre and G.Soots

From January 1963 to September 1968, the department of cardiovascular surgery of the Regional Hospital Center of Lille has implanted a cardiac pacemaker in 300 patients.

Patients

At the time of the first implantation, the sex-distribution for the 300 patients was:

- men: 204 (68%)
- women: 96 (32%)

The ages ranged from 11 months to 87 years. The baby is still alive and 12 years old. The median age (the age of both sides of which are found 50% of the given sample) was 67.5 years. This median age was 66.5 years for men and 69.5 years for women.

The most important clinical indication (65%) for pacemaking was Atrio-Ventricular Block or Sino-Atrial Block with Stokes-Adams attacks. The second one was Permanent Slow Pulse (35%) without syncope. There was no patient suffering from tachycardia or postsurgical Atrio-ventricular Block.

Surgical approaches

The first approach used from 1963 to 1965 was the left thoracotomy with the electrodes implanted on the left ventricle. Since June 1, 1965 following Furman, Chardack and Federico, the transvenous approach is often used. It allows implantation in patients aged of more than 90 years. The sub-xyphoïdian route appeared in 1966 (Bruck-Carpentier). The electrodes are implanted on the inferior side of the right ventricle, through the transdiaphragmatic way.

Follow-up period of pacing

Out of this total of 300 patients and 8 years after the first implantation 134 patients are dead and 59 are followed up by other clinics or do not answer to our letters.

107 patients are subjected to 8 years or more of permanent cardiac pacing. Those 107 records have been kept for this study. After 8 years of pacing, the sex-distribution is changed to:

- men: 77 (72%)
- women: 30 (28%)

Those patients have been paced for more than 10,272 months. The extreme limit is 157 months for one patient first implanted in March 1964. Our statistics are limited to 8 years of pacing, so the patient's group is homogeneous.

Operations and reoperations

662 interventions are pointed out: 107 first-implantations and 555 reoperations. The average interval between two operations is 15.5 months. Six patients have been operated for 3 times, 25 for 4; 22 for 5; 21 for 6; 10 for 7; 5 for 8; 7 for 9; 4 for 10; for 11; 1 for 12 times and 3 patients have been operated 14 times and the baby 19 times. Every patient underwent at least 3 operations. The median number was 6.2 per patient.

For the first implantation of the electrode, a myocardial approach was used in 29 cases (27%), and an endocardial one in 78 cases (73%). There were lead replacements during the follow-up period, so the distribution becomes after 8 years of pacing: myocardial leads in 25 cases (23%) and endocardiac leads in 82 cases (77%).

481 pulse generators were used, i.e. 4.5 per patient. The mean time between failures is 21.4 months. We can notice that 6 patients are now stimulated with an isotopic pulse generator.

Leads

176 leads have been implanted on 107 patients. The mean number is 1.6 per patient. At the end of the follow-up period, 50 leads (46,7%) have been replaced, 57 leads (53.3%) are still functioning after 8 years of pacing (fig. 1). Among these 57 leads, 44 had no fractures or displacements.

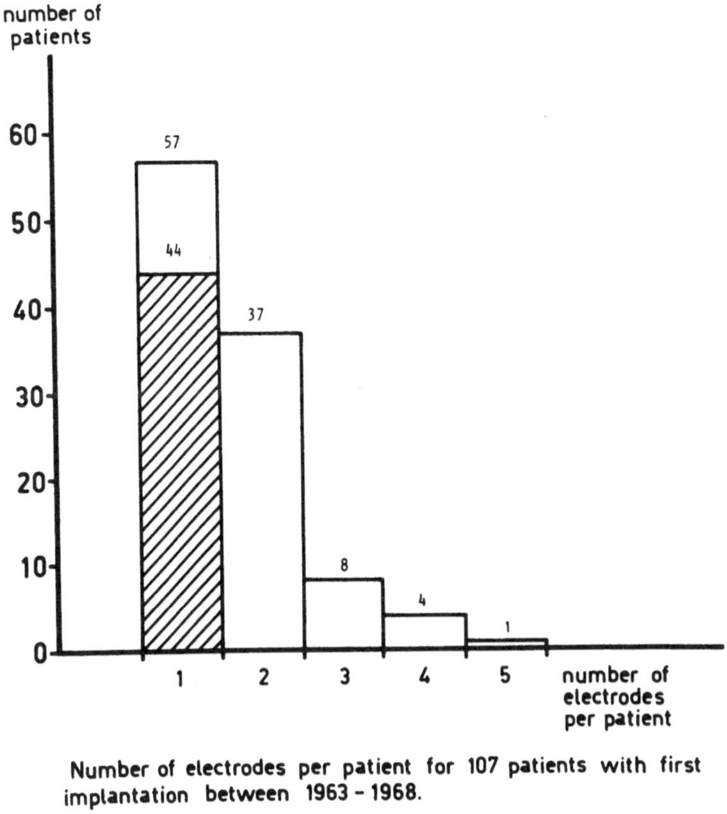

Figure 1. Number of electrodes per patient for 107 patients with first implantation between 1963-1968.

Fractures

17 first leads (12 myocardial and 5 endocardial) showed 28 fractures in 11 cases, and it was necessary to replace the lead. 4 fractures were observed on second leads. 48 myocardial leads were implanted, 29 for the first implantation and 19 for lead- replacement.

Those myocardial leads were fractured on different places.

– With the leads implanted in 1963-64 we noticed several ruptures at the transition from the ribs and at the zones with flexion, because of the rubbing of platinum spiralled wires. They do not always occur in areas of trauma.

– The intramural electrode itself is sometimes fractured in the case of an implantation on the left ventricle. We never observed an intramyocardial fracture of a lead implanted on the right ventricle.

– Two insulation fractures are also noticed, once a combination with a lead fracture.

The pacemaker replacements may increase the possibility of lead or insulation fractures near the pulse generator.

The fracture can usually be evaluated with ECG and X-ray examination. The electrode fracture is affirmed during the reoperation. The fractures of myocardial leads appeared during the four first years after the implantation. Two late fractures (79 months) are noticed on leads already repaired.

128 endocardial leads were implanted, 78 for the first implantation and 50 for lead-replacement. The fractures on the endocardial leads are usually revealed on the ECG. The breakage is not often seen on the X-rays. The reintervention confirms the cause of interrupted stimulation.

Displacements of endocardial leads

With the 128 endocardial leads we implanted, 47 lead displacements are noticed. The percentage of those displacements in function of time shows that 62% of them occur during the first month after the implantation, 75% during the first 3 months and 91.5% during the first year.

Two displacements happened 72 months after the implantation. The unipolar lead presented this abnormality after a pacemaker replacement, in both cases.

We separated unipolar and bipolar units. In our statistics 26 unipolar leads (20% of endocardial leads) had 11 displacements (42%) whereas 102 bipolar leads (80% of endocardial leads) only had 36 displacements (35%). It was necessary to replace the endocardial lead in 9 cases because of the repetition of this displacement. 4 patients had a new endocardial lead, the 5 others had myocardial leads. The rate of failures (fractures and displacements) for all leads is 9,23% per year (0,76% per month).

Threshold increase

Out of the 176 implanted electrodes, 9 cases of threshold increase are found (8 endocardial and 1 myocardial lead). The time when the threshold increase occurs is variable: from 1 to 53 months after implantation.

7 patients had another endocardial electrode, the last 2 were re-implanted with myocardial leads, through a left thoracotomy for one, and a myocardial extra-pleural implantation for the other. This myocardial unipolar lead was implanted

on the right ventricle and a threshold increase existed 18 months after the implantation.

The chronic thresholds are studied for 6 patients still paced with the original leads: 3 myocardial and 3 endocardial leads. Those thresholds measurements were measured after about 7 years of stimulation (shown in table 1). The chronic thresholds of endocardial leads are slightly higher than those of myocardial leads. This is one reason to implant long-life pacemakers with myocardial leads.

Table 1. Chronic thresholds for 3 myocardial and 3 endocardial leads after 7 years of pacing.

	Myocardial leads			*Endocardial leads*		
Pulse Duration	1,8 ms	1,8 ms	1,5 ms	1,5 ms	1,5 ms	1,5 ms
Voltage	1 V	1,3 V	0,72 V	1,10 V	1,24 V	1,53 V
Current	2,4 mA	1,2 mA	0,7 mA	3,12 mA	2,4 mA	3,8 mA
Energy per pulse	4,32 mJ	2,81 mJ	0,76 mJ	5,15 mJ	4,46 mJ	8,72 mJ

Infection

42 leads were infected; 38 had to be replaced. The infection appeared for 1 to 10 months after the first implantation in 6 cases. The other 36 leads were infected for 1 to 14 months after a reintervention.

4 infected leads were kept, but the pacemaker is exteriorised for several years in 2 cases.

It seems important to notice that in 9 cases, infection followed a reintervention for lead fracture or displacement. The infection followed a pacemaker replacement in 15 cases. Local problems may start with skin erosion and pacemaker protrusion especially with large pulse generators. It occurred 3 times with the baby.

Survival of implanted patients

The study that we have made represents a record on the treatment of slow pulse by cardiac pacemakers. The results are studied after 8 years of cardiac pacing. The follow-up of 241 patients whose eventual date of death is precisely known, permits us to calculate their survival curve. This curve includes 14% of pre- and post-operative mortality (3 months). The implanted patients' life expectancy is fairly parallel to the standard life- expectancy. After 8 years of cardiac pacing we notice that the survival is 44%.

Conclusion

The study of the causes of reoperations shows that there are 3 problems:

- For the follow-up period, the mean time between pacemaker failures was 21.4 months. It seems that the premature depletion of the pulse generators may be resolved by implanting new long-life batteries.
- Other defects of pacing in those 107 patients are due to lead problems. 8 years after the first implantation, only 57 patients (53.3%) are still paced with their original leads.
- The infection problems are increasing with the number of interventions. So it is necessary to decrease the number of reinterventions to decrease the infection rate.

The reliability of long-life pacemakers enhances the fact that the main problem is the electrode-lead problem: mechanical resistance, decrease of endocardial lead dislodgements and electrical stability of long-term thresholds.

LONG-TERM EXPERIENCE WITH AN ENDOCARDIAL SCREW-IN ELECTRODE

WILLY E. MEIER, I. BABOTAI AND Å. SENNING

The dislocation of endocardial electrodes is still a problem especially during the first postoperative period. Therefore in the last years different types of intravenous electrodes were created by different investigators all with the same purpose of better fixation of the catheter tip under a trabeculum of the right ventricle (Fig. 1).

In the surgical University Clinic A in Zürich we tested the Helifix-Electrode experimentally and the good results stimulated us to use it clinically.

The Helifix-Electrode is a cork-screw shaped electrode with a silicon-rubber isolated spiral wire. With a guide wire, which will be inserted through the electrode, the tip can easily be placed at the bottom of the right ventricle. This relatively stiff guide wire will then be replaced by a thin second wire by which the electrode will be screwed in between the trabecular network of the right ventricle, without perforation of the endocardium.

The tip of the electrode is in length 6 and in square 3 mm. The wire itself has a diameter of 0,5 mm and the whole surface is 30 mm^2. The length of the electrode is 105 cm for normal use.

In 8 dogs we implanted the electrode under X-ray control. The threshold was measured intraoperatively at the 14th, 21st and the 80th day. 3 months after implantation the dogs were sacrificed, the fixation of the electrodes macroscopically tested, and the tissue reaction histologically observed. All the electrodes were very well surrounded by a definitive fibrous tissue reaction.

Encouraged by the good findings we started using the electrodes clinically in February 1976 and implanted since this time the Helifix-Electrodes in 61 patients. For all of the implantations we took either the external or the internal jugular vein. Normally the impulse generator was implanted at the upper right abdomen. The threshold in every patient was measured. It was in mean 1.1 mAmp.

For further controls of the threshold a Vitatron MIP 42 RT pacemaker was implanted in 20 patients.

With this pacemaker the threshold could be measured after a period of 1 month, 5 months, and 11 months. Intraoperatively the threshold was mean 0.95

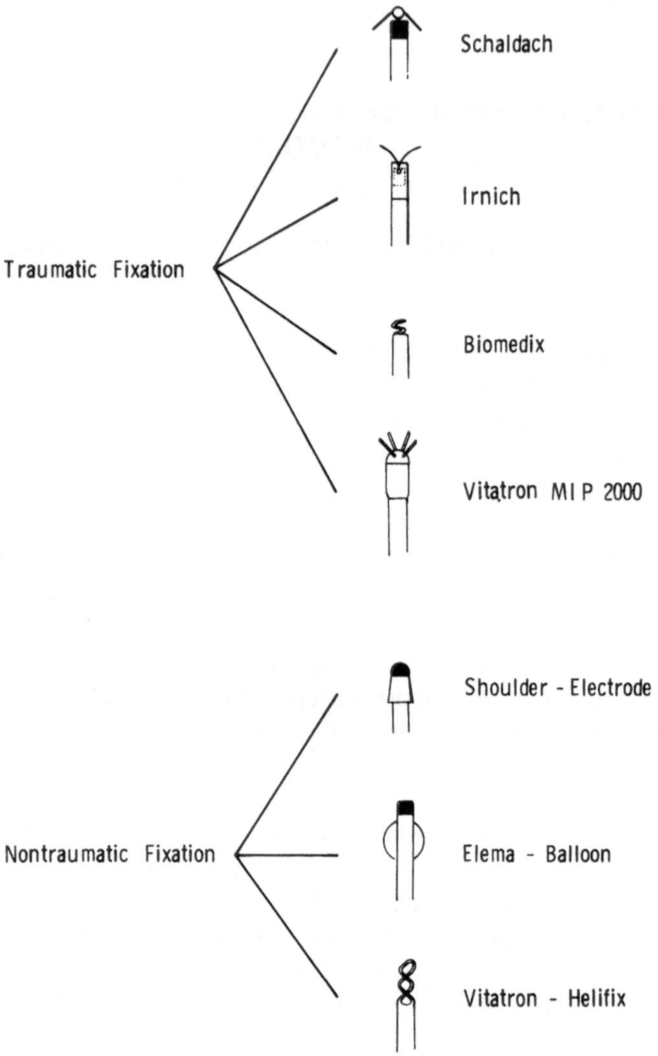

Figure 1. There are two groups of endocardial electrodes.
a) with traumatic fixation by perforation of the endocardium and
b) with non-traumatic fixation.

mAmp. The mean postoperative threshold rose after 1 month in 17 evaluated patients up to 3.3 mAmp; after 5 months, in 11 evaluated patients up to 2.9 mAmp; and after 11 months in 8 patients to 3.1 mAmp (Fig. 2). The pulse duration in all patients was 1 msec. In two cases (3,6%) the electrode was dislo-

Helifix - Electrode with MIP 42-RT Pacemaker	
Number of Implants	20
Mean Intraoperative Threshold (1ms Impulse duration)	0,95 mAmp.
Mean Postop. Threshold	
after 1 Month (n = 17)	3,3 mAmp.
after 5 Months (n = 11)	2,9 mAmp.
after 11 Months (n = 8)	3,1 mAmp.

Figure 2. Postoperative threshold control one, 5, resp. 11 months after implantation.

cated within 24 hours and the patient had to be reoperated and the electrode replaced.

In three cases we found an extreme elevation of the threshold and an exit block, so that the patients had to be reoperated also and the electrodes had to be screwed out and again fixed by screwing in at another place where the threshold was not so high.

Postoperatively the patients were mobilized on the first day if they were operated under general anaesthesia, and in the evening of the operative day, if they were operated under local anaesthesia with procain.

Due to our findings of the relatively high intra- and postoperative threshold we reduced the square of the wire to 0.4 mm. The Helifix-Electrode then at one half of the tip was isolated with silicon. The surface was reduced from 30 to 12 square mm. Some months ago we started a new series of experiments with the small electrode.

Five dogs were operated in the same manner as in the first experimental group. The threshold was measured intraoperatively and 11 days postoperatively. The results are encouraging. The comparison of the intraoperative measurement of the threshold shows that with the large surface the mean threshold was 0.78 mAmp. and with the small surface only 0.36 mAmp. (Fig. 3). Also in the postoperative follow-up, it seems that the small surface electrode will show better results than the big one (Fig. 4).

The Helifix-screw-in Electrode seems to be a reliable electrode with a minimum of complications. In the two observed dislocations we feel that the electrode was not fixed properly during the operation. No perforation of the right ventricular myocardium was seen.

Intraoperative Threshold Helifix

large (30 mm^2) and small (12 mm^2) Surface

30 mm^2		12 mm^2	
Dog No.	Threshold (mAmp.)	Dog No.	Threshold (mAmp.)
443	0.6	132	0.4
457	0.8	138	0.3
307	1.4	139	0.3
825	0.9	140	0.4
137	0.7	141	0.4
243	0.6		
553	0.5		
Mean	0.78		0.36

Figure 3. Comparison of intraoperative mesurement of the threshold using the Helifix electrode with large and small surface.

The first 20 patients we observed postoperatively for 5 days in the intensive care unit. They were mobilized very early and no dislocation except those two was observed. Now the patients are postoperatively controlled at the intensive care unit only for 24 hours, and then they are discharged to the normal ward.

We hope that we can avoid in the future the dislocation of the electrodes completely.

Postoperative Threshold Helifix

large (30 mm^2) and small (12 mm^2) Surface

30 mm^2		12 mm^2	
Dog No.	Threshold 14.postop. Day (mAmp.)	Dog No.	Threshold 10.postop. Day (mAmp.)
443	2.0	132	2.2
457	2.0	138	1.6
307	4.0	139	1.2
825	1.0	140	1.8
137	2.3	141	2.0
243	2.5		
553	2.5		
Mean	2.3		1.75

Figure 4. Comparison of postoperative measurement of the threshold using the Helifix electrode with large and small surface.

PERMANENT ENDOCARDIAL PACING WITHOUT ELECTRODE DISLODGEMENT?

J. BREDIKIS, A. DUMCIUS, P. STIRBYS AND K. MUCKUS

To decrease electrode dislodgement different endocardial electrodes with anchoring mechanisms have been suggested.

To improve electrode construction in our work the following main problems have been considered: (1). Reliable initial fixing in the endocardium. (2) Reducing the area of contact surface and threshold value.

A new original multi-edged electrode was constructed to achieve a maximal irritative effect at a minimal threshold. On the basis of morphological data a spreading tip electrode was created. Tissues grow into the spread spaces of this tip and ensure better stability. The contact end comprises a bunch of curved thin wires connected at the tip. In the open position this end reminds you of an ellipsoid with a longitudinal diameter of 4.6 mm, transversal 4.5 mm. The wire diameter is 0.25 mm. The contact surface area is 17.8 mm^2. This electrode creates a high electric field force in the heart. Then the "Biotronik" electrode with hooks has been modified in order to avoid blood penetration into the electrode. In 1974 we constructed a new original double-screw-in-electrode which differs from the other corkscrew types (fig. 1). The contact end consists of two sickle-shaped

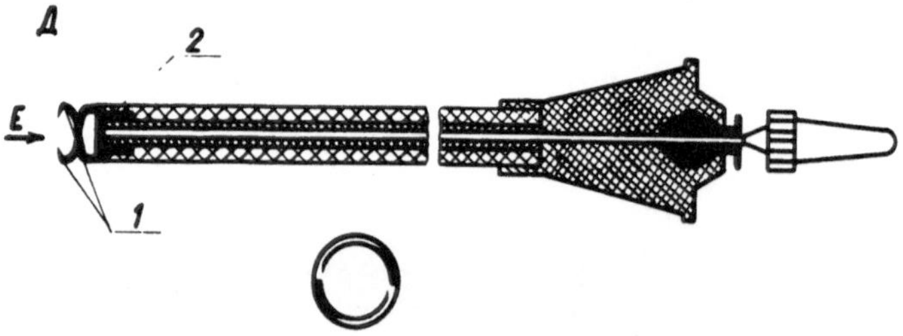

Figure 1. Double screw-in electrode
1. sickle-shaped hooks
2. silicon rubber insulation
3. stylet
E. front view.

hooks turned 180° (they are located one in front of the other). The sickle handle is 0.7 mm in length which prevents further hook penetration in the wall of the heart. Contact surface area is 10.4 mm^2. Resistance of the lead is similar to other Soviet electrodes and comprises 50 to 80 ohms.

We prefer silicon rubber for insulating permanent endocardial electrodes. Special biophysical experiments have been accomplished on perfused myocardium strips 2 × 2 cm under conditions close to those in living organism. A bipolar superficial electrogram was recorded by macro-electrodes from the endocardial surface. The threshold current, voltage and charge were determined.

It is important to note that in an energetic sense multi-edged electrodes are more effective than spherical electrodes with the same area of contact surface. The most effective electrodes in an energetic sense at impulse duration of 0.25 msec were found to be: spreading tip (17.8 mm^2), double-screw-in (10.4 mm^2) and wire hooks (18.7 mm^2) electrodes.

The double-screw-in electrode has useful features: a small and coarse contact surface, a multi-edged tip and good fixation. 35 double-screw-in endocardial electrodes were inserted into an atrial position and 28 into a ventricular position. We did not observe any displacement of such electrodes during the last two years.

The method of double-screw-in electrode insertion is rather simple. First of all the electrode is placed into a guide-catheter to a distance of 2-3 mm from its open end. The guide-catheter has a preshaped form depending on the place of insertion – right atrium or right ventricle. After that 4-5 rotations of the free end of an electrode are performed until by eye control it becomes clear that the contact end with sickle-form hooks begins to move. Later on under X-ray control optimal position of the guide-catheter is determined and the electrode is pushed out. In order to catch the endocardium with the sickle-form hooks all you have to do is to rotate the electrode 180°. Taking into account the elastic-spring properties of the lead we recommend to rotate the free end of the electrode 2 or 3 times. After having been convinced of the electrode fixation (by usual means) the guide catheter is removed. If the electrode position is not ideal, defixation by counter clockwise rotation 4 or 5 times must be performed. Defixation is not difficult. One can make a better position for the electrode without removing it from the heart.

Acute thresholds of the double-screw-in electrodes during the first 12 days increased a maximal average of 2.8 V. In two patients with ventricular electrodes during pacemaker replacement (after 18 and 28 months) the thresholds were found to be 1.8 and 2.0 volt. We now use double-screw-in electrodes more often, especially in atrial pacing. However we do not consider our investigations complete and it is still a question, whether or not permanent endocardial pacing can be performed without displacement of the electrodes.

DISCUSSION IV. STIMULATION ELECTRODES

Chairman: J.W. HARTHORNE *(Boston, U.S.A.)*

CHAIRMAN: While we are waiting for the speakers to come up to the podium, I would like to make a comment regarding the last paper concerning the helifix electrode, since recently we had experience in using this electrode in one patient. Personally, I have always been somewhat negative about the use of mechanical fixation leads, because it makes it exceedingly difficult to get the electrode out at a subsequent time, in case of infection for instance. But this particular patient last week was a rather elderly lady with chronic rheumatic heart disease, an immense right ventricle and tricuspid regurgitation. She had had four procedures done, during the preceding four months, with dislocation of multiple leads. In my judgement, this was absolutely the only electrode that we could fix within the right ventricle. It was very easy to fix it, to screw it into the trabeculae of the right ventricle. The threshold was somewhat high in different locations in the right ventricle. I would like to ask Dr. Meier: we found in this particular lady that the initial threshold recorded after implantation of the helifix lead was somewhat high. In the process of deciding to move to a new location, the threshold fell and by the time we were ready to move the electrode into a new location, it had arrived at a perfectly satisfactory level which we subsequently accepted. I wonder if there is not some mechanical irritation or damage to the endocardium that suggests that one should wait for a few moments before measuring the acute threshold in these leads.

W.E. MEIER *(Zürich, Switzerland):* We feel that from time to time, there are some patients where it is very difficult to find a good place with a low threshold. A lot of time is consumed in such cases. You can lose about an hour before you have found a point where the threshold is under one milli Ampere. I would not dare to look ten or twelve times before I found a very good place to screw in the electrodes. I think this is the mystery of the whole story.

R.G. GOLD *(Newcastle, England):* I was most interested, Dr. Harthorne, in your last remark, because we have noticed exactly the same thing.

Initially, with our experience of the Helifix electrode, we withdrew the patient's electrode in the first two cases because of exactly this rise in threshold which we considered unsatisfactory. But we have since put in eight electrodes –

only seven are actually shown in fig. 1 because the last one was only two days ago. We have noticed in four of them exactly what you described: that when you measure the threshold immediately after taking an endocardial ECG to confirm proper contact and showing a current of injury, you find very satisfactory thresholds of around 0,8 V. This is shown on the left-hand column of the fig. In one case the threshold was rather unacceptably high, at 1.3 V. Immediately after fixation, as you can see particularly in cases number 2, 4 and 5 and also in the

Pt. No.	Before fixation	Immed. after fixation	5 mins. after fixation	At implant
1	0.2	0.2	1.0	0.1
2	0.7	1.4	0.9	0.1
3	1.3	1.3	1.1	0.8
4	0.7	1.4	0.8	0.8
5	0.8	1.4	0.8	0.8
6	0.6	0.6	0.6	0.4
7	0.6	0.6	0.6	0.6

Figure 1. Vitatron Helifix Electrode threshold in volts.

patient that is not on this slide there was quite a dramatic rise in threshold up to 3 V. After five minutes in those cases the threshold had come down and at the time of the pacemaker implantation – I might mention that we use a 2-stage technique with a 48-hours delay before we implant the pulse generator – the threshold was perfectly satisfactory. The patient who went up to 3 V. took several hours to come down to 1.1 V. before I left for this symposium.

I would like to ask Dr. Meier whether he has measured the threshold at these various stages of the technique.

W.E. MEIER *(Zürich, Switzerland):* We found exactly the same as you found here. Our results are nearly the same as yours.

R.G. GOLD *(Newcastle, England):* Have you any explanation?

W.E. MEIER *(Zürich, Switzerland):* No, I have none. Maybe our electrical engineer, sitting near you, may have one. Dr. Babotai, do you have some comments?

I. BABOTAI *(Zürich, Switzerland):* No. Sofar we could not find an explanation.

A. VINCENT *(Nijmegen, The Netherlands):* We explain the decrease of the initial higher threshold, because of the hematoma which we provoke when placing this electrode. When in one patient we placed another and a third one within a 15-minute period, the threshold of the first electrode, which initially was the highest, decreased and therefore, we finally attached the first one to the pacemaker. Perhaps the explanation would be that even a non-traumatic Helifix makes a small hemorrhage which dissolves within a short time.

H.A. OUDE LUTTIKHUIS *(Zwolle, The Netherlands):* I would like to ask the three speakers on atrial electrodes: Did they do any hemodynamic measurements in the patients whom they gave atrial electrodes?

CHAIRMAN: The question is: Were hemodynamic investigations done of the relative merits of atrial versus ventricular pacing? Dr. Larsson, would you like to start off?

S. LARSSON *(Göteborg, Sweden):* I think it is very important to evaluate those patients before you decide to implant an atrial triggered pacemaker. You have to exclude angina pectoris and I think it is important to perform an exercise test. Of course, there should be normal atrial activity.

With demand pacemakers and alternating sinus- and pacemaker-induced ventricular contractions changes occur in the atrial pressure, as with Valsalva manoeuvre, and cause considerable changes in the aortic pressure particularly in patients with rigid vessels. Simple haemodynamic studies with pressure measurements in the right atrium and the brachial artery showed very great variations in pressure. As a result the cerebral blood flow becomes irregular and this may cause very unpleasant dizziness. However, we do not routinely perform invasive haemodynamic studies in these patients. In patients in whom we have changed from ventricular demand pacing to atrial synchronous ventricular pacing the patients have expressed themselves spontaneously considerable subjective improvement.

CHAIRMAN: I presume the question meant especially cardiac output. We have measured cardiac output with both ventricular and atrial pacing. The average increase in cardiac output is about 20% to 40% between atrial pacing and ventricular pacing at similar rates. These are patients with fairly poor ventricular function. We have elected to do this in people with poor function but with intact A-V conduction.

In fact we have had patients who had atrial pacers that had to be converted to ventricular pacers and seen a dramatic loss of function with an increase in congestive heart failure. So there may be a very marked increase in cardiac output in a patient with poor function, when you use an atrial pacer.

W.E. Meier *(Zürich, Switzerland):* We found nearly the same. You can expect a cardiac output increase in a patient by stimulating the atrium or implanting atrial synchronized ventricular stimulating units of about 30%. It depends on the state of myocardium. If you have a patient who has congestive heart failure, you can even find a higher increase.

H.A. Oude Luttikhuis *(Zwolle, The Netherlands):* Did you investigate your patients at rest, or during exercise, or both?

Chairman: Only at rest. The results are fairly similar throughout the world though and people who have studied this – and our own experience has been the same – have found that the range of improvement in cardiac output between atrial versus ventricular stimulation has been between 10 and 40%, the average being 23%. The magnitude of improvement depends somewhat upon the P-R interval. In patients who have first-degree heartblock, the increment in cardiac output may not be appreciated until one normalizes the P-R interval by using A-V sequential pacing. But there is fairly definitely an improvement in cardiac output by normalization of the atrial-ventricular synchrony.

F. Pizarda *(Boston U.S.A.):* I have a question regarding the ventricular fixed electrodes. I was wondering if you have had any problems of arrhythmias with these types. I recently had a patient in which a Biotronic lead was used and we had sensing problems with the pacemaker with concealed systoles, which were not apparent on the surface E.K.G. The phenomenon has been speculated way back in the '30s and '40s and was also demonstrated by Massumi in a case report.

I was just wondering if you had any problems with your larger group of patients in which the fixing electrodes have been used?

Chairman: Would you care to respond to that: particular arrhythmias related to fixation of leads in the heart.

W.E. Meier *(Zürich, Switzerland):* Sofar we have had none.

Chairman: Thank you. Well I would also like to ask our various panelists who have spoken on atrial pacing about the type of generator they employed. I believe it is the feeling of most that the frequency of the pacemaker has to be programmable, as it is desirable to control the cardiac stimulation rate. Another point as shown by Dr. Ellestad very nicely is the recycling phenomenon that occurs with atrial pacing in using a demand pacemaker when the P-R interval is prolonged, because the resulting QRS complex falls outside of the refractory period of the standard demand pacemaker. This means that, with future devices, we should have some external control over the refractory period, so that we should be able not only to control the rate, but to externally program the refractory period also. Dr. Ellestad, were most of your patients treated with programmable devices, or was there some fixed rate?

M.H. Ellestad *(Irvine, U.S.A.):* Yes, almost everyone had a programmable device, with a few exceptions and in those that we did not use a programmable device, we usually wished later that we had. I believe it is very important to be able to control the rate but I know there are some experts in this field who feel entirely differently about this. When you are involved with these patients year after year, there comes a time when you want to have a different heart rate. In most patients, a programmable rate for atrial pacing is going to be essential.

Chairman: Thank you, Dr. Ellestad. We saw today what I think is the first slide of the pathology of a coronary sinus lead. I have been trying to get one of these slides for about ten years, without success.

The other observation was made that no one has seen an example of perforation of the coronary sinus by a coronary sinus electrode and I am somewhat embarrassed to report that we have just had our first experience last week. This was with a temporary coronary sinus lead, using what is known in the United States as a Zucker electrode. It is an electrode through which one can infuse fluid. Although it is a rather dangerous kind of electrode, it is useful in positioning in the coronary sinus because one can confirm the position by injection of contrast agents through the electrode. Our patient was a very sick lady with an acute myocardial infarction, with pulmonary edema, ongoing unstable angina, who had an intra-aortic balloon pump put in and showed a variety of atrial and ventricular tachyarrhythmias. We had a coronary sinus electrode put in for overdriving and she did rather nicely. She was scheduled to have a ventricular aneurysmectomy the following day, when her pressure fell progressively over the course of three hours. At the time of opening the pericardium, the surgeon was surprised to find a tinted pericardial infusion consisting of 5% dextrose and water which had been infused through the coronary sinus electrode, that had perforated through the back wall of the heart from the coronary vein. So it is extremely important in using coronary sinus leads and also with ventricular electrodes to avoid infusing fluids through those electrodes. The same has also been reported with central venous lines attached to infusion systems which have migrated into the ventricle.

M.H. Ellestad *(Irvine, U.S.A.):* I would like to appeal here to the manufacturers to design us a temporary coronary sinus lead that is soft and a-traumatic, because we end up using things like ventricular catheters and other stiffer leads. We really need a temporary soft, pliable coronary sinus lead.

G.D. Green *(Glasgow, Scotland):* Could I ask Dr. Lefèbvre about the figure of 15.5 months which I think she quoted as the mean time between implant and replacement. An incredibly short time, that presumably is weighted by some of the poor earlier results in the early 1960's. I wonder if she has a more up-to-date figure which excludes those presumably bad earlier results which we all had. Because if we are still talking about this sort of short time between operations, then we are in a terrible state in a time that technology seems to advance so much. Mr. Greatbatch is talking about batteries which last ten years or more and the electronic reliability is incredibly good, but it does seem that there are very important other factors which we ought to know more about.

Secondly, the lead failure of 9.2% a year. Were these uni-polar or bi-polar leads and what happened to the patients? Did they all come in as emergency admissions and did any of them die?

CHAIRMAN: The question I think has come up in the minds of others but a brief comment from Dr. Lefèbvre can possibly solve the problem.

M.F. LEFÈBVRE *(Lille, France):* In our statistics, the mean time between pacemaker replacement was short – 21,4 months – but we must not forget that these are old statistics, including pulse generators implanted more than ten years ago.

For comparison we calculated the mean time of functioning of the pulse generators replaced in 1975. This was 28 months.

Concerning the second question of Dr. Green you have to realize that the rate of failure, in our statistics – 9.23% per year – includes all the leads implanted during 8 years of follow-up (a bipolar lead represents one unit). If we separate unipolar and bipolar leads, the rate of failure is 10,33% per year for unipolar leads and 8,63 per year for bipolar leads.

CHAIRMAN: The question, if the replacement is due to battery depletion only, is a pertinent one. It has concerned me through the years, because Dr. Parsonnet – perhaps he would like to defend my quoting his statement – has said in the past that in his own experience 30% of the invasive procedures for pacemaker systems have been for non-battery related conditions and that lead system failure, circuit failure, infections, erosions, etc., account for a significant proportion of reoperations in patients with permanent pacemaker systems. If this is the case, then one-third of the reoperations are done for non-battery related conditions. Are we outstripping ourselves with the improved technology of long lived devices?

P. JONES, *(London, England):* Some of us must be confused, particularly those of us concerned with atrial pacing by the rather conflicting statements of Dr. Larsson, who considered that perhaps only 1% of patients were suitable for atrial pacing and the statement of Dr. Ellestad, who suggested that perhaps all patients might be considered for atrial pacing.

In this context, I think it is relevant that very few of our speakers on atrial pacing have indicated precisely what their reasons were for instituting atrial pacing. If it is for hemodynamic reasons, would it perhaps be justifiable to suggest to patients a hemodynamic study before instituting atrial pacing? Have the speakers also noticed a high incidence of thromboembolic disease in sinus node disease?

CHAIRMAN: I think the questions have been touched upon in various aspects, but I gather that the primary point of the question is what is the difference between the 1% of the population, as Dr. Larsson quoted, who are suitable for atrial pacing and the larger proportion seen in Long Beach, California? I know from a previous report from Dr. Ellestad's colleague, Dr. Messenger, that Long Beach is referred to as "Wrinkle City" – it is an old-age population of retired individuals. Possibly, there is a difference in the age.

S. LARSSON *(Göteborg, Sweden):* I implanted atrial triggered pacemakers because of the hemodynamic advantages. It has been shown that an optimally timed atrial systole is of major importance when the ventricular filling period is short. Particularly in diseased hearts, the atrial systole appears to be of significant benefit in improving the ventricular function. I think that indications and the necessary conditions for atrial synchronous ventricular pacing are present in roughly 10-15% of pacemaker patients.

M.H. ELLESTAD *(Irvine, U.S.A.):* We have done the limited hemodynamic studies that I mentioned, but there have been some excellent studies. Dr. Starr in Portland did some beautiful studies on their post-operative patients and showed conclusively – and this has been repeated in other laboratories – that the atrial component in people with diseased hearts is a very critical and a very important condition. Therefore, it would seem to me to be desirable to pace from the atrium wherever possible, because you get a better cardiac function. If you do not have a good way to do that, you should then use what I consider the second-best approach and that is from the ventricle. I do not believe that you have to justify in each individual case a hemodynamic improvement, because this has been well documented in the literature and it has been universally found in our own experience, where we have treated patients with severe intractable congestive failure with atrial pacing. Those where we have measured cardiac output have shown hemodynamic increases and they have also shown dramatic improvements in their clinical course.

M. KLEINERT *(Hamburg, F.R. Germany):* The reasons for permanent atrial pacing in our group were only hemodynamic ones, because you can find in patients with sinus node syndrome, firstly, in a very high degree – up to 90% and more – if you pace the ventricles a retrograde conduction, and secondly, we have found in this group also a tendency to systemic hypotension. Both are reasons why we stimulate the atrium in these patients. We have not done, up to now, hemodynamic studies by measuring the cardiac output.

CHAIRMAN: We have heard an interesting dialogue this afternoon, contrasting different groups' experience with different electrode systems. I think they would all admit that the ideal lead system has not yet been developed and that the future will demonstrate a tendency towards systems employing atrial pacing, A-V synchronous pacing or atrio-ventricular sequential pacing. All of us look forward with enthusiasm to the continuing experience of these groups that have done some of the pioneer work. Thank you all.

Section V

THE CHOICE OF THE PACEMAKER-ELECTRODE COMBINATION

THE PACEMAKER-ELECTRODE COMBINATION AND ITS RELATIONSHIP TO SERVICE LIFE

W. IRNICH AND U. GEBHARDT

Introduction

In the past there were repeated complaints that the service life of implantable pacemakers was too short and that as a result pacemaker patients had to be operated on too frequently. This has led to two main developments in recent years. On the one hand, new energy sources have been developed which have a larger capacity and are more reliable than the well known mercury oxide cell. On the other hand, the current needed by the pacemaker itself and by the heart has been drastically reduced (1).

We are now in a position to implant pacemaker systems which are likely to last longer than the patient. The question of which pacemaker system is best suited to which patient can be answered very simply. The ideal pacemaker system is the one which requires no further surgical intervention. A lot of questions remain, however, as to how to reach this aim. This paper tries to outline the principles whereby the overall complication rate can be reduced to such a degree that the majority of pacemaker patients have the chance that they need undergo only one surgical operation, namely the first implantation.

Complications in pacemaker therapy

Table 1 shows a synopsis of all complications which occurred in 1976 in our clinic. All reasons for surgical intervention were related to the average number of our living patients in 1976. By far the most prevalent reason was battery depletion with 9.4% per year. It is followed by "electrode breakages" with 3.9% per 100 living patients per year.

"Medical complications" such as infections, perforations of pacemakers or electrodes through the skin, malpositioning of the electrode within the sinus coronarius occurred in 2.6% per year. Other "technical defects" such as insulation and adapter defects, cracking of the epoxy resin etc. happened in 2.1% per year. "Late threshold elevation" with 1.3% per year and "late dislodge-

Table 1. Complications in pacemaker therapy (383 living patients)

	related to 100 living patients per year	*related to the total number of defects*
Exhaustions	9.4	46.3%
Electrode breakage	3.9	19.2%
Medical complications*	2.6	12.8%
Other technical defects**	2.1	10.3%
Late threshold elevations	1.3	6.4%
Late dislodgements	0.5	2.5%
Electronic defects	0.5	2.5%
Total	20.3	100%

* Infection, perforation, malpositioning (s.c.)
** Insulation + adaptor defects, cracking epoxy resin.

ments" with 0.5% per year were present. "Electronic defects" occurred in only 0.5% per year corresponding to a mean time between two failures of 1.75×10^6h. If all "late" complications are taken as 100%, 46,3% of all surgical interventions were due to depleted energy sources though the mean implantation time was 34.6 months (minimum 17, maximum 64 months). All electrode complications together came in second place with 28.1%, followed by technical defects and medical complications with 12.8% each. Thus, energy and electrode problems roughly form three quarters of all complications. The ideal pacemaker system in terms of energy source and electrode could reduce today's complication rate to one quarter. Therefore, to look for adequate energy sources and better electrodes will be essential for the future. The energy problem is now solvable, leaving the electrodes as by far the weakest link in the chain of the pacemaker system. Roughly one third of all pacemaker patients who have a pacemaker for 10 years will have an electrode breakage if the mechanical strength is not improved in the future.

"Early complications" are summarized in Table 2. Our interventions because of threshold elevations and dislodgements within one month after implantation reached 11.3% related to the total amount of electrodes implanted in 1976.

Table 2. Early complications (within 1 month after implantation)

Threshold elevation	6.8%
Dislodgement	4.5%
Total	11.3%

Life expectancy of pacemaker patients

If the survival rate of pacemaker patients is investigated, it should be divided into male and female groups. We found in our patients that the 50% point differed by more than two years with 5 years for male and 7.2 years for female (see Figure 1). As there were the same number of patients in each group, the mean 50% point is 6.1 years which is in good agreement with the results from other groups.

It could be concluded from those findings that pacemaker longevity should be of the order of 6 years. However this conclusion is not very logical because about

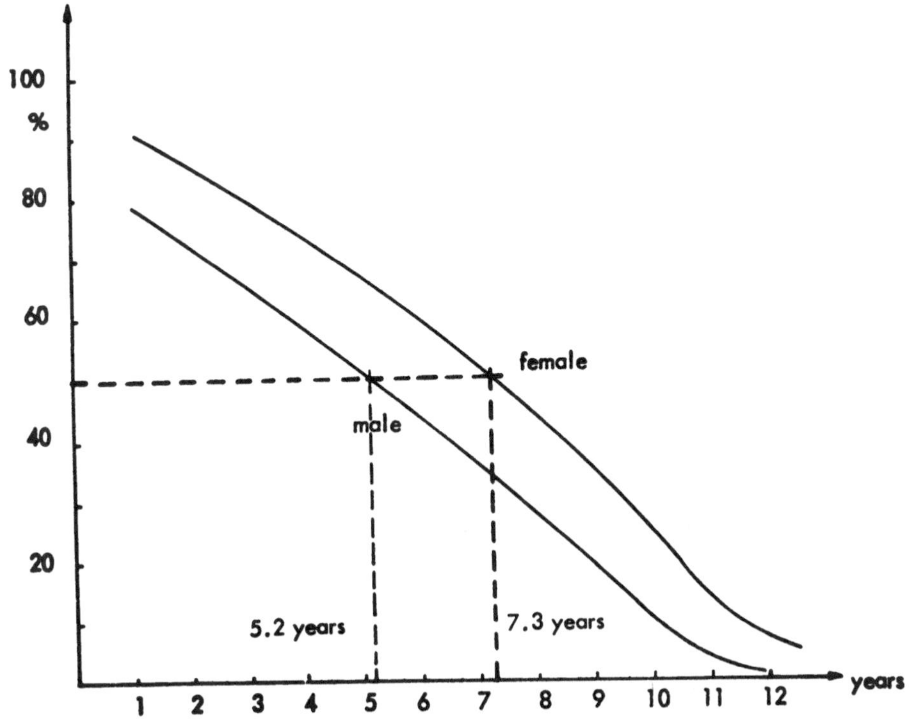

Figure 1. Survival rate after implantation.

50% of all patients will by then have undergone a second operation because of exhaustion of the batteries. The exchange rate is, consequently, only lowered from 80% with a two years pacemaker to 50% with a six years pacemaker, which corresponds to a reduction of 63%.

To investigate the life expectancy of pacemaker patients and to draw conclusions from it with respect to the power sources needed for the corresponding pacemaker, we compared the life expectancy of our deceased patients with that of the normal population in the Federal Republic of Germany (2).

Figure 2 shows the result for female, Figure 3 that for male patients. It can be seen that the normal expectancy curve is only reached by a few patients in the

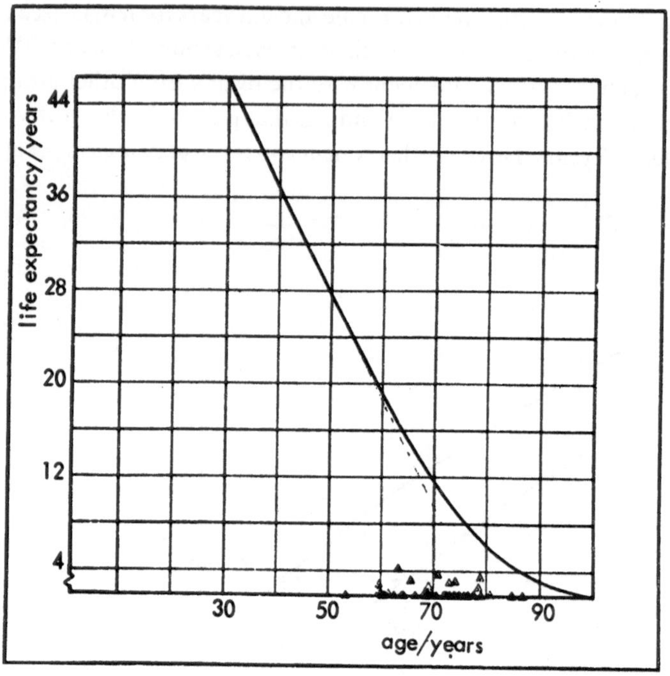

Figure 2. Normal life expectancy compared with life expectancy of our deceased patients (female).

range above 75 years. Especially the younger patients are positioned far below the curve.

There are two reasons to explain this:

1. The younger patients who have died so far represent the most unfavorable cases. We have to wait some time to know whether a 30 years old female pacemaker patient will ever reach a life expectancy of 45 years.

2. The prognosis for younger patients seems to be more unfavorable than that of the older. This is indicated by the fact that the mean age of our deceased patients (69.1 years) is lower than that of our living patients (69.7 years).

Figures 4 and 5 show the general life expectancy compared with that of our still living patients demonstrating that only a few patients in the 75 to 85 years range reached and exceeded the curves. If it is taken into consideration that the life expectancy of pacemaker patients is restricted because of their coronary disease and for other cardiac defects, it seems to us to be not unrealistic that the supposed life expectancy of pacemaker patients is about 70% of that of normal subjects (3). The few patients who exceed this reduced curve (32 out of 522 patients) are best taken into account by adding two years to the 70% curve. No living or deceased

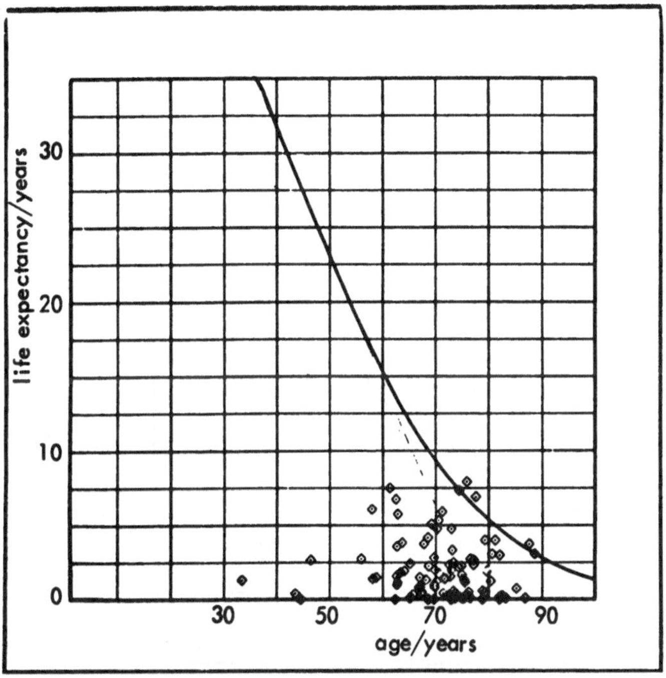

Figure 3. Normal life expectancy compared with life expectancy of our deceased patients (male).

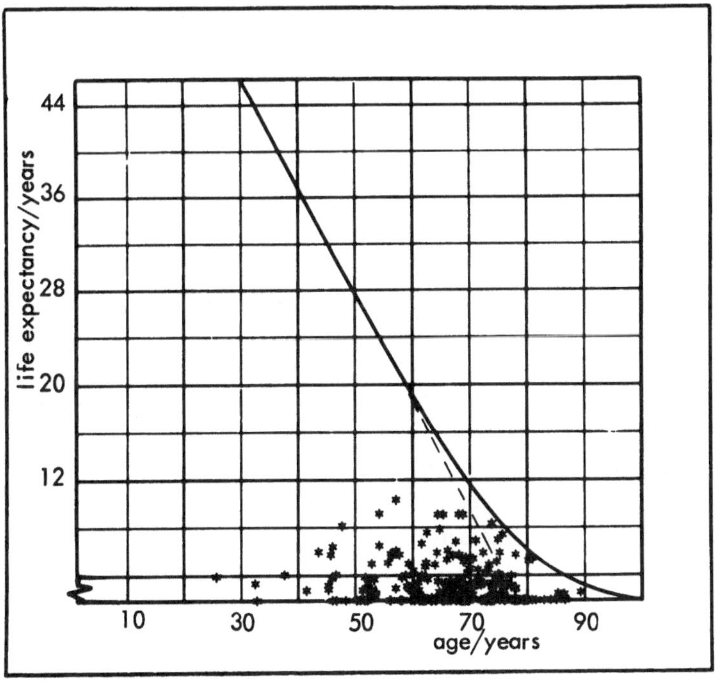

Figure 4. Normal life expectancy compared with that of our living patients (female).

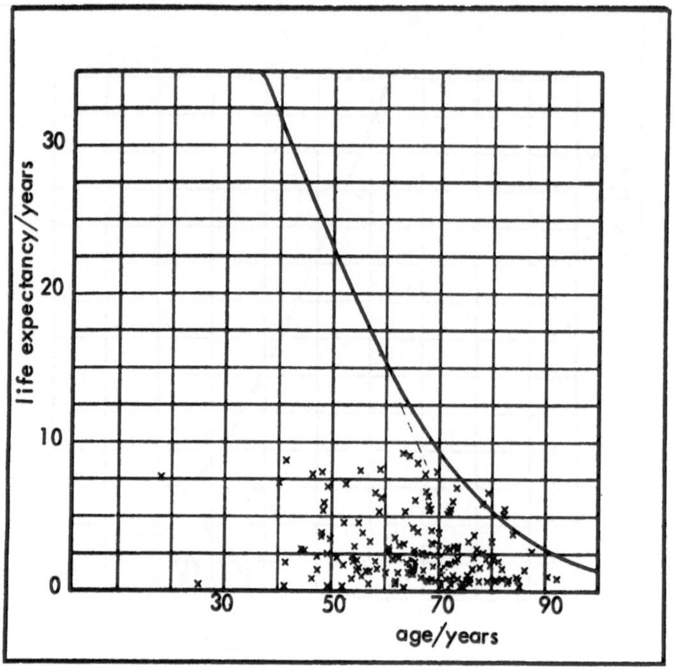

Figure 5. Normal life expectancy compared with that of our living patients (male).

patient of our group has exceeded this life expectancy curve so far.

Figure 6 can be used to estimate the probable maximum life expectancy of pacemaker patients as a function of age at implantation (3).

Energy sources and service life of pacemakers

In the light of Figure 6 we can now postulate that it is necessary to have pacemakers with different service lives corresponding to the age of the patient at initial implantation. This is the optimum procedure because it offers the patient a high probability of living out the rest of his life without needing an exchange operation while at the same time being an economical method of treatment. In 1976 the costs for pacemakers in West Germany amounted to approximately 100 million DM. To save only 1% means a saving of the order of one million DM.

We calculated the ranges of service lives of different demand pacemakers with different energy sources which are given in Table 3 for 4 types of lithium bat-

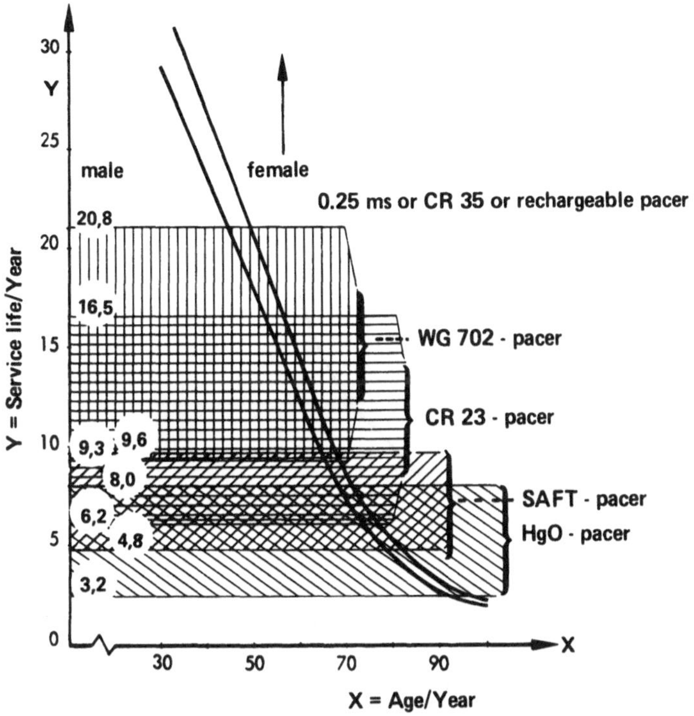

Figure 6. Maximum life expectancy of pacemaker patients as a function of implantation age.

teries. This should be compared with the service life of mercury oxide pacemakers which have an expectancy of 38 to 96 months (3 to 8 years) (3). All ranges are overlapping; service lives of up to 300 months (25 years) seem to be possible today.

Table 3. Estimated service life of different lithium energy sources

SAFT Li 210	58 ≤ *89* ≤ 130 months
Catalyst Research CR 23	87 ≤ *133* ≤ 185 months
Wilson Greatbatch 702 E	111 ≤ *180* ≤ 249 months
Catalyst Research CR 35	200 ≤ *250* ≤ 304 months

In Figure 7 the age distribution for our female and in Figure 8 that for our male patients are given along with an indication of which power source would be adequate after consideration of our life expectancy curve for pacemaker patients. Even without nuclear power sources it can be seen that it is possible today to give the majority of patients a pacemaker that he will not outlive. For patients aged below 45 years for male and 51 years for female, rechargeable or 0.25 ms pulse duration pacemakers are needed.

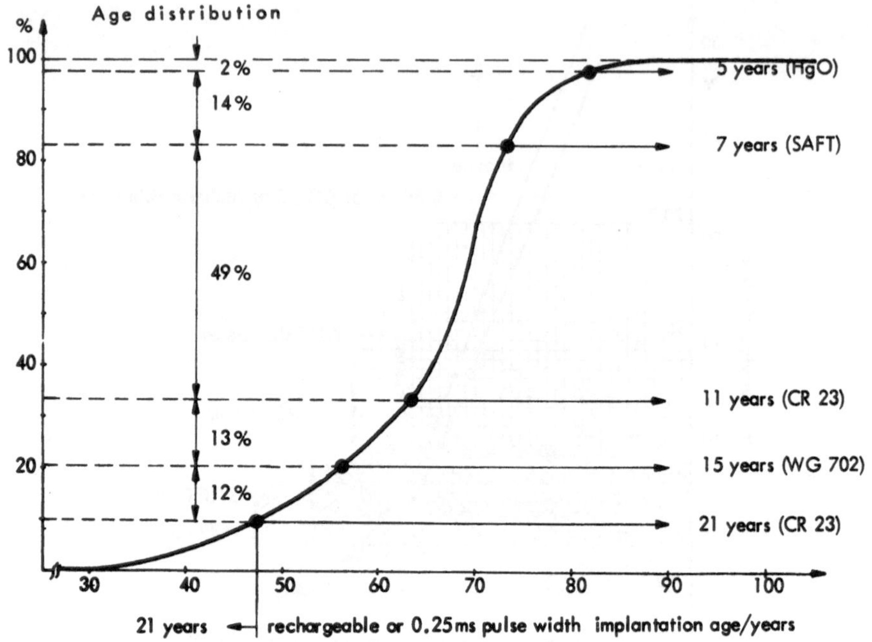

Figure 7. Age distribution and correlated energy sources in relation to implantation age (female).

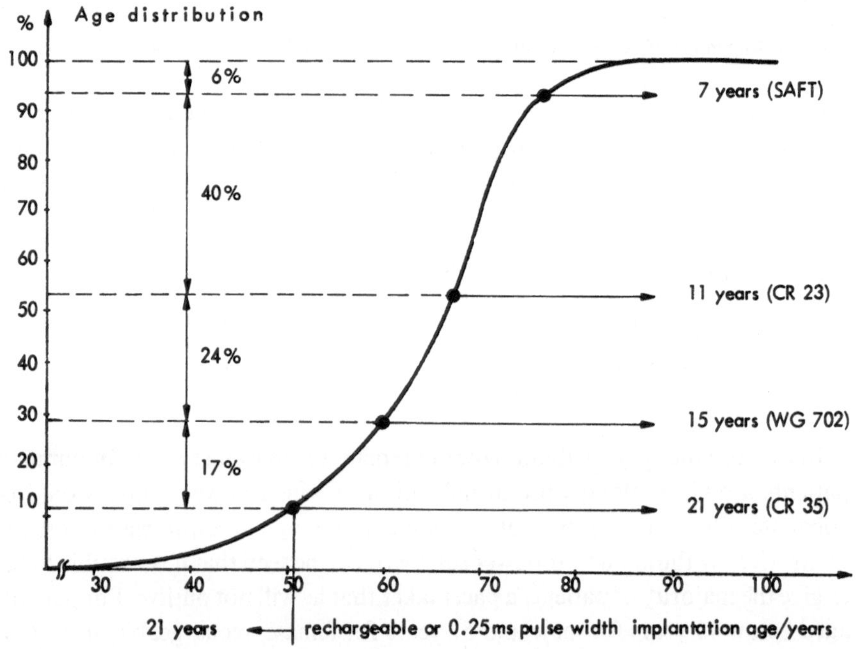

Figure 8. Age distribution and correlated energy sources in relation to implantation age (male).

Table 4 shows a synopsis of 5 different power sources, their mean function time and the estimated market share derived from Figures 7 and 8. The eleven-years-pacemaker, regardless whether it is reached by the CR 23 battery or another, has the largest market share with 45%. A 5 years pacemaker is, with only 2%, a nearly insignificant type which could be replaced by the cheapest lithium type.

Table 4. Power source, implantation age, and suggested market share. For patients aged below 46.5 years (male) and 51 years (female) rechargeable or 0.25 ms pulse duration pacemakers are needed.

source	*capacity Wh*	*service years*	*market share male*	*female*	*total*
HgO	5.4	5	2%	0%	1%
SAFT	4	7	14%	6%	10%
CR 23	6.2	11	49%	40%	44.5%
WG 702	9.8	15	13%	24%	18.5%
CR 35	10.9	21	12%	17%	14.5%

Properties of electrodes with respect to service life

Lots of investigations have proved that with smaller electrode sizes the current consumption of pacemakers can be markedly reduced so yielding longer service lives. (4, 5, 6).

Two mechanisms are responsible:

1) The impedance increases with smaller surface area.
2) The so-called chronaxie time is diminished which means that the pulse duration can be reduced without significant loss of safety margin (6).

Figure 9 shows the relationship of surface area and impedance. If the lead resistance is subtracted from the total circuit impedance the remaining "transition impedance" is nicely correlated (correlation coefficient 0.91) according to the following equation:

$$\left(\frac{1}{Z_t/K\,\Omega}\right)^2 = 0{,}375\ A/\text{mm}^2 - 0.443 \qquad (r = 0.91)$$

with Z_t = transition impedance, A = surface area (valid for 0.5 ms pulse duration).

According to the above equation a normal electrode with a lead resistance of 70 to 90 Ω has an impedance of 500 Ω with 17 mm^2 or 700 Ω with 8.5 mm^2. A similar relationship was already postulated by us for ball-shaped electrodes in 1969 (7).

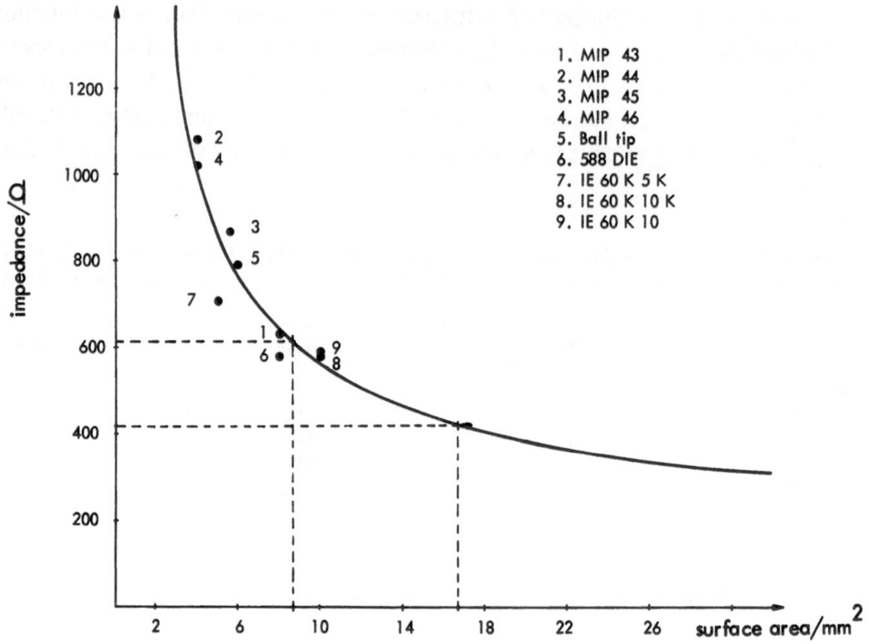

Figure 9. Relationship between transition impedance and surface area of electrodes.

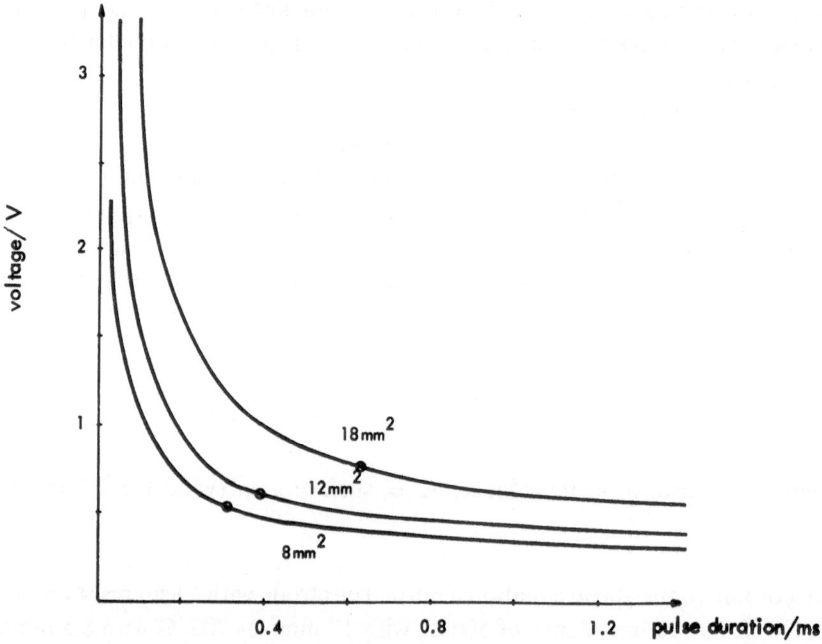

Figure 10. Strength duration curves for three different surface areas (acute measurements). The circles indicate the corresponding chronaxie time.

Figure 10 shows the decrease in chronaxie time from 0.62 ms for 18 mm^2 surface area to 0.39 ms for 12 mm^2 and to 0.31 for 8 mm^2. The curves show averaged values from measurements made by Kleinert and coworkers (8). It is reasonable to have a pacemaker pulse duration in the vicinity of the chronaxie time. These remarks are quantitatively only valid for constant voltage pulses. However, this tendency is true for constant current too.

There is no evidence that smaller electrodes and reduced pulse duration will increase the early and late complication rates. We have combined small area electrodes with 0.25 ms pulse generators at initial implantation in 36 cases yielding "early" complications in 3 cases corresponding to a complication rate of 8.3%.

The current saving effect with reduced pulse duration is remarkable. Table 5 shows two examples, one for mercury oxide and one for lithium SAFT batteries.

Service lives with 0.25 ms pulse duration are prolonged up to 170% for HgO and up to 214% for lithium compared with those of 1 ms pulse duration and 500 Ω load.

Table 5. Dependence of service life on pulse duration t and electrode impedance (500 Ω and 700 Ω)

	service	*t/m s*	*life/months* 500 Ω	*700 Ω*
1. Example: Vitatron (HgO)	MIP 42	1	57	64
	MIP 42	0.5	74	81
	MIP 42	0.25	93	97
2. Example: Biotronik (SAFT)	IDP-44 L	0.9	84	99
	IDP-54 L	0.5	111	131
	IDP-94 L	0.25	155	180

A solution to the problem of dislocations may be found in the future by electrode tips which can be anchored. At the last pacemaker symposium in Tokyo at least three new transvenous versions were introduced. We think this method to be important because late dislocations too could be avoided. Figure 11a shows a hooking electrode anchored within the atrium. There was initially a generous loop. 15 months later the X-ray (figure 11b) was taken. Surprisingly the loop had nearly disappeared. A comparison of both pictures showed that approximately 5 cm of lead length had disappeared (figure 11c). We don't know whether the correction of an adapter failure or the sinking of the pacemaker itself was the reason for the retraction. Clearly, however, any anatomically caused elongation between the tip of the electrode and the fixation site in the vein, or any tension, may lead after implantation to a late dislodgement, or in its unrecognized form to a late threshold elevation.

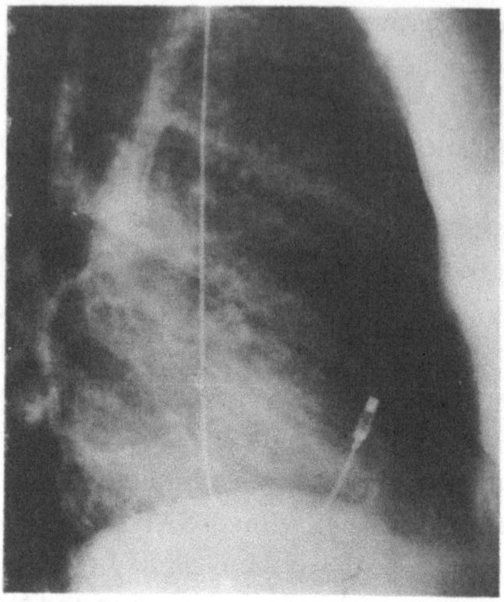

a.

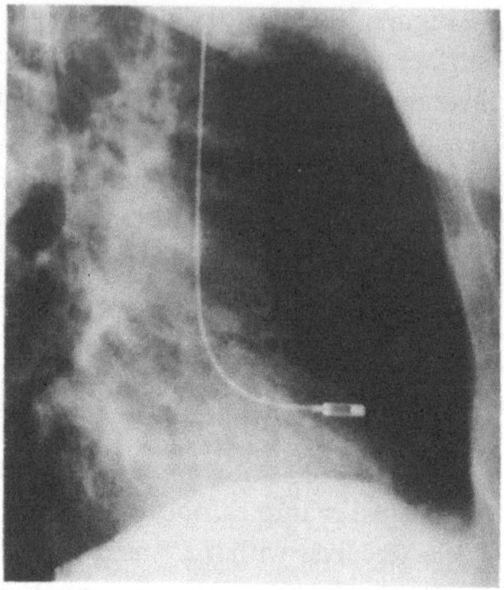

b.

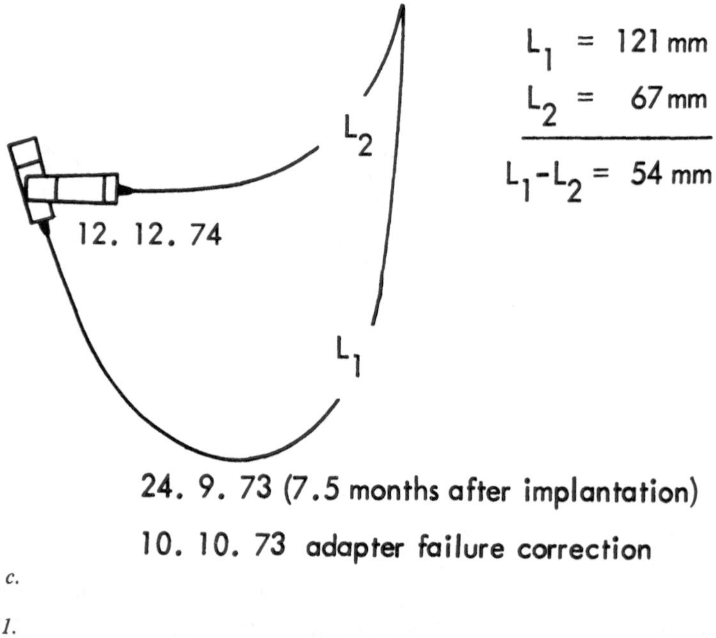

c.

Figure 11.
a. Atrial hooking electrode 7.5 months after implantation.
b. Atrial hooking electrode 22 months after implantation.
c. Comparison between fig. 11a) and 11b).

The problem of electrode breakages was investigated extensively. Of the 15 cases we experienced in 1976, all were broken in the vicinity of the pacemaker. Of 85 cases investigated, we found more than 94% to be in the vicinity of the pacemaker. We were astonished by this because this part of the lead is not exposed to flexing or torsion as it would be within the heart. Possibly bending or stretching beyond the elastic limit is the reason for our frequent breakages in the pacemaker pocket. The mean time between failures of 0.22×10^6h is far below the results obtained by manufacturers. Moreover, the probability of breakage is not a function of time which means that an old electrode has no higher probability of breakage than a relatively new one. We thought the incidence of breakage to be dependent on the number of surgical operations performed but that proved statistically not true.

We feel that the today's transvenous single coil leads are no longer adequate with respect to long life pacemakers as was already shown with Table 1. More flexible and more stretchable leads with electric redundancy are needed to reduce this most prevalent technical complication. Redundancy is today only incorporated in the Elema 588 electrode which, at the same time, is also unbreakable. It has the disadvantage that it is not stretchable and it is difficult to position. Two other manufacturers have now two or threefold coiled leads which are more flexible but don't have that excellent redundancy of the Elema electrode. In this respect further efforts should be made to solve the problem of the weakest link in today's pacemaker system.

Conclusions

The ideal electrode should have the following features:

1. Small size (< 10 mm^2) to reduce current consumption by increasing the impedance and decreasing the generator's pulse duration,
2. Anchoring properties to reduce early dislodgements and, by generous loops, later ones too,
3. A multicoil flexible and redundant lead to reduce the chance of late dislodgement as well as to avoid breakages.

If such an electrode were to be combined with a pacemaker which is not outlived by the patient, the overall complication rate would be drastically reduced. This would not only benefit the patient but would also remarkably reduce costs, an advantage which will gain increasing importance in the future.

References

1. Irnich, W., Schrittmachertherapie Heute, Med. Welt (in press).
2. Statistisches Jahrbuch 1975 für die Bundesrepublik Deutschland. Editor: Statistisches Bundesamt, Wiesbaden, Kohlhammer, Stuttgart-Mainz 1975.
3. Irnich, W., Gebhardt, U., Ein Beitrag zur Auswahl von Herzschrittmachern. Biomed. Tech. 22, 106-114 (1977).
4. Furman, S., Garvey, J., and Hurzeler, P., Pulse duration variation and electrode size as factors in pacemaker longevity. J. Thoracic Cardiovasc. Surg. 69, 382-389 (1975).
5. Wirtzfeld, A., Himmler, Ch., Lampadius, M., Schmuck, L. and Prämer, H., Verlängerung der Funktionszeit implantierter Herzschrittmacher durch Reduzierung der Impulsdauer. Dtsch. med. Wschr. 100, 1683-1687 (1975).
6. Irnich, W., Engineering concepts of pacemaker electrodes. In: Advances in pacemaker technology. M. Schaldach and S. Furman editors. Springer-Verlag, Berlin, Heidelberg, New York 241-272 (1975).
7. Irnich, W., Der Einfluß der Elektrodengröße auf die Reizschwelle. Elektromedizin 14, 175-177 (1969).
8. Kleinert, M., Irnich, W., Beer, P., Vergleichende Untersuchungen des Reizschwellenverhaltens nach Implantation verschieden groszer Herzschrittmacherelektroden. Z. Kardiol. 66, 151-157 (1977).

THE CHOICE OF THE PACEMAKER-ELECTRODE COMBINATION: CLINICAL IMPLICATIONS IN PAROXYSMAL ARRHYTHMIAS

Sergio Dalla Volta, Ildebrando Maragno and Andrea Nava

Advancement in the engineering and technology of pacemakers has led to the introduction of a new generation of pulse generators, which have smaller size, are better tolerated by the patients and promise more reliable and longer life.

The ease of transvenous pacer insertion access, the very small risk and the good clinical results of chronic stimulation, particularly in fixed blocks and bradycardias, have prompted a more aggressive consideration of clinical indications of permanent cardiac pacing (1).

The advances in engineering are determined by the need for more sophisticated devices (2) to meet new clinical indications, such as paroxysmal blocks and related conditions.

The optimal combination of pulse generator-electrodes in chronic pacing is intended not only to overcome the previous short useful life of the pacing system (sources of energy, leads, cost) but also, of increasing importance, how the final choice affects the life of patients in terms of morbidity and mortality (and perhaps discomfort). This choice must be directly related to the progress in engineering and to the resulting clinical applications (3).

We have decided to present in this paper our experience, with a selection of cases in whom long-term internal stimulation has produced or created an iatrogenic pacemaker pathology.

We do not intend, here, to discuss the electrical and pathophysiological problems of arrhythmias produced during the life of a normally functioning pacemaker, presented by our group elsewhere (4).

The importance of new factors in the replacement of generators is demonstrated by the increase, in the last five years, of "choice" as a cause of replacement in about 20% of cases in two large institutions, our University Hospital and the Newark Beth Israel Medical Center, (5), where more than 1500 cases (our experience is now of about 2000 first implants in fourteen years) were treated.

Choice of pacemakers

The more important problems related to the choice in permanent pacing for paroxysmal conditions will be discussed in the text.

The choice of a pacing system can produce clinical effects depending on several technological, engineering (2) and medical conditions (1).

The choice of *pacing mode* is usually limited to the non competitive models of pulse generators, developed in order to avoid competitive rhythms and hazards of ventricular ectopic beats and tachyarrhythmias.

For patients in permanent block, the mode has proved reliable, safe and, in 50% of cases (1), capable, without other treatment, of normalizing the patients' life; in patients with paroxysmal block abnormal iatrogenic conditions have been observed.

The preselected impulse delivery rate is a major cause of concern, since in many cases a pacing frequency above 60 beats per minute prevents in patients, who need to be paced intermittently, the appearance of spontaneous firing. Suppression of the natural pacemaker produces obvious hemodynamic consequences (absence of atrial contraction and loss synchronism of the atrial and ventricular systole) (vide infra). Moreover a high rate (68-72) means an earlier exhaustion of the generator, as the more elevated the impulse firing, the higher the energy consumption and lesser the inhibition capacity.

A *fixed asynchronous generator* presents some advantages, such as lower cost, longer duration, higher reliability; indications for the fixed mode are exceptional in paroxysmal dysrhythmias because reversion to normal sinus rhythm is the rule.

Duration of generators; a long life can be obtained either through a better conservation of energy drained from the battery, or employing longer life batteries (2).

The first goal can be achieved with the use of small surface area electrodes; with adjustable variable output generators; with the development of low current drain electrodes and components; with a selective replacement of the generator immediately prior to the exhaustion of the battery and not from the average manufacturer-recommended time of failure; changing some characteristics of the impulse, such as reducing the frequency, etc.

The second goal means exploration of new sources of energy (chemical (7), biological and nuclear (8)) to power cardiac pacemakers.

How much the improvement in the procedures of quality control will introduce clinical problems when a large clinical application will be available, is uncertain.

The *characteristics of the stimulus* are considered in terms of the minimal amount of energy required to stimulate permanently and safely in a given subject: a short duration stimulus means higher stimulation threshold.

The type of follow-up is relevant to the patient's mobility. The pacemaker control is usually accomplished by:

a) analysing the changes in frequency of stimulation;

b) changing the non competitive mode to the fixed mode, with augmented impulse delivery frequency through an electromagnet; c) with the aid of the photo-analysis (9). No system is currently totally safe and defects (and hazards to patients) may still occur that were not properly diagnosed.

Choice of electrodes

Endocardial approach is the logical technique for most patients with paroxysmal dysrhythmias.

The multifacet aspect of dysrhythmias requires accurate positioning, following a detailed electrophysiological study: both must be done by experienced cardiologists.

The advantage of the *unipolar system* (10, not universally accepted Ed.) is based on the need of less current for operation of (voltage) controlled pacemakers; the large electrodes are more suitable for R wave sensing even in presence of small intracardiac signals.

The size of electrodes (10) provides important advantage in term of density of current per square millimeter; offers difference in the stimulation threshold and in sensing the cardiac signals. The ratio of the current threshold to the surface area of the electrode and to the current density cannot be emphasized enough in patients with potentially severe stimulation-induced arrhythmias.

While we did not consider an important parameter namely the *shape* of the electrode, the *connection* to the generator can be relevant at the time of generator changes because of the possibility of fractures of some models.

Criteria for optimal stimulation

Paroxysmal dysrhythmias are cases for whom a *low frequency impulse* pacemaker (56 to 60 impulse per minute) is appropriate. The three major clinical indications are:

a) the sick sinus syndrome;
b) the bradycardia-tachycardia syndrome;
c) vagal crisis generated by multiple factors but with a common symptom of *syncope*.

Before committing the patient to a pacemaker for these disorders some general considerations must be discussed. The frequency of the paroxysmal episode is variable and in our experience a rapid deterioration of the conduction trouble toward a stable block is not very common. Moreover several antiarrhythmic drugs are usually required.

The low frequency of impulse seems to have in these cases several advantages: it enhances the duration of the system; prevents dangerous hemodynamic changes that a frequency of 70-74 can induce and reduces the hazards of arrhythmias.

"Tailoring" (2) the pacemaker to the patients is a real need in this field of arrhythmias. An autoprogramming pacemaker would have the possibility both to track ventricular ectopic beats and to induce the overdrive-suppression of myocardial focus. A patient-activated generator with an automatic change of impulse amplitude in order to track the stimulation threshold, is needed to expand with confidence the electrical stimulation of an increasing number of intermittent arrhythmias.

The importance of maintaining the *maximal cardiac output*, for opposite reasons, in young men (to change the output according to changes in physical activity) and in senior age (to avoid a frequency increase with a critical and well tolerated long-term bradycardia) are shown by our experience with prefixed rate in a group of patients, during cardiac catheterization, at rest and exercise, with and without digitalis administration (1) (table 1 and 2).

Table 1.

	Rest	*Exercise*
Freq. (b/min.)	72	72
Cardiac Output (L/min.)	4,6	4,8
Cardiac Index (L/min/m²)	2,6	2,8
Right Atrium	4	5
Right Ventricle	39-5/18	35-5/8
Pulmonary Artery	41/10-18	35/14-20
"Left Atrium"	13	11
Left Ventricle	180-8/12	150-6/9
Femoral Artery	180/70	150/80

Table 2.

	Rest	*Exercise*	*Digoxine (0,25 mg)* *Rest*	*Exercise*
Right Atrium	6; ± 2	14; ± 2	5; ± 2	12; ± 2
Right Ventricle	40-6/10	50-7/12	40-5/8	48 7/11
Pulm. Artery	40/18-25	50/21-27	40/17-21	49-20-25
Left Atrium	14; ± 3	18; ± 4	12; ± 2	17; ± 2
Fem. Artery	150/80-95	160/90-100	155//80-94	155/85-95
Cardiac Index (L/min./m²)	2,9 ± 0,3	4,4 ± 0,3	2,8; ± 0,2	4,9; ± 0,2

Problems in stimulation of paroxysmal blocks

The above discussed considerations are founded on hemodynamic and electrophysiological studies.

The *loss of atrial systole* and the *atrio-ventricular asynchronism* must be studied relative to the hazards of syncope-inducing arrhythmias. Moreover a relatively high presetting of impulse delivery can induce a number of *re-entry dysrhythmias*.

The logical answer to these problems seems to be the use of generators with reduced impulse rate, enabling the patient to run on his own endogenous pacemaker, except during the paroxysms. The possibility of a change of a paroxysmal arrhythmia to a permanent block however, must be carefully examined.

Developments in engineering of pacemakers, leading to programmable and reprogrammable generators, can be expected and will be the future answer to these problems.

Clinical problems from preselected frequency

Three major *clinical conditions* have been observed by our group in recent years, in patients stimulated for paroxysmal arrhythmias with preselected rate (70 to 72 impulse) of stimulation: angina pectoris, cardiac failure and cerebral vascular insufficiency. The two first conditions are not rare; the third is unusual. However the change of the generator to a lower frequency (58 to 60) was necessary in all cases to overcome the problem.

Angina pectoris was observed in patients with angiographically proven diffuse stenosing lesions and reduced collateral circulation. Cardiac frequency was less than 45 during the episodes and between 55 and 62 in between. Pacemaker stimulation was followed by appearance or the increase of anginal pain, which proved to be frequency-dependent. A decrease of the pacer rate from 72 to 60 was associated with the disappearance of angina.

The most plausible explanation seems to be a critical increase during pacing of the preload, (11) which, in patients with a fixed coronary reserve and reduced ventricular compliance was sufficient to produce the cardiac pain.

Attacks of *cardiac insufficiency* were precipitated in at least ten old patients with chronic bradycardia and paroxysmal syncopal episodes, when the cardiac frequency was raised to 72 by stimulation. The presence of sinus rhythm or of atrial fibrillation was not related to the appearance of cardiac failure. Again the reduction of preload, even for small changes of cardiac frequency, seems to be the triggering mechanism of the episodes (12).

Conclusion

The extraordinary progress of the technology of pacing has tremendously expanded the horizons of clinical applications for chronic stimulation. In medically oriented pacing centers, the new indication has switched to a number of paroxysmal arrhythmias, in which sinus rhythm is often present and the trend toward complete block infrequent.

These new indications involve consideration of problems of the pacemaker function in terms of safety, need of autoprogramming, accurate assessment of the pacemaker function, optimal indications for any case, and a preliminary careful electrophysiological study.

"Tailoring" the system to the patients' needs is no more a dream, but will be a reality in the near future if the clinician will prompt the manufacturer to develop more sophisticated devices in term of a physiological approach to a group of high risk patients.

References

1. Dalla Volta, S., Indicazioni e fisiopatologia della etiolazione cardiaca permanente. *Rel. Congr. Cardiol. Osped. Pozzi Ed. Roma* (1974).
2. Hauser, R.G., Giuffre, V.W., Newer developments in pacemakers. *Medical Clinics of North America.* 60, 2 (1976).
3. Walter, W.H., Mitchell, J.C., Rustan, P.L., Cardiac pulse generators and electromagnetic interference. *JAMA* 224, 1628 (1973).
4. Dalla Volta, S., Nava, A., Scarparo, M., Arrhythmias induced by normally functioning synchronous pacemakers. In "*Cardiac Pacing*," Hilbert J. Th. Thalen Editor, *Van Gorcum, Assen*, (1973).
5. Parsonnet, V., Permanent pacing of the heart: 1952 to 1976. *Amer. J. Cardiol.* 39, 250 (1977).
6. Center, S., Nathan, D.A., Wu, C.Y. et al., The implantable synchronous pacemaker in the treatment of complete heart block. *J. Thorac. Cardiovasc. Surg.* 6, 744 (1963).
7. Greatbatch, W., Lee, J.H., Mathias, W. et al., The solid state lithium battery. A new improved chemical power source for implantable cardiac pacemaker. *IEEE Trans. Biomed. Eng.* 18, 317 (1971).
8. Greatbatch, W., Bustard, T., A $Pu^{238}O_2$ nuclear power source for implantable cardiac pacemakers. *IEEE Trans. Biomed. Eng.* 20, 232 (1973).
9. Thalen, H.J.Th., Berg, J.W., Photoanalysis of electrode function. *Proceed. Conf. "Advances in Cardiac Pacemakers," New York* (1968).
10. Thalen, J.H.Th., Van den Berg, J.W., Van der Heide, J.N., Nieveen, J., The artificial cardiac pacemaker. *Van Gorcum, Assen*, (1970).
11. Ross, J.Jr., Afterload mismatch and preload reserve: a conceptual framework for the analysis of ventricular function. *Progr. Cardiovasc. Dis.* 18, 255 (1976).
12. Guyton, A.C., Determination of cardiac output by equating venous return curves with cardiac response curves. *Physiol. Review* 35, 123 (1955).

THE CHOICE OF THE ELECTRODE AND PACING METHOD FOR EMERGENCY CARDIAC PACING

A.H. Sheikh-Zadeh, H. Pour Kalbassi, M. Ataii and M.J. Tabaee-Zadeh

The first successful cardiac resuscitation by external transthoracic pacing was reported by Zoll in 1952. This was followed by other reports and proved an impetus for the development of subsequent techniques. (2-3-4-5-6-7).

In cardiopulmonary arrest either primary or secondary (after ventricular fibrillation) rapid and safe implantation of a pacemaker can be lifesaving. Artificial cardiac pacing can be instituted as an emergency by several methods:

1. External transthoracic pacing.
2. External transesophageal pacing.
3. Internal blind transvenous pacing.
   a. Normal pacing catheter.
   b. Floating or semifloating catheter.
   c. Balloon pacing catheter.
4. Direct percutanous transthoracic pacing.
   a. Needle.
   b. Special catheter.

These methods must be used only as a stop-gap emergency followed by stable transvenous electrode placement. By external transthoracic pacing using two electrodes similar to what Zoll reported, cardiac resuscitation can be carried out. For this purpose 75-150 V/1-2 m Sec is required (8). Up to 1955 Zoll reported 25 successful cases using this method (4). This method is quick and simple, but complications such as skin burns, severe pains, contraction of chest muscles, electrical leakage and occasional ventricular fibrillation occur (9). In an experimental study using one unipolar electrode in the esophagus and the other on the chest, Zoll was able to pace the heart in dogs before applying external transthoracic pacing to man (10). Later on, using bipolar electrodes in the esophagus, pacing of the atrium, ventricles and even cardioversion was accomplished by this method (11, 12). The advantage of this method is the simplicity, quickness and the lack of electrical leakage (13). The success rate of this method is 60% for ventricular and 77% for atrial pacing (11, 13, 14). A bipolar catheter is introduced into the mouth or nose and advanced 40-50 cm in the esophagus. Under ECG monitoring the catheter is pulled back gradually until ventricular activation is observed. If the electrode catheter is pulled further back, atrial pacing can also be achieved. Disadvantages of this method are the requirements of high current 15-2Oma, esophageal lesions, poor patient tolerance and vagotonia due to stimulation of the pharynx. (11, 12).

With the development of the floating and semifloating catheter and also the balloon catheter it is possible to insert the catheter through the subclavian vein or other routes without fluoroscopy. External cardiac massage can be performed simultanously (15, 16, 17, 18, 19). This method has the advantage of low voltage requirement and lack of electrical leakage, but the success rate is only about 60 to 80 per cent (20). Even in experienced hands this method is time-consuming and the venous puncture is not without complications (21, 22).

Direct stimulation of the heart with passage of a proper needle through the 5th or 6th left intercostal space was reported by Thevenet (23).

Later Lillehei used a 20 Gauge needle through the 6th intercostal space aimed towards the xyphoid process. Through this needle a wire was passed which could directly stimulate the heart (24, 25). Following these reports various other methods came to use for direct ventricular or atrial stimulation (26, 27, 28, 29, 30, 31). This method used in emergency cases and in cardiopulmonary resuscitation is simple and quick.

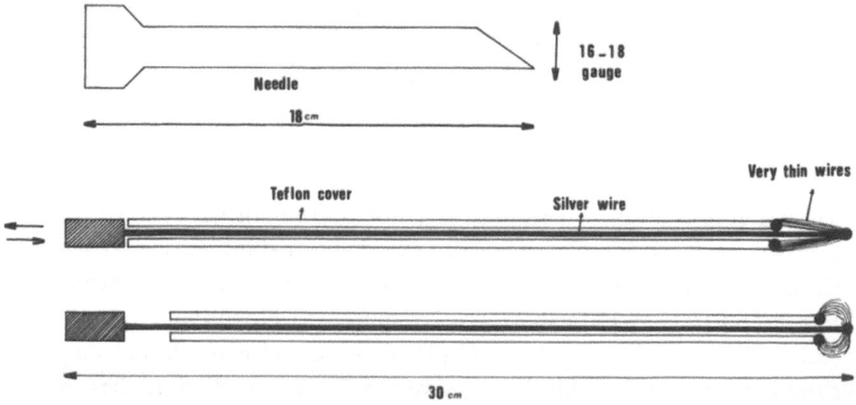

Figure 1.

The complications of this method are pericardial tamponade, pneumothorax and laceration of the coronary arteries 8). Considering the complications in each of the above methods we have developed a new electrode catheter to reduce the above mentioned complications. In this method the subxyphoid approach is used. Thus the possibility of pneumothorax and laceration of the coronary arteries is greatly reduced. Also, since this electrode catheter is more flexible, external cardiac massage is possible.

The new method described below uses a catheter 30 cm long consisting of a central wire which is teflon covered except for 18 mm on both ends. The wire is freely movable in this cover. At the distal end, there are thin wires fixed to the tip at one end and to teflon cover at the other end. Pulling the central wire makes the wire end bulge like an umbrella and pushing it makes them straight. This is designed to make a better contact with the myocardium. Removal of the catheter is also facilitated. The catheter can pass through a 16-18 gauge needle (fig. 1).

The needle is inserted through the subxyphoid region according to the method described for pericardiocentesis (32) and pushed into the ventricular chamber. The catheter is inserted through the needle, the needle is removed and the catheter left in the heart. By withdrawing the central wire, the thin wires open up and pulling back the electrode make a better and stable contact with the ventricular wall. Our clinical experience with this method is limited and further investigation and follow-up will be needed.

References

1. Zoll, P.M., Resuscitation of the heart in ventricular standstill by external electric stimulation. *New Eng. J. Med.*, 247, 768 (1952).
2. Zoll, P.M., Linenthal, A.J., Norman, L.R., treatment of Stokes-Adams disease by external electric stimulation of the heart. *Circulation*, 9, 482 (1954).
3. Zoll, P.M., Linenthal, A.J., Norman, L.R., Paul, M.E., Gibson, W., Use of external electric pacemaker in cardiac arrest. *JAMA*, 159, 1428 (1955).
4. Zoll, P.M., Linenthal, A.J., Norman, L.R., Paul, M.E., Gibson, W., External electric stimulation of the heart in cardiac arrest. *Arch. Intern. Med. (Chicago)*, 96, 639 (1955).
5. Zoll, P.M., Linenthal, A.J., Norman, L.R., Paul, M.H., Gibson, W., Treatment of unexpected cardiac arrest by external electric stimulation of the heart. *New Eng. J. Med.*, 254, 541 (1956).
6. Zoll, P.M., Linenthal, A.J., Zarsky, L.R.N., Ventricular fibrillation-treatment and prevention by external electric currents. *New Eng. J. Med.*, 262, 105 (1960).
7. Zoll, P.M., Paul, M.H., Linenthal, A.J., Norman, L.R., Gibson, W., The effects of external electric currents on the heart. *Circulation*, 14, 745 (1956).
8. Kitchen II, J.G. and Kaster, J.A., pacing in acute Myocardical Infarction – Indication, Methods and results. Innovations in the diagnosis and management of acute MI, *Davis Philadelphia* 1975.
9. Weinstein, J., Goui, J., Mazzara, J.T. et al., Temporary transvenous pacing via the percutaneous femoral vein approach. *Am. Heart. J.* 85, 695 (1973).
10. Zoll, P.M., Historical development of cardiac pacemakers. *Prog. Cardiovasc. Dis.* 14, 421 (1970).

11. Montoyo, J., Angel, J., Valle, V., et al., Cardioversion of tachycardia by transesophageal atrial pacing. *Am. J. Cardiol* 32, 85 (1973).
12. Vergara, G., Hildner, F.J., Schoenfeld, C.B. et al., Conversion of supraventricular tachycardia with rapid atrial stimulation. *Circulation* 46, 788 (1972).
13. Burack, B. and Furman, S., Transesophageal cardiac pacing. *Am. J. Cardiol.* 23, 469 (1969).
14. Lubell, D.L., Cardiac pacing from the esophagus. *Am. J. Cardiol.* 27, 641 (1971).
15. Kimball, J.T. and Killip, T., A simple beside method for transvenous intracardiac pacing. *Am. Heart J.* 70, 35 (1965).
16. Harris, C.S., Huriburt, J.C., Floyd, W.L. et al., Percutaneous techniques for cardiac pacing with a platinum tipped electrode catheter. *Am. J. Cardiol.* 15, 48 (1965).
17. Vogel, J.H., Tabari, K., Åverill, K.H., et al., A simple technique for identifying P. waves in complex arrhythmias. *Am. Heart J.* 367, 158 (1964).
18. Swan, H.J.C., Ganz, W., Forrester, J., et al., Catheterization of the Heart in man with use of flow-directed balloontipped catheter. *N. Engl. J. Med.* 283, 417 (1970).
19. Schnitzler, R.N., Caracta, A. and Damato, A.N., "Floating" catheter for temporary transvenous ventricular pacing. *Am. J. Cardiol.* 31, 351 (1973).
20. Meltzer, L.E., Kitchell, J.R., Current Concepts of cardiac pacing and cardioversion. A symposium. Charles Press, *Maryland* 1971.
21. Escher, D.J.W., Types of pacemakers and their complications. *Circulation* 37, 119 (1973).
22. Campo, I., Carfield, G., Escher, D.J.W., Furman, S., Complications of pacing by pervenous subclavian semi-floating electrodes including 2 extraluminal insertions. *Am. J. Cardiol.* 26, 627 (1970).
23. Thevenet, A., Hodges, P.C., Lillehei, C.W., The use of a myocardial electrode inserted percutaneously for control of complete atrioventricular block by an artificial pacemaker. *Dis. Chest* 34, 621 (1958).
24. Thevenet, A., Hodges, P. and Lillehei, W.C., The use of a myocardial electrode inserted percutaneously for control of complete atrioventricular block by an artificial pacemaker. *Dis. Chest.* 34, 621 (1968).
25. Lillehei, W.C., Morris, J.C., Bonnabean, R.C., et al., Direct wire electrical stimulation for acute post-surgical and post-infarction complete heart block. *Ann. N.Y. Acad. Sci.* 111, 938 (1966).
26. Jennings, E.R., Hightower, J.A., Addison, B.A., The percutaneous insertion of an intracardiac electrode in the treatment of complete heart block. *Am. Surg.*, 29, 553 (1963).
27. Levy, L., Albert, H.M., Therapy of complete heart block complicating recent myocardial infarction. *JAMA*, 187, 617 (1964).
28. Portheine, H., Menges, G., Beitrag zur Technik der temporären Elektrostimulation des Herzens, *Med. Klin.*, 60, 98 (1965).
29. Roe, B.B., Intractable Stokes-Adams disease. *Amer. Heart J.*, 69, 470 (1965).
30. Roe, B.B., Katz, H.J., Complete heart block intractable asystole and recurrent ventricular fibrillation with survival. *Am. J. Cardiol.*, 15, 401 (1965).
31. Ross, J., Harkins, G.A., Percutaneous introduction of cardiac pacemaker electrode. *Lancet*, 2, 1109 (1959).
32. Gostman, M.S. and Schrirer, R., A pericardiocentesis electrode needle. *Br. Heart J.* 28, 566 (1966).

ROUND TABLE

ROUND TABLE DISCUSSION. THE CHOICE OF THE PACEMAKER-ELECTRODE COMBINATION

Chairman: H.J.TH. THALEN *(Groningen, The Netherlands)*
Panel members: M. BILITCH *(Los Angeles, U.S.A.)*
S. DALLA VOLTA *(Padova, Italy)*
R.G. GOLD *(Newcastle, England)*
R. HARDJOWYONO *(Groningen, The Netherlands)*
W. IRNICH *(Aachen, F.R. Germany)*
C. MEERE *(Montreal, Canada)*
M. MURTRA *(Barcelona, Spain)*
V. PARSONNET *(Newark, U.S.A.)*
J.G. SLOMAN *(Melbourne, Australia)*
C.J. WESTERHOLM *(Uppsala, Sweden)*
A.H. SHEIKH-ZADEH *(Tehran, Iran)*

CHAIRMAN: Let us bring things a bit together. Werner Irnich told us about the best energy source and ideal electrode. But before we go on discussing the pacemaker and the electrode, I think it is good to make some comments about the life expectancy of the patients. According to Irnich: to reach with a pacemaker life expectancies of a normal related age group, the best patient is a female patient who is old and the worst one is a male patient, who is young.

However Irnich is an engineer and parameters like sex and age fit nicely into a computer program. But, as a doctor you also have to look after other factors like disease etc. Perhaps Dr. Parsonnet can start this Round Table discussion with some comments in this respect.

V. PARSONNET: As a physician, of course, I am interested in what the risk is to the patient. We have looked at the number of operations a patient would have to have, if he had lived three years. For 100 consecutive patients who lived 36 months, 30% of them required another operation for something other than pulse generator failures. So the figures look a lot like Irnich's and show us a substantial problem.

I am concerned a little bit about your estimates of life expectancy only because you have not looked at it yet from the point of view of the original diagnosis. Quite clearly, the prognosis of a patient with complete A-V dissociation is going to be somewhat different than that of a patient with a sick sinus syndrome. I hope that someday you will break that down and analyse it in that way as well.

We have looked at the cumulative survival figures of our patients and it is interesting that 17% of our patients are alive after 16 years. The number of patients does not go down to zero. It is an asymptote somewhere out there. We have to design pacemakers – if we are all talking about the ideal system – for every patient, but I do not know how we can select which patient is going to last ten years or seventeen years, ahead of time. All we know is that a certain number do live that long and we all have to have a pulse generator and electrode leads that will last as long as our longest living patient. That presents quite a problem for our 20-year olds, but we have to face that too and I think it is achievable.

CHAIRMAN: Thank you Dr. Parsonnet. I think, Dr. Warren Harthorne reported his own results at the Tokyo meeting. Patients with congestive heart failure seem to do very poorly and it seems that patients with total A-V block do very well when they are paced. That explains most probably why we have, of the earliest series which included mostly patients with total A-V block, still some patients going. We had in the Groningen clinic five patients who got their pacemakers in 1962 and two of these are still alive. Is there someone else here who wishes to comment on pacemaker types and life expectancy?

R.G. GOLD: Our problem is that three quarters of our patients are over the age of 60, several of them are over the age of 70, some over the age of 80 and I have two over the age of 90. Now, with the present economic climate, we find it quite unjustified to put in the much more expensive lithium-cell pacemakers until the forecasts of the members of the previous panel come true, and the price of the lithium-cell pacemaker comes down to that of the mercury-cell. So what we have had to do is to look at how to get the best possible life out of our mercury series of pacemakers and we have approached this largely by trying to minimize current consumption of the unit. We have done this in two ways.

The first way has been to use a fixed-rate pacemaker with an adjustable pulse width, the Medtronic 5931. We have put this into 8 patients over the past $17\frac{1}{2}$ months and we have progressively reduced the pulse width. Now 6 patients are paced at a pulse duration of 0.2 ms and the remaining two at a pulse duration of 0.25 ms. If the calculations that Medtronic has supplied are correct, then we should be operating at a current drainage of something like 4 microamps into a 500 ohm load, at a pulse duration of 0.2 ms. All of these patients are paced quite satisfactorily. This required no particular choice of electrode and only one of these electrodes is really what one could call a low surface area electrode. The second way has been to use a 0.5 ms current limited pacemaker. The trend seems to have been that now most pacemakers under about 1 ms pulse width are not current limited. We have chosen to combine current limitation with a half millisecond pulse width and we have implanted this system into nine patients over the past eleven months. Again, we have had no pacing problems and the thresholds, as measured with the Vitatron Pacing Analyzer at the follow-up visits, have become stable. Current limitation has been observed at least for the first 0.1 ms of the impulse in these patients. I would welcome the opinion of our physicist colleagues as to whether a combination of current limitation and narrowing of the pulse width is the way of getting the optimum life out of these pacemakers, short of having to change the electrodes in some of these patients who have already got large-surface area electrodes in them for some years.

CHAIRMAN: Who would care to comment on that? Should we have a programmability in impulse duration and in output, so that we can get a long lifetime out of these pacemakers?

W. IRNICH: The problem with a programmable impulse duration is that you can measure the impulse duration at a threshold level, but you do not know what the safety margin is. That is to say, if you double the impulse duration at threshold level you cannot say: we now have a 100% safety margin.

R.G. GOLD: May I come back on that one? I did not mention that we took these patients down to the minimum possible impulse duration of 0.15 ms. with this particular pacemaker. Even now the longest one – which has been going for 17½ months – still shows capture at 0.15 ms. and we felt justified to pace him at 0.2 ms.

CHAIRMAN: I think this is one solution although you still do not know your safety margin in these cases also because you did not reach the threshold level. Another thing we have to think about and Dr. Gold brought it up, is would you select for a certain group of patients a special type of pacemaker, of which you know that it goes longer although it might be a little bit more expensive? This is to say: do you select for your patients pacemakers after their life expectancy?

M.BILITCH: We do not make that distinction in Los Angeles.

CHAIRMAN: How about Italy?

S. DALLA VOLTA: Yes, we do.

CHAIRMAN: Dr. Gold. Do you select lithium pacemakers for your younger patients?

R. GOLD: Yes, we implant lithium pacemakers into our younger patients.

Indeed, the younger the patient, obviously, the longer lived pacemaker it is that we look for. But in patients in their '70s, we feel that we have got to concentrate on a pacemaker that has a realistic life of perhaps three or four years.

CHAIRMAN: Thank you. We learned that some patients live a longer and some live a shorter time with a pacemaker compared to their normal age groups. We also learned that in some countries, there is more pacemaker selection in that respect. Irnich also stated that you should combine a small electrode with a lithium unit. But when you have more energy, is it still reasonable to select smaller electrodes? Would not 12 mm^2 be sufficient? You even spoke about one of 5 mm^2.

W. IRNICH: If you combine a small-area electrode with a lithium battery, you have the advantage of very small units. You may say, with a 3.5 Ah. battery, we have energy enough to stimulate, even with a 40 square millimeter electrode, for ten years. But to have a small-area electrode and a small-capacity battery in a small pacemaker, I would say, is a better system than a big one.

CHAIRMAN: So the smaller electrode, in the long term, will also give us smaller pacers because we need less energy. But smaller electrodes might have also other features. Dr. Parsonnet, you did some research on ventricular fibrillation and smaller electrodes. I would like your comments in this respect.

V. PARSONNET: We did study that because we were interested in using the small electrodes, originally to save energy and extend the pacemaker lifetime. When you analyse acute and chronic stimulation thresholds for four different size electrodes, you will see that the stimulation thresholds for small electrodes, expressed in current, are extremely low, both acutely and chronically. Now, if you look at the fibrillation threshold – the current needed for fibrillating the heart with a single impulse – you will find that they all are in the same order of magnitude. Therefore, if one uses a small electrode with a very low stimulation threshold, the safety margin for the danger of producing ventricular fibrillation accidentally by stimulation in the vulnerable period, is very great. So there is a small dividend here, a safety dividend in using little electrodes that was not entirely expected when we started this work.

CHAIRMAN: In the early years of pacing, there was a lot of discussion about the ventricular fibrillation threshold. It would seem that small electrodes have also the advantage that the incidence of ventricular fibrillation could be lower. I want to go to Dr. Westerholm from Sweden. He found some disadvantages with small-surface electrodes, as related to the late stimulation threshold. Perhaps he can make some comments about his experiences.

C.J. WESTERHOLM: We get about 250 new patients every year. I use the Siemens

Elema 588 electrode. During 1974 and 1975, we used a 8 mm^2 small-surface electrode, together with a 0.5 ms impulse generator, in order to save as much energy as possible. However, we noticed an increasing number of cases with late exit block; that is, after more than half a year after implantation. It was 7% among 500 patients and we thought that the combination of small-surface electrode and short impulse duration was the reason for this exit block.

During 1976 and 1977, we have implanted 150 large-surface electrodes of 47 square millimeters, together with half millisecond lithium impulse generators of different marks and we have seen no exit block.

In all of these 650 cases, the same surgeon has performed the operation, with the same technique. The large-surface electrode is very easily positioned, gives a good sensing signal from the QRS complex and is durable for a long time. The oldest one we have is fourteen years old. From these data we have drawn the conclusion that there are two choices. Either the combination of small-surface electrodes and 1.0 millisecond impulse duration, or large-surface electrodes and 0.5 ms. impulse duration. From our point of view, we prefer the last combination, because this electrode is easier to handle.

CHAIRMAN: Thank you. This is a complication I, personally, have never heard of before. We are not aware of it, either, in our clinic. Has someone of this panel experienced late dislocation and exit block when he used small-surface electrodes, that the did not see when he used the larger ones. Let us talk about elektrodes of over 15 square millimeters. Claude, did you see this complication?

C. MEERE: On the contrary, we found just the opposite. That the thresholds tend to be lower with the chronically implanted small electrodes than they are with the big ones.

CHAIRMAN: Has someone in the audience seen difficulties like late exit block with small-surface electrodes?

J.W. HARTHORNE: There is an inverse relation to the frequency of perforation of intracardial electrodes relative to the size of the tip. Virtually all our myocardial perforations occur with unipolar lead systems. So I would just submit, without any documentary evidence, that the exit block situation seen with a small-surface electrode is not a manifestation of the small-surface area, but possibly the smaller caliber of the lead tip. Is the lead that you are using identical to the larger surface area and its other physical characteristics? Do they have the same diameter? Is the shape of the flange the same?

C.J. WESTERHOLM: When we implant these electrodes, we use a special technique. We turn the patient 90 degrees and we do not use any additional catheters or stylets. We "drop the electrode down" and we have never had any perforation.

CHAIRMAN: Do you think it could be a perforation or the penetration that causes the trouble?

C.J. WESTERHOLM: It is very difficult to explain this phenomenon, because, if you look at the X-ray, the electrode has the same position. It must come from a microdislocation.

J. MEIBOM *(Copenhagen, Denmark):* I would like to make a short comment, because we use exactly the same electrode as Westerholm. On the basis of 100 implantations of this electrode type, we have found that over 15% of this electrode perforates the heart. There is no doubt about that. This special electrode is inconvenient as far as the shape of the electrode is concerned. If you change to an electrode type called "K," you do not have this complication. But with the electrode Dr. Westerholm described, we had over 15% more perforation.

CHAIRMAN: Is there someone in the audience who has experience with this electrode? Hans Lagergren?

H. LAGERGREN: I happen to have some experience with that electrode. It has the same diameter as the larger area type and is identical in shape. It never perforates if handled rightly. But I do agree that you sometimes see unexplainable late exit blocks, however with electrodes of both sizes. I think that is due to an infarction in that area and not really due to dislocation or other things.

CHAIRMAN: Thank you. So that would mean that we cannot generalize about small-surface electrodes. To prove that late dislocation problems are related to the 588 Siemens Elema electrode, Dr. Westerholm would have to implant some other types of small-surface electrodes to evaluate if he finds trouble with them also. We here seem to think that small-surface electrodes have big advantages. It has been mentioned by Vic Parsonnet that the risk of ventricular fibrillation is lower. It has also been mentioned that we can have longer lasting pacemaker systems and even smaller pacemakers. However, dislocation is a problem in pacing. I think we should consider fixation mechanisms and I am very happy that Warren Harthorne, at last, implanted an electrode that needed some sort of fixation, because he was troubling everybody saying he had no dislocations at all, just perforations. But after his experience with the Helifix electrode we can feel less frustrated. There are various anchoring principles to diminish the dislocation ratio. I would like to give the floor to Dr. Hardjowyono of our department of Thoracic Surgery at the Groningen University. He does most implants in our clinic and has a lot of experience with electrode placement, especially the Siemens Elema balloon type.

R. HARDJOWYONO: Since the end of 1974 until now, we have been implanting about 130 Siemens Elema catheter electrodes with the balloon fixation mechanism. Up to now, we are satisfied with the results, as reported earlier by our colleague, Dr. Oude Luttikhuis in Tokyo (Vth International Symposium on Cardiac Pacing 1976) and in Amsterdam (European Congress on Cardiology, 1976). In our whole series we found a dislocation ratio of 4%. All of these cases except for one, showed rupture of the balloon some weeks or months after implantation. Our conclusion after using 130 balloon catheter electrodes, is that a fixation can be achieved with this system, while traumatic lesion of the endocardium with this fixation method is avoided. We also use this method in cases where the transvenous implantation of a usual electrode type had failed. Another benefit for the patient is the early mobilization, just after the operation he is permitted to get up and walk. This early mobilization permits also a shorter hospitalisation.

The balloon in our experience should be filled with 0.4 to 0.6 cc urografine 10%, to visualize it, while on the other hand to prevent any rupture or emptying due to higher osmolarity of the contrast fluid.

The balloon is anchored in the heart between the trabecular muscles. After implanting a balloon catheter electrode, you must pull it to try the fixation. If you can give a gentle pull without dislocation of the electrode, then you can be sure that the electrode is well positioned and, if necessary, to find a good stimulation threshold, I never hesitate to implant such a catheter at a non-ideal place in the right ventricle.

CHAIRMAN: Why we are discussing this electrode is that it has one of the features that I think should be mentioned when speaking about an anchoring electrode: it should anchor in a different place than the place where it stimulates the heart, so that the tissue reaction of the fixation is not at the place where the stimulation is going to occur. Dr. Sloman, you have also experience with this type of electrode and you have reported your early experiences. Do you have some late results?

J.G. SLOMAN: We presented our data of about 50 patients at the meeting in Tokyo in a very optimistic way. Since then, we have found it necessary to replace the generators in 8 of these patients as the generator had become exhausted. In these 8 patients who required a new generator, we were able to remeasure the threshold. On the figure you see at the left-hand side the initial thresholds which were all acceptably low, but on the right-hand side, where we outlined the thresholds at replacement of the generator you can see that we had much increase in threshold; I now believe that this was in some way related to fibrous tissue formation around the more complicated tip of the catheter. In the right-hand part of the slide, the mean increase in threshold is compared with 8 people with standard, ordinary, non-balloon-type electrodes. Although I am very impressed and very pleased with the fixation of the balloon catheter, I think that we have to keep an open mind on the fact that the method of fixation may give later problems e.g. high thresholds and therefore the balloon at this stage, is not a proven instrument and cannot be recommended to all who have problems in fixation.

CHAIRMAN: I want to ask you a question regarding this figure. Two of the 8 thresholds go very high. But the other ones are not that bad, they are in the area of about two volts. Do you think this is unacceptable? Do you have these results also with other types of electrodes?

J.G. SLOMAN: No, I really do not have a good control group. The suggestion is, that the increase in threshold may be related to the balloon and when it bursts – because they all burst – there is a change in position and a higher threshold. When we have reimplanted we will have better data to present our 50 cases.

CHAIRMAN: Dr. Hardjowyono, I believe we have not found, so far, extremely high thresholds in this group. We followed them also. Have you any more on this?

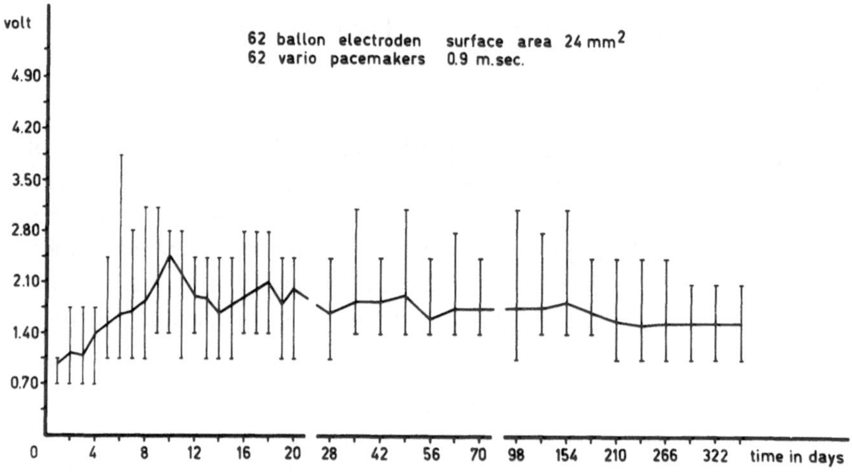

Figure 1.

R. HARDJOWYONO: We see in fig. 1 the follow-up results of 62 balloon-catheter electrodes combined with Siemens Elema Vario pacemakers of 0.9 ms. You can see that we have not so many higher thresholds afterwards like the patients of Dr. Sloman.

CHAIRMAN: Thank you, Dr. Hardjowyono. I really think that we have been warned, so we will look very critically at what is happening when we replace these units. So far we did not replace too many of them. Dr. Meere wants to make some comments.

C. MEERE: I would like to make some remarks concerning displacement of electrodes. One of the possible ways to decrease displacement is to try to develop new models of electrodes, fancy things with hooks, balloons and so on. The other way would be to try to avoid that kind of implantation in certain patients, who have pulmonary hypertension, right-sided chronic heart failure, tricuspid insufficiency and go by another route. This is what we are doing at the Montreal Heart Institute. We do not want to favor such kinds of electrodes. Maybe this is the weak point of my statement, because we have no sufficient statistical data on these electrodes.

CHAIRMAN: Let us put the question about dislocation in a somewhat different perspective. Now we have pacers that go longer, should we not implant pacemaker electrodes that produce less dislocation. Just think about the corkscrew electrode. I have the impression that the corkscrew is getting somewhat more popular in the United States where we see fewer transvenous electrodes and more of these corkscrew types. Is that true?

M. BILITCH: I think perhaps Dr. Parsonnet could comment on this. There is no question in the United States that there has been a move towards myocardial electrode implantation. I believe that the percentage of sales of the companies that have both kinds of electrodes available has markedly increased in the myocardial electrode area. This is becoming more popular. I am not sure that is a solution to the problem; it is only a fact.

CHAIRMAN: I mentioned the United States because I got the impression that, in the United States, except for some clinics, a lot of thoracic surgeons are doing the implants, whereas in Europe and other parts of the world a lot of cardiologists are doing this. I think this could determine greatly the selection of the electrode. Vic, do you think there is an increase in corkscrew electrode implantation now, in the United States, in regard to the transvenous catheter electrodes?

V. PARSONNET: I have not got good data on it. The last time we did a survey has been for the Tokyo meeting. The percentage of myocardial electrodes was 5% of this sample of 164 centers that reported. One gets the impression that it is going up, because of the people who talk about it quite loudly and all over the place. But I am happy to see the persistence of the transvenous enthusiasts in Europe. I am enthusiast, even though, as you will hear from Mike Bilitch and Sey Fruman and myself later on, our transvenous dislocation rate is somewhat higher than we like, but we think that is perhaps because of slight laxity in attention to technical detail. I can not see why we should have dislocation rates of over 4 or 5%.

Experience with some of these electrodes including the Helifix, with which I also had a marvelous experience the way Dr. Harthorne had, may result in that we will stay with transvenous implantation which, after all, is the most a-traumatic to the patient and that is a very important goal for all of us.

I would like to make a comment. It has been reported in public meetings – so there is nothing secret about it – that Medtronic says that 40% of their lead sales now are myocardial leads. Even if one half – on the premise that most surgeons put in two leads – is still 20%. It has obviously gone up.

CHAIRMAN: I agree with you. I had also that figure in mind. Well, this is where we stop with the electrodes. In conclusion we can summarize that small electrodes have some big advantages and that the disadvantages seem very limited. It is up to everybody to draw his own conclusions from what has been said here and to select the electrode that fits best in his system. I just want to go now to the various types of pacemakers. Dr. Bilitch is working with a variety of pacemaker types. When you look at the types of pacing, Mike, what kind of pacemakers are you using the most?

M. BILITCH: We have a study in progress, in the United States, which involves three medical centers in New York, Newark (N.J.) and Los Angeles. I would like to show you what our results have been for the last 30 months. This particular data is from new patients; that is to say, those who have first-time implantations. As you can see in Table 1 we have implanted in 838 new patients the following pacemaker system: 96% ventricular-inhibited pacemaker systems; 0.6% ventricular-triggered and 0.4% ventricular-fixed rate, so that the total experience

Table 1. Types of pacemaker systems used* 7-1-74 through 12-31-76

Mode	*Number*	%
VVI	804	95.9
VVT	5	0.6
VOO	3	0.4
DVI	5	0.6
AAI	21	2.5
TOTAL	838	100.0

* One pulse generator with a tracking pulse (Edwards) has been classified as VV1. The tracking pulse is of full amplitude but short (15 milliseconds) duration; this interval is considered to be too short to produce an effective stimulus.

is vastly in favor of fairly conventional types of ventricular pacing. We have 2,5% which are atrial-inhibited and only 0.6% which are bifocal.

Of the 844 electrodes (Table 2) that we have implanted in these 838 patients, 797 are in the right ventricle, 9 in the coronary sinus, 14 in the atrial appendage

Table 2. Lead implantations – new patients (844 leads in 838 patients) 7-1-74 through 12-31-76

Endocardial (820)			*Myocardial (24)*	
Right ventricle	*Right atrial*		*Ventricular*	*Atrial*
	C.S.		*A.A.*	
797				
9	14	21	3	

C.S. = Coronary sinus
A.A. = Atrial appendage.

and only 24 are trans-thoracic myocardial electrodes; 21 ventricular and 3 atrial. With respect to the ones that were placed transvenously, there were 71 that had malposition. (Table 3)

Table 3. Lead manipulations n = 844 (in 838 patients)*

Malposition	71
Infection &/or erosion	4
Fracture	8
High Threshold	4
Other**	11
Total	98

* 838 patients had 98 manipulations
** 2 elective mode changes
1 mechanical
1 possible arrhythmia
1 set screw problem
1 inadequate sensitivity
1 muscle twitching
1 false sensing
1 connector problem
2 insulation breaks

Incidentally, we described malposition rather than displacement because I believe that in many instances, we really do not know what has happened. This question has come up already: Has the electrode perforated? Has it moved a small distance? What has occurred? What is interesting if we look at those 71 interventions in 59 patients, is that 38 of these were manipulated one time whereupon the pacing was satisfactory. (Table 4) All of these electrodes that we are

Table 4. Right ventricular malposition n = 791 patients*

Manipulated one time	38
Manipulated two times	3
Replaced (new endocardial)	7
Manipulated one time then replaced	4
Epicardial	3
Manipulated one time then epicardial	3
Manipulated two times then epicardial	1

* 59 patients (7.5%) had 71 interventions

talking about are conventional electrodes in the sense that they are available for general distribution; there is nothing unique about them in that sense. They vary in surface area and configuration and so forth. This says that if we are very careful about the placement of the electrode, our incidence would be very small.

CHAIRMAN: I have a question in connection with the first slide. You showed the various circuits you are using. Is there recently a trend to use a broader variety, or is it about the same over the years?

M. BILITCH: This is the last 30 months, up until the end of December 1976. We have not broken these down into specific time periods. I do not believe we would have anything that would be statistically significant at the moment because of the numbers being so small. On the basis of the experience that we have all had I suspect that there will be some shift. My personal view is that I do not believe it will be very dramatic.

CHAIRMAN: So we see from this data that a ventricular on-demand unit most probably with a programmable rate, would be covering a wide range of the units that we are going to implant now and in the future.

Let us now look at the energy source. We are using lithium batteries more and more now. Dr. Sloman has a long-time experience with lithium units and he will present some data.

J.G. SLOMAN: Since 1972, we have progressively changed over to Lithium powered pacemakers. We have a total of 257 patients who have had various types of lithium units inserted (Table 5). The first unit was put in in December 1972. This model was a CPI 702 C. We put three of those in and the experience now is

Table 5. Lithium anode pacemakers [Experience Royal Melbourne Hospital December 1972 – February 1977]

Lithium Iodide (702)	67
702C 3	
702P 7	
702E 57	
Lithium Silver Chromate (Li 210)	70
Lithium Iodide (752, 755, 742, C.R.C.)	120
	257

about 50 months and there has only been one failure. The one where the rate fell six beats per minute in three years. This is the only battery failure of 257. The other two patients have had some fall in their heart rate, but we are continuing to observe them. Historically, the second was the 702 P. We have put in 7 CPI units with this battery. The follow-up period again is almost four years and no failures have occurred. The 702 E was the next battery.

We have 57 of those with an experience so far of 30 months. None of these have failed. I would like to end up on a very optimistic note, as far as my comments are concerned. With our 257 patients with lithium units put in, we have only had one definite battery failure.

CHAIRMAN: Because of the good results with the lithium batteries we almost are forgetting the nuclear units. Dr. Parsonnet, who has a lot of experience in that respect can give some comments.

V. PARSONNET: Two quick comments. One is that our experience with lithium is identical to Dr. Sloman's, but I want to remind you that in our lithium patients 20% have had reoperations for something other than the power source. The other is the nuclear pacemakers – I have a personal experience of 112 of them. We have had no battery failures for the follow-up period, and one component failure. So, it is also a highly reliable unit, with a highly reliable battery and it may have a place in pacing in about 10 to 15% of the patients.

CHAIRMAN: We have discussed the patient, the electrode and the pacemaker. Our time is almost up. However, before we stop, I would like to ask all panel members the choice of electrode and the choice of pacemaker for long-term pacing. First Dr. Murtra, what are you using in Barcelona?

M. MURTRA: As you can see in Table 6 the pacemakers are the on-demand R-wave blocked types with lithium batteries and for the electrodes we have used endocardial monopolar small-surface electrodes. We select the mercury powered pacemaker only when it is a socio-economic problem or when the patient is over 75.

Table 6.

Pacemaker-electrode combination
Pacemaker
R-Inhibited ventricular demand
Long-life lithium batteries
Hermetically sealed
Fairly small weight and size
Round smooth edges
Simple connections
Reasonable price
Electrode
Endocavitary monopolar electrode lead
Small surface electrode

CHAIRMAN: Werner, you are not a physician but a physicist, and you know more than us about a lot of pacing aspects. What do you use, small-surface or large-surface electrodes? And this goes for all the members: lithium or mercury oxide and, if possible some percentages please.

W. IRNICH: We are now using small-area electrodes, that is to say 5 mm^2 in surface. I would even like to have 4 or 3 mm^2. As to the choice of pacemakers we are using 3 different types of pacemakers with respect to energy source. 18% of them are powered by mercury oxide. Of the remaining 82% two thirds are with lithium batteries whose service life is anticipated to be 10 years. The rest are lithium pacemakers functioning still longer.

S. DALLA VOLTA: Endocardial approach, small-surface electrodes. If I had a choice, I would prefer lithium, but our experience with lithium has only been for the last years. So by now mostly we will use pacemakers with a mercury battery.

V. PARSONNET: For permanent pacing: mostly small electrodes, mostly lithium powered sources with hermetically sealed cases, some nuclears. We would prefer to have almost everything programmable.

J.G. SLOMAN: We are using small-surface electrodes with lithium power source. I do not mind the manufacturer, but we prefer a 752, 742 or 755 lithium-iodine battery. I think those are by far the best batteries that are available at the moment. No old-fashioned pacemakers.

R.G. GOLD: Obviously low-surface area electrodes are first choice. But if they fail or cannot retain a stable position, then a Helifix electrode, which I have found very satisfactory. As far as lithium pacemakers are concerned, they are obviously a first choice, but subject to the price limitations and the patient's age, as I mentioned earlier. I do not have any particular favorite at the moment.

M. BILITCH: I have no further comment.

C. MEERE: We use 40% lithium pacemakers, nowadays, at the Montreal Heart Institute, with small-surface electrodes and, once in a while, we use small lithium pacemakers, not for the purpose of longevity but for the purpose of avoiding skin erosion. About 90% are transvenous electrodes and the rest epicardial electrodes.

C.J. WESTERHOLM: Endocardial electrodes and small lithium pacers.

CHAIRMAN: Would you use large-surface electrodes? Are you scared of small-surface ones?

C.J. WESTERHOLM: No, no small-surface ones.

R. Hardjowyono: I like lithium pacemakers. They are small and I am a surgeon and I like to make a nice small pocket.

Chairman: It seems that – with the exception of Dr. Westerholm for the electrode size – the choice of the ideal pacemaker-electrode combination for this panel is the lithium powered R-wave blocked (programmable) pacemaker with a small-surface electrode.

This uniform opinion closes our Round Table and also the first day of the Colloquium.

I thank the panel members and the audience for their contributions.

Section VI

PACEMAKER IMPLANTATION: SURGEON AND/OR CARDIOLOGIST

THE COOPERATION IN MANAGEMENT OF PACEMAKER PATIENTS

K. Steinbach, G. Joskowicz and A. Laczkovics

The cooperation between surgeons and cardiologists in the management of pacemaker (PM) patients is a result of historical evolution. The cardiologist is responsible for the selection of patients for this treatment, the follow-up and technical problems, the surgeon on the other hand, is responsible for the implantation of the PM system and the test of the reliability of new electrodes.

Now, I don't want to give a detailed survey of cardiac pacing but one has to mention that the cardiologist was the first who was confronted with the problem of bradyarrhythmias and applied electrostimulation instead of inadequate medical treatment. So it is not surprising that the cardiologist Zoll for the first time tried to treat bradycardia by external stimulation in 1951. External electrostimulation, however, was not effective as a long-term treatment. Consequently, surgeons applied this therapy since initially only an epicardial electrode was used which required surgical intervention. Thus, the cooperation between surgeons and cardiologists started in many centers and has continued until today. This cooperation remained even when transvenous application of the PM electrode was used, which made only a simple surgical intervention necessary. The fact that the implantation of a PM electrode passed the experimental stage and became a clinical routine made it necessary to establish diagnostic methods to improve the selection of patients, optimal systems and the follow-up in regard to the function of the PM and other medical problems of the patients. All these activities are best performed as a team. The program of this symposium illustrates that surgeons and cardiologists share research and clinical routine. Of course, you should not forget the role of the bio-engineer incorporated in this team whose help makes the solution of multiple problems possible.

In order to demonstrate this distribution of efforts, I would like to give some examples of the cardiologists' activities in this team at our center in Vienna.

Preoperative diagnostic procedures

Besides programmed electrostimulation and His bundle electrocardiography the long-term follow up of ECG can be applied for the evaluation of patients with total AV-block. However, the automatic analysis of the ECG still creates a major problem. Recently, we developed the so-called 'Multipass scanning system' which solves the problem of the tremendous amount of data which are analyzed during repeated runs (Fig. 1).

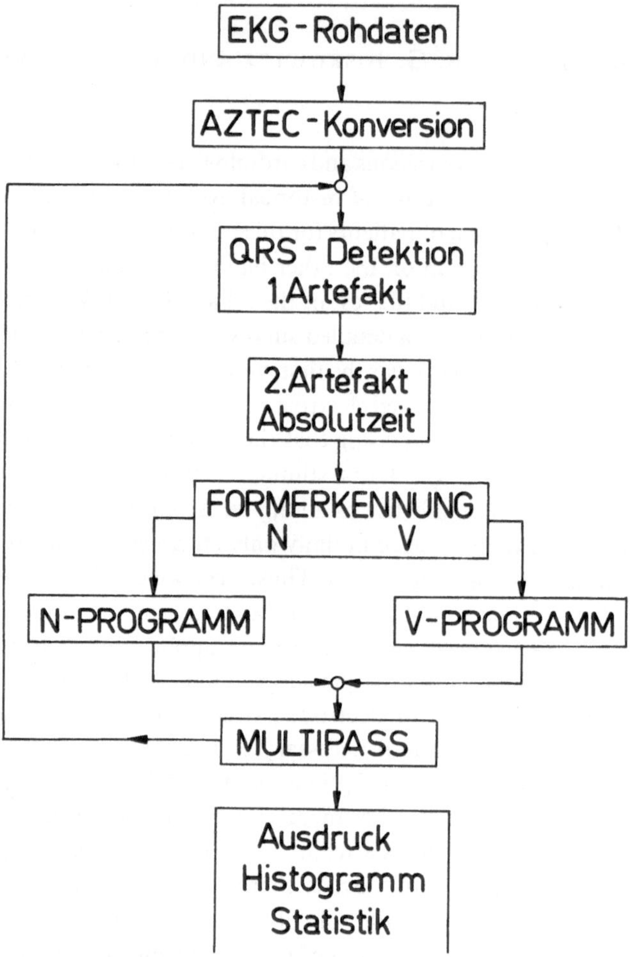

Figure 1. Scheme of computerized arrhythmia analysis (explanation see text).

Long-term supervision of the ECG could be improved so that at the first run amplitude and width of the QRS-complex can be determined and first artefact detection can be performed. During a second run another artefact detection and form analysis is performed. According to the area of the QRS-complex they are defined as N (normal) or V (widened). They are then analysed by a special program.

Follow-up

The control of PM patients was improved in the late sixties by measuring the impulse width and interval. We have been using this method in Vienna since 1969 and were able to prolong the function of the pacemakers dramatically. We could replace batteries on elective basis rather than routinely (1). In addition, the analysis of the PM impulse provides information about changes in the resistance in the patient's circuit. The resistance can be calculated from the exponential decrease of the PM impulse if the capacity of the condenser at the PM exit is known. The equation is $\tau = R \times C$. By utilizing these parameters, we were able to detect an incomplete defect of the electrode indicated by an increase of the resistance and an isolation defect indicated by a decrease of resistance.

On the other hand it could be demonstrated that in patients with lower resistance the function of the same PM type was significantly shorter than in patients with a higher resistance (Fig. 2), (2).

In the past there have been discussions whether a decrease of the impulse duration below 0,8 msec might be hazardous for the patient. In order to solve this problem, we used PM systems with percutaneous variable impulse duration. We calculated the impulse duration for this PM type based on a safety level of 50% and 100% current over the threshold (3). In contrast to systems controlled by an amplitude in which the safety interval is directly related to threshold, this is not the case in systems with variable impulse duration. Assuming that changes of the threshold mostly influence the rheobase, it is possible to relate the threshold measured in time to an equivalent rheobase (4). After multiplying this value with the safety factor defined for amplitude-controlled systems one is able to reconvert in the time domain and to fix the appropriate safety margin. In 118 patients where this PM system was implanted during a follow-up period of 44 months we tested the reliability of this calculation. No exit block was observed (5). In addition to PM control by the patient himself, the transtelephone follow-up is more and more used. The system developed in our laboratory has the advantage of being able to transmit even the impulse interval by a low time prolongation before the modulation of the signal (6).

I did not intend to describe these examples of various activities of the cardiologists in the diagnostic aspects and follow-up of PM patients in order to stress the importance of one center rather than to describe the function of the cardiologists in this team. I am convinced that it is the cardiologists' task to perform the diagnostic procedures and the follow-up of PM patients. Together with the surgeon the cardiologist should test the applicability of new PM systems and electrodes. For instance it is of clinical importance to solve the problem of reduction of energy drain by decrease of amplitude and pulse width. It is necessary to calculate for each electrode type the maximal threshold in which a low output pacemaker can be used. We found for instance a rheobase of 3,63 mA for an electrode with a 24 mm² surface of the tip (7, 8). Another phenomenon of

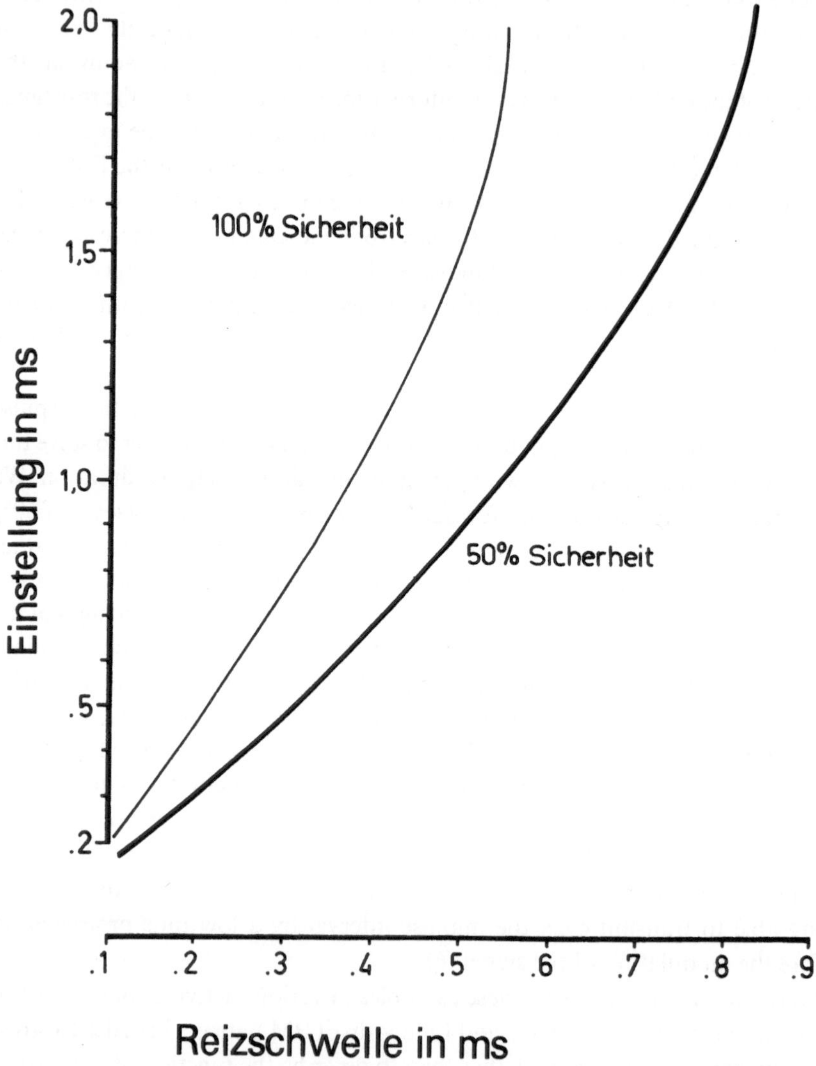

Figure 2. Fixing of a pulse width system in function of threshold and a safety margin of 50% and 100% respectively.

clinical importance is the polarization around the electrode tip. This electrochemical reaction has been investigated extensively. In accordance with other centers we found a loss of energy consumed by this reaction in the range up to 30% and a significant difference in the velocity depending on surface and material of the electrode tip (9). We have tested Schwan's formula in vivo by analysing the action potential which was derived through the intracardiac electrode. The calculation of the imaginary portion of the resistance in the patients' circuit by a fast Fourier transformation gives an exact information about the amount and velocity of the polarization (10).

Finally, the long-term follow-up is another very important and also time-consuming activity but the only way by which complications of PM therapy can be observed and life expectancy of the patients evaluated. Careful observation of these patients can detect possible dysfunction of PM in time and prophylactic replacement can be undertaken. In order to have an exact follow-up of our patients we control them at our clinic in regular intervals. If the patient does not show up for these check-ups we get in touch with him by letter and if this is not succesful we get in touch with his family doctor. We therefore have an exact record of the causes of death in our patients, in 68% of our patients an autopsy was performed and from the other patients we get the information through the family doctor (11). We therefore were able to clarify the cause of death in 97% of our patients. The mortality of the patients dying suddenly outside of the hospital is of course of special interest and was in our material 9%. Half of them had a fixed rate PM and half synchronized PM. This is in agreement with the results of Zoll from previous years and may indicate that competition between idioventricular rhythm and PM is not as dangerous as we learned from the pharmacologists (12). On the other hand the energy need for the synchronization unit in the last years was reduced under 10 μA so the only reason for the use of anachronous PM might be the lower price.

I have tried to demonstrate that at our center the cooperation between the cardiologists and the surgeons is necessary and has proven to be effective: The cardiologists being in charge for the selection of the patients for implantation using sometimes highly specialized methods such as His bundle electrocardiography or long-term monitoring and careful follow-up postoperatively, the surgeon performing the implantation of the electrode system either in one session or in two if research questions are under investigation. This cooperation seems to be necessary in a center where 1200 operations per year are performed and over 700 patients are regularly controlled. It may be possible that in institutions with a low number of patients the task can be managed either by the surgeon or cardiologist alone.

The team effort in the field of PM therapy also seems to be required since both the surgeons and the cardiologists are engaged in other activities within their speciality. I hardly can believe that there is one surgeon or cardiologist who deals exclusively with PM therapy.

References

1. Lahoda, R., Steinbach, K. & Weissenhofer W., Die Beurteilung des Funktionszustandes chronisch implantierter Schrittmacher. Wr. Ztschr. f. Inn. Medizin, 51, 545 (1970).
2. Steinbach, K., Joskowicz, G., Weissenhofer, W. & Brunner, H., Fortschritte in der Meβtechnik bei der Schrittmachertherapie. Herz Kreisl. 6, 208 (1974).
3. Furman, S., Denize, A., Escher, D.J.W. & Schwedel, J.B., Energy consumption for cardiac stimulation as a function of pulse duration. J. Surg. Res. 6, 441 (1966).
4. Joskowicz, G., Steinbach, K. & Domanig, E. jr., Practical application of a power-controlled pacemaker. ESAO I, 74 (1974).
5. Steinbach, K. & Joskowicz, G., Erfahrungen mit einem zeitgesteuerten Schrittmachersystem. Wr. Klin. Wochenschr., 87, 371 (1975).
6. Pfundner, P. & Steinbach, K., Die EKG-Überwachung des Patienten auβerhalb des Krankenhauses. Wr. Zeitschr. f. Inn. Med. u. ihre Grenzgebiete, 53, 343 (1972).
7. Steinbach, K. & Joskowicz, G., Verkürzung der Impulsdauer zur Energieeinsparung bei der Schrittmachertherapie. Acta Med. Austriaca, 3, 13 (1976).
8. Unger, F. & Steinbach, K., Objectification of the Increase in Stimulation Threshold in Electrostimulation of the Heart. Electromedica, 2, 63 (1974).
9. Greatbatch, W., Electrochemical Polarization of Physiological Electrodes Med. Res. Eng. Vol. 6, 2 (1967).
10. Joskowicz, G. & Steinbach, K., Die Bedeutung der Polarisationsphänomene bei der meβtechnischen Erfassung der elektrischen Stimulation des Herzens. Zeitschr. f. Kardiol. 63, 811 (1974).
11. Unger, F. & Steinbach, K., Long-time results in cardiac pacing. Atti del V Congr. Naz., 208 (1974).
12. Steinbach, K., Stellwag, F. & Unger, F., Langzeitergebnis bei der Schrittmachertherapie. Acta Med. Austriaca 2, 15 (1975).

THE TEAMWORK IN PACEMAKER IMPLANTATION

A.J. DZIATKOWIAK AND J.W. KOZLOWSKI

With introduction of the transvenous electrodes and implantable units in the early sixties and with rapid development of artificial cardiac pacing, a new period started in pacemaker therapy which appeared to be one of the most efficient methods of treatment in clinical practice. Now it is quite impossible to create a cardiological department or coronary care unit without a pacemaker section. We are still of the opinion that permanent pacing should be performed only in the experienced centers which have the ability to perform at least 50-100 new implants per year. Some years ago mostly surgeons have been dealing with pacemaker treatment. Now it spreads to the cardiologists but the teamwork is necessary for efficient results and for avoiding as much as possible the percentage of complications, errors and difficulties. Only the cooperative efforts and the application of the latest findings can provide the patient with optimal aid, thus leading to a considerable improvement in therapeutic possibilities.

Based on our experience in pacemaker treatment for over 13 years we would give some methodological remarks to the important question, how to organize the pacemaker teamwork.

During the years 1964-1976 we performed 1804 pacemaker procedures to 481 patients with cardiac rhythm disorders in the Institute of Cardiology, Medical Academy Lódź, Poland, using various types of pacemakers and electrodes (Biotronik, Cordis, CPI, Devices, ELA, Elema, General Electric, LEM, Medtronic, Vitatron) as well as diverse operative techniques. Till 1969 all implantations were performed at the Department of Cardiac Surgery; since 1970 the cardiologists started with permanent pacemaker applications.

At present our pacemaker team consists of 2 skilled cardiologists, 1 surgeon, 1 anesthesiologist, 1 radiologist and 1 electronic engineer, who are closely cooperating in pacemaker implantations (1). We would place considerable emphasis on the elasticity of cooperation and supervision with no competition in the team (Figure 1). The participation in pacemaker teamwork is shown in Table 1. We do not suggest all 6 persons should be occupied at the implantation. The main procedure and the final decision to make use of a particular piece of equipment or to select the application route rests with the cardiological staff. The surgeon usually takes part in this procedure as the stand-by specialist for solving

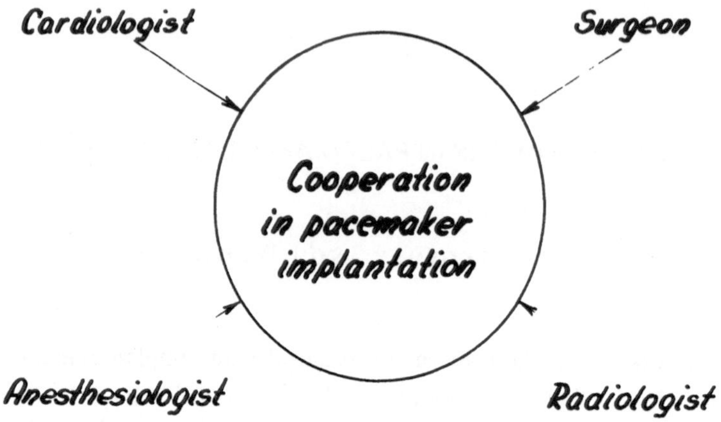

Figure 1. Elasticity of cooperation and supervision with no competition.

Table 1. Participation in pacemaker teamwork.

	Selection	Emergency	Programmed	Complications	Follow-up	Research
Cardiologist	+++	+++	+++	++	+++	+++
Surgeon	+	+	++	+++		++
Anesthesiologist		++	+			
Radiologist			+	+	+	
Electronic					++	+++

some urgent surgical problems, he is usually treating the complications and takes part in research studies as well. Although the whole staff is well-trained and experienced in emergency cardiology and resuscitation we used to have also our anesthesiologist standing by as well as a radiologist to avoid electrode malplacement during the operation. (2). This clearly indicates that the physicians are working together, but also the engineer is increasingly involved in the successful treatment of the patient.

Table 2. Ability and expertise of the pacemaker team.

	Cardiologist	Surgeon	Anesthesiologist	Radiologist
Pathology of conduction disturbances	+ + +	+ +	+	
Knowledge of current pacing systems	+ + +	+		
Indication and selection of pacemaker and route of impl.	+ + +	+ + +	+	
Comprehension of antiseptic and aseptic rules	+ + +	+ + +	+	+
Capability in small surgical procedures	+ + +	+ + +	+	+
Major surgical procedures /ECC/	+	+ + +		
Diagnosis and management of intraoperative malfunctions	+ + +	+ + +		+ +
Evaluation and treatment of complications	+ + +	+ + +		+
Reimplantation	+ +	+ + +		

From Table 2 one can see that the ability and expertise of the pacemaker team are based upon the cardiologist and surgeon who take part almost equally in the final results. Although in contrast to pervenous implantations, the application of myocardial (also sutureless) and epicardial wires is done usually by the surgeon, the cardiologists attend every operation not only for ECG monitoring, measuring the stimulation threshold or intracavitary potentials but also as the surgical assistant. Pacemaker reimplantations and replacements are performed equally by the surgeon or/and cardiologist (3).

This kind of cooperation we found to be desirable to avoid the main complications which, as it is shown in Table 3 are dependent mostly upon the operator.

It is to be hoped that owing to our experience and cooperation we were able to decrease now the percentage of complications to a very low level and so for example in our clinic: electrode dislodgement in the last 2 years has been observed only in 7 cases (3%), infections in 4 patients (1,5%), exteriorization of the generator in 1 male patient and no case of any other serious complications.

Table 3. The team-dependent most common factors of pacemaking complications.

	Operator	Co-workers
Electrode dislodgement	+ + +	
Perforation of ventricle	+ + +	
Uncorrect placement of electrode	+ + +	+
Haematoma	+ + +	
Infection	+ + +	+ +
Sepsis, endocarditis, pulmonary embolism	+ + +	+ +
Thrombophlebitis	?	?
Exteriorations /wire, generator/	+ + +	
Disconnection	+ + +	

That assures us that an experienced team and close cooperation help to promote proper pacemaker treatment and to obtain good results in pacing. In conclusion the ideal pacemaker implantation is performed with:

1. Proper indications for permanent pacing
2. Correctly selected type of pacing system
3. The most convenient approach and route of implantation
4. Implantation performed by the well-trained, experienced and stable team
5. No hospital and late complications
6. Short hospitalizing period (up to 7 days).

References

1. Goldman, B.S., Noble, E.J., Macgregor, D.C., Morrow, J.D., Convey, H.D., Heller J.G., Taylor, K.W., Conceptual development of a university pacemaker centre. In: Thalen, H.J.Th., (ed.), *Cardiac Pacing* – Proceedings of the 4th International Symposium, Van Gorcum Co., Assen – The Netherlands, p. 465, (1973).
2 Parsonnet, V., Permanent pacing of the heart – a comment on technique. *Am. J. Cardiol.* 36, 268 (1975).
3. Bilitch, M., Myocardial and endocardial pacing systems – an appraisal. In: Schaldach, M., Furman, S. (ed.), *Advances in Pacemaker Technology*. Springer Verlag, Berlin, Heidelberg, New York, p. 91, (1975).

WHO SHOULD IMPLANT A PACEMAKER SYSTEM, CARDIOLOGIST OR SURGEON?

J. Warren Harthorne,* John McDermott* and Karen B. Peterson*

The question, 'To pace or not to pace' stated by the theme of this symposium has gained increasing significance and implication. The electronic wizards, conceived in the aerospace industry and delivered in the competitive 'think tanks' of pacemaker manufacturers' Research and Development Departments, have given us every manner of circuit design for simulating or even improving on the normal heart's conduction system. There is little question that the future will witness a return to the use of atrial triggered ventricular systems in the vast majority of patients with heart block. Automatic conversion of atrial or ventricular tachyarrhythmias through biologic programmability is already a reality for temporary pacing systems and only awaits the perfection of a dependable atrial electrode before such devices will be ready for permanent implantation.

It is curious that, after twenty years of developing the technology to provide effective cardiac stimulation, the question 'To pace or not to pace' can be asked. Certainly in the majority of instances, pacing produces profound and dramatic benefits to the recipient.

There are several aspects of the question to be considered. Assuming that the insertion of a pacemaker is deemed proper, should the device be implanted by a surgeon, a cardiologist, or a team of both? During the last World Survey of Cardiac Pacing prepared for the Tokyo Meeting, Dr. Victor Parsonnet found that the vast majority of permanent pacemakers implanted in the United States were performed by surgeons (about 75%) or surgeon-cardiologist teams (about 23%). In only 5% of instances was the procedure performed solely by a cardiologist. Thus, the onus of tradition presents somewhat of a stumbling block to the cardiologist who chooses to carry out these procedures without surgical collaboration.

During the past twelve years, all permanent pacemaker implantations performed at the Massachusetts General Hospital in Boston have been performed by internists with subspecialty training in cardiology and cardiac catheterization. Over one thousand primary implantations and two thousand generator changes have been performed and encompass all varieties of atrial, atrioventricular

* Cardiac Unit, Massachusetts General Hospital, Boston, Mass., USA.

synchronous, atrioventricular sequential, ventricular synchronous, and ventricular demand devices. The purpose of this presentation is to discuss our own methodology and results.

Methods

All permanent pacemaker implantations are performed in a laboratory established for that purpose. It would be presumptuous to quote guidelines for such a laboratory in other institutions having differing needs and requirements but a brief description of our own facility may be of interest to those who anticipate establishing such a room in their own institution.

Until 1974, all permanent pacemaker procedures had been performed in the Cardiac Catheterization Laboratory. These procedures were traditionally performed at the end of the regular schedule of diagnostic procedures so as not to defer the angiographic caseload and subsequent film processing. With the annual growth of coronary angiography, the time allotted for pacing procedures became deferred until later each day. The physical environment within that facility rendered impossible the maintenance of a sterile operating room environment and necessitated the establishment of the present Pacemaker Laboratory.

The room set aside for this purpose is 12 by 18 feet and rectangular in shape. The only renovation needed to convert the room from a secretarial to a laboratory facility suitable for pacemaker implantation was the installation of a standard operating room scrub sink, additional electrical outlets with central ground and a small ceiling-mounted, movable operating room light. The room is air conditioned with a filtered exhaust system. Renovation costs were kept below $ 5,000. Standard monitoring devices, a portable C-arm General Electric Fluoricon Model 10359 portable fluoroscope and mobile fluoroscopic Graf Bix table complete the equipment. A 4 by 6 foot storage rack for sterile minor packs and instrument trays occupies one corner. A six-drawer lateral file cabinet for patient records, pacemaker generators, leads, replacement parts, etc. occupies another corner along with an emergency resuscitation cart.

The procedures are performed entirely by internists who have had subspecialty training in cardiology and catheterization under supervision by the senior author (J. Warren Harthorne, M.D.). A laboratory technician with four prior years of experience in a busy hemodynamic laboratory completes the 'team.' It is most essential that the Pacemaker Laboratory technician does not change from one procedure to another since constant exposure to a wide variety of differing pacemaker systems and types of implants is necessary to establish confidence and familiarity with subtle but important electronic and mechanical differences between various commercial systems. A pleasant, reassuring (and entertaining!)

personality minimizes patient apprehension since procedures are performed under local anesthesia.

Technique

The general procedure is similar whether a permanent ventricular, atrial or atrio-ventricular sequential pacemaker is being implanted. Most patients have already been made aware of the need for the procedure by their own physician before being visited by a member of the implanting team on the night prior to the procedure. A thorough discussion of the procedure, customary operating time, risks, postoperative complications and usual hospital stay and follow-up schedule is provided. General anesthesia is discouraged and has been used in only three of over three thousand procedures. Patients are kept 'n.p.o.' for eight hours before the procedure. Premedication is provided only for apprehensive patients. Oftentimes a temporary pacemaker is already in place or may be inserted according to individual considerations but is no longer considered essential in all patients.

The implanting physician follows a standard hospital prescribed scrub technique using Betadyne inpregnated scrub brushes. All personnel are masked and gowned with underlying 0.50 mm lead aprons. The area for proposed pacemaker insertion is selected with several considerations in mind. When possible, considerations of the patient's right- or left-handedness or hobbies or occupations requiring the predominant use of one arm or the other are taken into account. (In a population of elderly, ill patients, one is often left to take whatever space on the patient's chest wall is 'left over' after the usual intravenous lines, Swan Ganz catheters or temporary electrodes have been inserted). The upper chest including the jugular area of the neck of whichever side is selected is carefully prepared with surgical soap, Surgical Prep Solution (containing 70% alcohol) and Ether. Sterile towels are applied to map out the selected area. Care is taken by the operator not to touch the sterilized area of skin until after a sterilized adhesive plastic drape (Steridrape, Minnesota Mining and Manufacturing) has been applied. Following infiltration with 0.5% Lidocaine, an incision is made parallel to the delto pectoral groove and the cephalic branch of the axillary system is dissected 'free' in the groove created where the medial border of the deltoid muscle meets the pectoralis. About 85% of patients will have a cephalic vein adequate for use. In the remainder the ipsilateral external (or internal) jugular vein will suffice. On infrequent occasions, it has been necessary to dissect out the axillary vein – a somewhat formidable procedure for the average internist! A small venotomy is made after the vein has been ligated distally and smooth tipped forceps inserted to spread the margins. The electrode to be used is introduced and will usually pass easily to the right atrium. Occasionally difficulties are encountered due to tortuosity or even thrombosis of vessels. These can usually be overcome by slight withdrawal of the electrode stylet allowing the tip to be prolapsed or 'knuckled' past the obstruction. A tight curve in the stylet, deep inspiration, and soft profanity often help. When alternative venous routes are unavailable, the senior author has succeeded in thrombectomizing clotted axillary-subclavian venous systems or dilating stenotic segments of veins by progressive passage of tapered tipped catheters of increasing calibre over a wire guide.

Once the right atrium has been reached, the fluoroscope (sterilely draped) is positioned over the patient. (Whenever the incision does not require direct access, it is kept covered with a sterile towel to minimize contamination). Passage of the electrode from the right atrium is facilitated by using stylets of varying curvature created by drawing them across the operator's finger. Once the ventricle has been entered, final positioning is usually best achieved with a straight stylet or one with a gentle curve. The stylet is withdrawn slightly so that the very tip remains flexible during positioning. Delicacy in lead handling is essential. One 'works' the flanged tip into the trabeculations of the right ventricle rather than simply ramming it into the apex in the hope it will 'stick.' Multiple attempts in differing positions may be necessary before the operator is confident of a stable position. Confirmation of the latter is aided by observation of lead position during gentle withdrawal. (The stylet should be removed). When the lead is properly positioned it can be 'lifted up' off the floor of the atrium without motion of the tip. Occasionally a gentle tugging sensation by the heart can be appreciated.

Proper determination of stimulation threshold cannot be discussed in detail here beyond noting that it *must* be performed at the pulse width of the pulse generator to be used. Acceptable thresholds vary according to the surface area and shape of the lead in use but are generally below 1.0 m.a. and often below 0.5 m.a. Our own procedure includes stimulation at the full output of the testing device to detect diaphragmatic contraction which may be troublesome to the patient later on. Re-positioning of the electrode is done until a position is achieved which has physical stability, acceptable threshold and lack of diaphragmatic contraction within the output range of the device to be used. The endocardial signal strength is also of essential importance in ensuring proper demand functioning and can be determined with most commercially available test devices.

Once acceptable position is achieved, the lead is anchored at its point of entry into the vein using a tapered silastic butterfly to avert suture kinking of the electrode. Sufficient lead is left within the heart to provide a smooth gentle curve across the tricuspid valve. (Excessive amounts of electrode produce buckling, kinking, or actual loops and encourage dislocation and clot formation.)

A pocket ('three fingers wide, three fingers deep') is created deep to the subcutaneous tissue but anterior to pectoralis fascia and the pacemaker with attached lead inserted. Meticulous attention is paid to bleeders prior to closure with 3/0 Dexon subcuticular and 5/0 nylon skin sutures. Betadyne ointment is applied and a small dressing which is left undisturbed for five to seven days. Drains or flushing the pocket with antibiotics are not employed. All patients remain in bed on a cardiac monitor for thirty-six to forty-eight hours and then ambulate freely. Temporary electrodes, if present, are often left in place for one or two days but are always removed under fluoroscopy. Antibiotic coverage is administered only for primary insertions and consists of one of the semisynthetic penicillin derivatives (oxacillin, cloxacillin, dicloxacillin) in an oral dose of 2 grams daily for five to seven days after the procedure.

Results

As noted in the introductory remarks, approximately one thousand primary transvenous pacemaker insertions and two thousand generator changes or revisions have been performed during the past twelve years. No deaths have occurred coincident with any of these procedures. Postoperative hospital mortality remains around 1% due to related illnesses (recent myocardial infarction, refractory congestive heart failure, cerebral vascular accident, etc.). Immediate operative complications are infrequent and relate primarily to penetration of the right ventricular myocardium with resultant erratic pacemaker performance. This affects approximately 5% of implants and is seen almost solely with unipolar electrodes. Actual physical dislocation of the electrode out of the heart is a rare event with increasing experience. Hematoma formation within the pacemaker pocket continues to occur in 5 to 10% of procedures mostly in the elderly and in those patients on anticoagulants for other reasons (prosthetic valves, pulmonary thromboembolism, etc.). Aspiration or surgical drainage is seldom required unless wound dehiscence threatens. Sepsis has not been a problem, occurring almost exclusively as a secondary consequence of pacemaker erosion or wound dehiscence due to hematoma (three cases). No instance of endocarditis has been recognized following a procedure performed in our laboratory. Late erosion of the pacemaker generator or various segments of the extrathoracic electrode remain a continuing problem especially among long-term survivors. There seems to be no 'common denominator' to account for these occurrences which have affected young and old alike. In general, such erosions are more common in the thin and elderly subject and usually occur at points of mechanical stress along corners, edges, or protuberances of the pacemaker generator and its lead system. The process seldom occurs following the initial pacemaker implant and is more commonly witnessed after one or several generator changes suggesting that avascularity of the implant site may play a role. Individual aspects of the patient's lifestyle doubtlessly contribute. Two of our patients with repeated multiple erosions have been witnessed by their families to scratch the implant site constantly until erosion occurred. Another elderly patient, a noted international sailor, struck the area of the pacemaker during a fall at sea. An alcoholic derelict plunged down a flight of stairs striking the pacemaker on a projecting corner. An elderly butcher in his 90's presented in the Emergency Room with what appeared to be an ugly erosion and an idioventricular rate of 30/minute. Chest x-ray revealed total absence of the pacemaker system. Subsequent investigation revealed that the patient, in a fit of despondency, had removed it with a kitchen knife! The introduction of smaller, more physiologically shaped pulse generators of low specific gravity will help to minimize these occurrences. We have not employed a dacron pouch around the pulse generator as a routine but did not believe it to be of help in a limited experience.

Discussion

The foregoing dialogue has concerned itself primarily with the technique and results of permanent pacemaker implantation as practiced at the Massachusetts General Hospital by cardiologists and has not addressed the question 'To pace or not to pace' and who should perform the procedure – physician or surgeon.

Table 1.

1.	Results of Pacing vs. Medical Treatment
2.	Prognosis of Patients after Pacemaker Implant
3.	Economic Cost of Pacing
4.	Moral issue in the Elderly or Demented

Table 1 illustrates various aspects of pacemaker insertion which may be considered. Most authors report improved longevity and survival curves following successful institution of cardiac pacing in contrast to earlier reports of patients with heart block treated medically. Certainly the improved *quality* of life provided by cardiac pacing seems sufficient to justify the procedure without regard to survival statistics. The prognosis of patients following institution of pacing has been studied at the Massachusetts General Hospital (Fig. 1) and indicates that 50% of such patients are dead within about five years. Recognition of this segment of the patient population through clinical descriptors plays an important role in selecting and matching the pulse generator appropriate for the

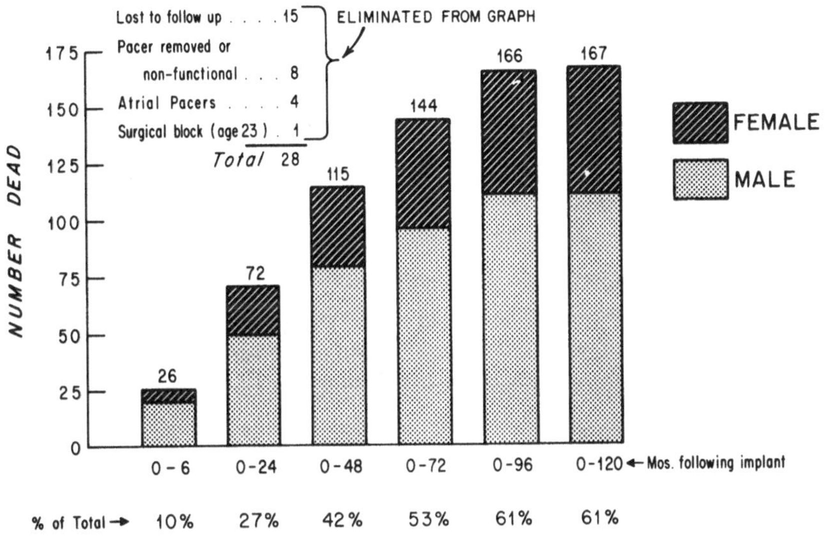

Figure 1. Chronologic mortality of 272 patients with endocardial pacers implanted from 7/65 to 12/71.

patient's projected needs. The escalating costs of medical care necessitate some awareness by the implanting physician of cost effectiveness. The economic cost of cardiac pacing to the individual patient varies widely. A single pacemaker, implanted once, which lasts just slightly longer than the patient would be the cheapest. Repeated interventions for generator replacement escalate the overall cost and risk to the patient and lower the cost effectiveness ratio. In 1975 it was estimated that the average cost per pacemaker stimulus was 0.0054 cents. While we as physicians should not place a value judgement on the cost of health maintenance, we should recognize that a generous segment of our patient population will fail to survive long enough to benefit from recently introduced, longer-lived and costlier pacemaker systems.

The question of whether the procedure should be performed by a surgeon or cardiologist or a team consisting of both is a local issue to be resolved at each individual institution. An adversary approach should never be allowed to develop since willing surgical assistance may, on occasion, be desirable. In our own institution the ultimate result of nearly three thousand procedures appears to justify the continuation of cardiologists performing the procedures. There may be some cardiologists and internists who, like me, have felt a sense of intimidation by the aura of mysticism and eminence that surrounds our surgical colleagues. The reader may find some consolation in the final illustration.

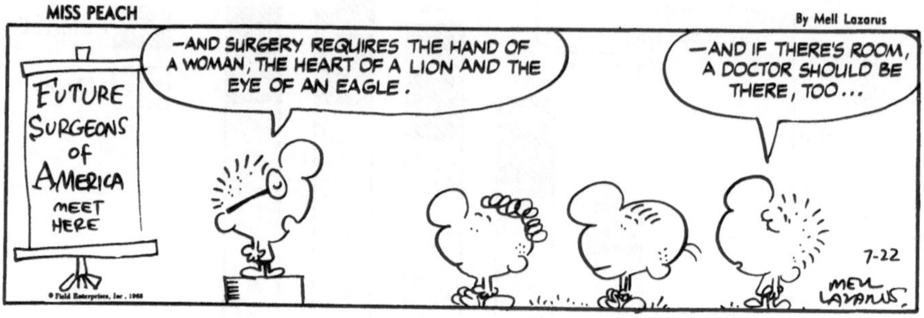
MISS PEACH
By Mell Lazarus
FUTURE SURGEONS of AMERICA MEET HERE
—AND SURGERY REQUIRES THE HAND OF A WOMAN, THE HEART OF A LION AND THE EYE OF AN EAGLE.
—AND IF THERE'S ROOM, A DOCTOR SHOULD BE THERE, TOO...
7-22
MELL LAZARUS

Figure 2. A cartoon Miss Peach by Mell Lazarus. Courtesy of Mell Lazarus and Field Newspaper Syndicate.

THE SURGEON, WHO SELECTS AND IMPLANTS?

SEYMOUR FURMAN

Dr. Harthorne and I agree that the question raised is not so much whether a pacemaker implant should be done by physician or surgeon, but whether the person performing the procedure is properly trained, skillful, and makes the proper measurements and decisions during the course of the procedure. The operator will be compelled to make critical decisions concerning the patient's welfare and the adequacy of the implant. Despite all technical assistance, the final decision will be his or hers.

The first and most important skill is that in performance of the surgical portion of the procedure. He must be able to make an incision, control both venous and small arterial bleeders, and then develop a pocket for the pulse generator in the subcutaneous tissue of the chest. He must be able to appreciate the need for sterility, for careful handling of tissue, and the secure tying of knots. He must be able to deal with thick, well-vascularized skin and with thin, tenuous, poorly vascularized skin so common in elderly patients. The operator must also be able to approach all of the veins used, the cephalic, the external jugular, and the internal jugular. Certainly, approaching the internal jugular involves avoidance of the carotid artery and the recurrent laryngeal nerve and obvious skills which go beyond those required for the more easily approached vessels. The operator who implants via the transvenous route must also be able to recognize the rare failure of that approach and be prepared and able to go to thoracotomy implant.

During the procedure, a number of measurements must be made to ascertain that pacing will be satisfactory. The stimulation threshold must be measured and the operator must be certain that the thresholds are satisfactory and compatible with the output of the pacemaker to be used. The procedure must be performed with fluoroscopy with two projections, AP and lateral. The signal from the heart which will trigger the pacemaker must be measured for its adequacy. In the unusual instance a position with a satisfactory stimulation threshold but a poor signal may be found. The operator must then select a generator of conventional output and high sensitivity. He must also be aware that the sensing characteristics of unipolar and bipolar electrodes are different and that measurement of the bipolar signal may show inadequate sensing and yet that conversion of bipolar to unipolar may restore sensing.

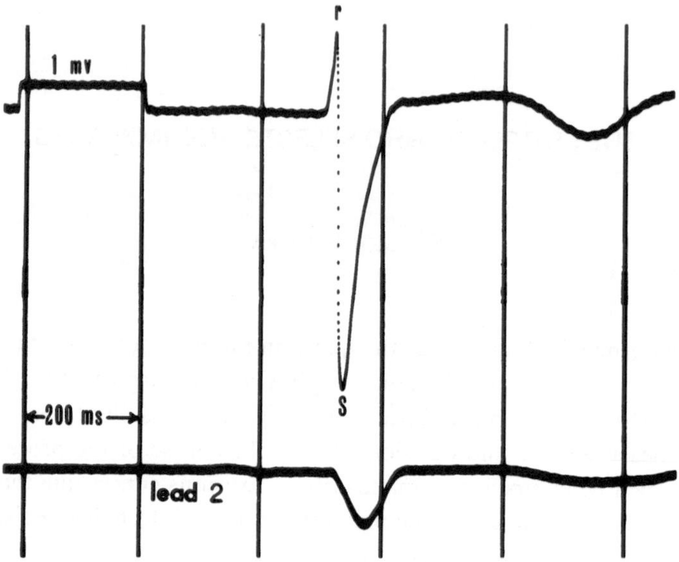

Figure 1. The endocardial electrogram via the electrode. The portion that provides the triggering amplitude is the intrinsic deflection (ID), in this illustration the rs vertical segment, which achieves adequate amplitude and slew rate (dv/dt) to trigger the pulse generator. In this instance the ID occurs at the beginning of the lead 2 QRS complex so that sensing of that complex by the pulse generator occurs at the anticipated time.

Looking carefully at the signal from the ventricle after electrode implantation, the unipolar signal is dominated by the intrinsic deflection, a sharp, positive-negative deflection of the depolarization wave as it passed the electrode (Figure 1). In our recordings, we always record the electrogram and a peripheral electrocardiogram simultaneously so that events caused by the electrogram can be timed against the ECG, which is recorded after implantation.

It is this intrinsic deflection, first described by Wilson in the 1930's and only now receiving its proper recognition in pacemaker technology, which triggers the generator. The intrinsic deflection may be adequate or inadequate to trigger the generator and may be early or late compared to the peripheral ventricular complex and in the case of a bipolar electrode two intrinsic deflections may be present as the depolarization wave front passes by both intracardiac electrodes. The initial ventricular complex at implant consists as well of an elevated S-T segment and almost always no T wave. The operator must recognize deviations which indicate poor tissue contact or ventricular perforation. The chronic unipolar signal is similar in amplitude and rate of rise of the intrinsic deflection but the S-T segment is isoelectric and the T wave is now visible as a negative deflection. If displacement of the electrode occurs during the implant procedure he must know that there is a variety of electrodes which grip the endocardium and which can be used to aid in the resolution of the problem. The implanter by the thoracotomy route must be aware of the same threshold and electrogram problems.

The implanter of cardiac pacemakers must be able to read an electrocardiogram and determine whether pacing and sensing are satisfactory. He must be aware of the meaning of such terms as hysteresis and must distinguish "late sensing," a normal event, from poorly sensed beats (Figure 2). There are now five

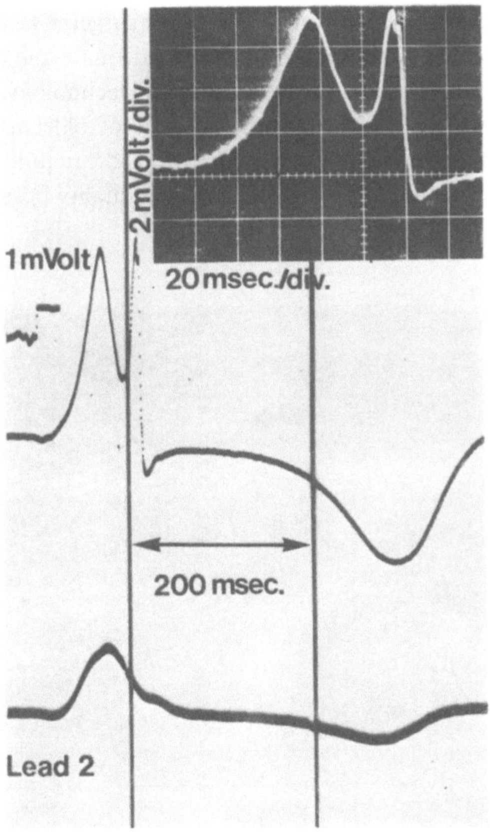

Figure 2. The intrinsic deflection (ID) of this electrogram occurs near the end of the lead 2 QRS. As the pulse generator will be triggered by the intrinsic deflection, sensing will be "late" compared to the onset of the QRS complex. This circumstance indicates no malfunction.

different pacing modes each with its strengths and weaknesses. The implanter must know when one or another pacing mode is indicated, what benefits and complications may be expected or feared. There are a variety of programmable pacemakers now becoming available. The implanter must know when output programmability will be useful and know its capabilities. He must also know when rate programmability is desirable and how to use it.

In short, the techniques and technology of electrical stimulation are now highly sophisticated. The implanter, whether surgeon or physician, must meet similar standards: adequate surgical skills for safe implantation, electrophysiologic comprehension, bioengineering knowledge to understand thresholds, electrograms, sensitivity, and the ability to interpret the electrocardiogram and the roentgenogram (Figure 3). Whoever implants the pacemaker must know whether it is indicated. As with any physician or surgeon, he must recognize that the maximum knowledge of his field is barely adequate and that in the presence of rapidly developing therapeutic indications and technology, constant attention to what is new as well as careful maintenance of older and well-established principles are mandatory. Two persons meeting these requirements, approached from different disciplines, will provide an equal quality of service.

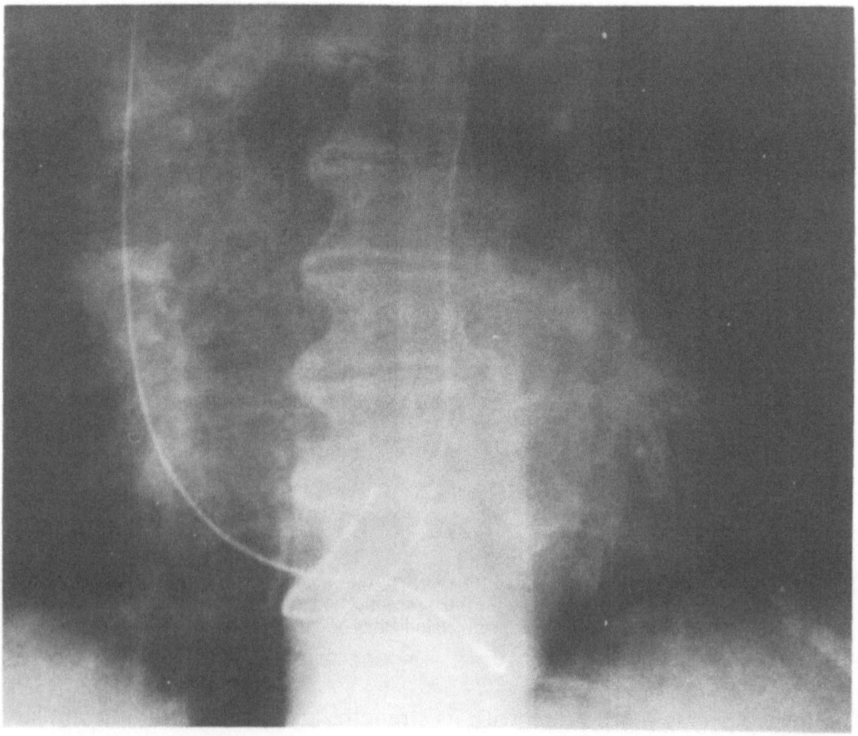

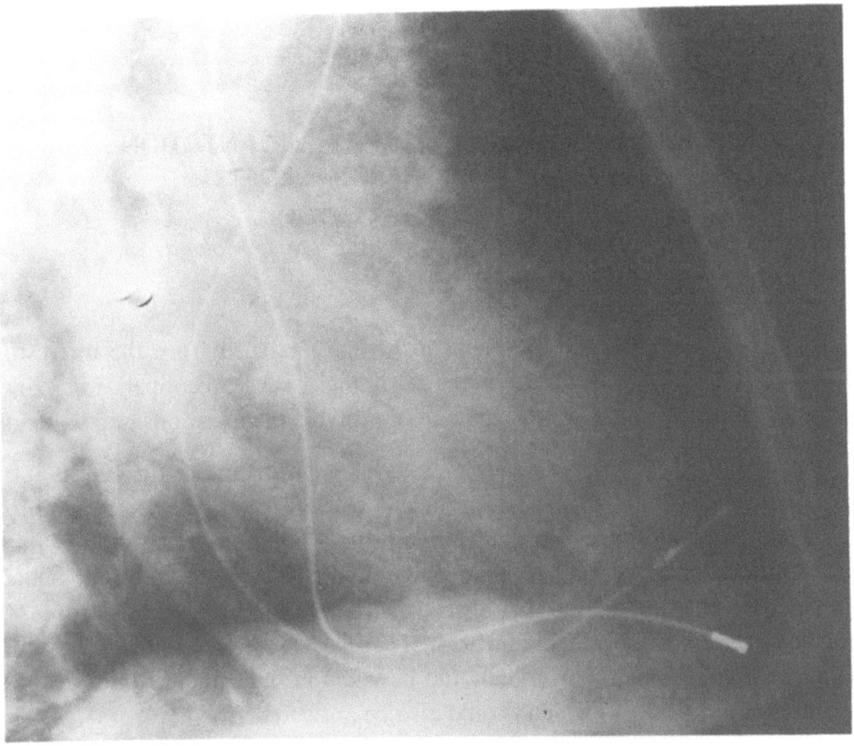

Figure 3. These films indicate the need to interpret the chest film. (A) Postero-anterior projection of a temporary electrode appearing anomalously in the mid-cardiac silhouette. The situation is clarified in (B) the lateral projection in which the seemingly displaced electrode is posterior in the coronary sinus, diagnostic of persistent left superior vena cava.

DISCUSSION VI. PACEMAKER IMPLANTATION: SURGEON AND/OR CARDIOLOGIST

CHAIRMAN: A.J. DZIATKOWIAK *(Lodz, Poland)*

CHAIRMAN: Ladies and Gentlemen. We have learned from the interesting presentations various opinions on the cardiologist-surgeon cooperation. Now I would like to ask you from the audience, have you any questions or comments?

J. NIEVEEN *(Groningen, The Netherlands)*: I heard from Dr. Furman that the cardiologist and the surgeon can perform a pacemaker implantation, a woman or a man can do this procedure. I would like to ask the speakers what they think about the room in which these procedures should be performed. Is it absolutely necessary to have these done in a specially sterilized surgical operating room? Or is it also possible to do them in a normal cardiac catheterization room. And, in the affirmative, what measures should be taken in the catheterization room? I think this is a problem which should also be answered.

CHAIRMAN: I see that Dr. Furman wants to answer these questions.

S. FURMAN *(New York, U.S.A.)*: I think that the procedure should be performed in a special room, as far as possible. While the cardiac catheterization room which is appropriately prepared before each case and properly maintained in the interval is adequate, it is not as satisfactory as a room equipped with a special air flow system, a special air lock and all of the other materials for strict sterility which, I believe, must be maintained as if it were an operating room. At my institution, the surgeons are trained in this approach, but the cardiologists do not have satisfactory training in sterility. Therefore, a surgeon must establish the technique. Finally, there is a variety of recordings that must be made, whether they be done by the cardiologist or surgeon and they include signal and threshold measurement, etc.

CHAIRMAN: Thank you Dr. Furman. Dr. Harthorne wants to add something to that subject.

J.W. HARTHORNE *(Boston, U.S.A.)*: We have actually done it both ways. For about eight years, we used the main catheter laboratory. The biggest deterrent, I think, in using the catheter laboratory was the lack of availability of the room. It was usually tied up for catheterization procedures until 3, 4, 5 o'clock in the afternoon. The permanent pacemaker implantations tended to be "second-class citizens" as far as when they could be done. We found ourselves staying on until 8, 9 10 o'clock at night getting the procedures accomplished. Also, there was a great deal of traffic through the catheter laboratory, which was very difficult to cut down on. So, the availability of the pacemaker laboratory has been one of convenience, but in fact it has not altered the results of the procedure. For reasons which are totally difficult for me to understand, we have had very, very few problems of sepsis and the sepsis problems we have had, have been predominantly secondary to erosions or repeated interventions. We have had no problems with sepsis with a primary insertion, regardless of where the procedure was done.

CHAIRMAN: Thank you. Any other questions from the audience?

L.L. KOSSAKOWSKI *('s-Hertogenbosch, The Netherlands):* Gentlemen, I have heard four speakers this morning talking about surgeons and cardiologists. One of you – I think it was Dr. Furman – said that in the background there may be a bio-medical technician and he was the one who really wants to burden all the surgeons or cardiologists with the technical knowledge. Our hospital team is composed of one surgeon, one cardiologist and one clinical physicist who really advises the surgeon who does not have the technical knowledge required for placing an electrode. In this way we also do not burden the cardiologist who has a lot of things to think about. I would like to ask the panel what it thinks about the new specialization which has come into most of Western Europe and the United States. I mean the clinical physicist.

CHAIRMAN: Someone who wants to answer this question?

J.W. HARTHORNE *(Boston, U.S.A.):* I am not sure I understand entirely all the aspects of your question. The team concept, I think, is very important to encourage and we certainly do depend heavily upon our biomedical engineers for advice regarding new products. When I promote the concept of a cardiologist implanting pacemaker devices, he is backed up by a three-dimensional team consisting of the knowledge that a surgeon is willingly available if trouble arises. We have not had to call upon him in many years, but we know that he is there to help us if we get into trouble. We also know that if we get into a situation which is difficult for us to understand, electronically, we can call upon the department of Medical Engineering with their more sophisticated knowledge and equipment and bail us out. So, I think that your question is appropriate: that most teams implanting pacemaker devices should have the availability of electronic expertise, if they need it. We do not generally need it in the average routine implantation. We also depend upon them for the evaluation of new products. We will never use a new product, a new pacemaker device, unless it has been evaluated by our medical engineering department.

CHAIRMAN: Thank you. Dr. Steinbach, what is your opinion?

K. STEINBACH *(Vienna, Austria):* I agree that team work is necessary, in principle. But I think nobody is authorized to set down regulations or rules for each center, because it mainly depends on the number of the operations and patients who have to be controlled. I also cannot imagine that one person can be a specialist in all the surgical procedures, technical matters, all the follow-up methods. I would think that in a center where the number of implantations is more than 20-30 a year, there has to be a team. If I report the figures from Vienna, where 1200 operations a year are performed in the Surgery Department and 700 patients are regularly controlled, I can hardly believe that one surgeon or a cardiologist can do all this work.

The other argument is that the cardiologist and the surgeon, in my opinion also have to be involved in other activities within their speciality and cannot spend all their time on pacemakers.

CHAIRMAN: Thank you. Dr. Furman, what is your opinion?

S. FURMAN *(New York, U.S.A.):* I believe that you are quite right, Dr. Steinbach. All of us have a large group of colleagues who assist us. However, when the operator (notice, I have not said surgeon) is operating, he or she must recognize difficulty and know when that difficulty requires assistance. Therefore, the responsibility of decision is ultimately in the operator's hands.

CHAIRMAN: Thank you. I would like to ask you... Sorry, Dr. Kossakowski wants to have a word – please go ahead.

L.L. KOSSAKOWSKI *('s-Hertogenbosch, The Netherlands):* I would like to comment, on behalf of the patient. There is a lot of damage done to the patient by lack of knowledge on the part of the cardiologist or surgeon. You know yourself that in a couple of years 1200 patients have died, have been electrocuted in hospitals in the United States, until Congress did something against it.

S. FURMAN*(New York, U.S.A.):* I believe this statement to be untrue and I believe that making such a statement is raising an issue which is inflammatory and incorrect.

CHAIRMAN: Thank you very much gentlemen. The temperature of our discussion raised a bit up which is good, but we have only two minutes to go and I would ask you to be so kind as to put your questions briefly first whereupon we will try to answer them as concisely as possible.

J. MEIBOM *(Copenhagen, Denmark):* I agree very much with Dr. Harthorne and Dr. Furman that it is not important who has to perform the procedures. It depends on tradition. I want to mention that in our hospital in Copenhagen, it is the cardiologist who performs the primary procedures. The surgeon is responsible for the major part of the procedure, during the exchange of the generator. That is not so fortunate. Simply because it is the youngest thoracic surgeon who performs this procedure. I also want to emphasize the presentation of Dr. Kozlowski about the team work in pacemaker implantation that as far as we have seen it in Copenhagen, it is very important to emphasize the cooperation between doctors – what type of doctors does not matter – and nurses and technicians. Without perfect cooperation among personnel in such groups, you will never have a good pacemaker treatment.

Last question I want to ask Dr. Steinbach how one measures the capacity, as mentioned in his slides.

CHAIRMAN: May we have the question from the next speaker first?

B. DODINOT *(Nancy, France):* Do you think, Dr. Furman, when you implant the pacemaker at an acute phase, you must always have an S-T elevation or not? And if not, do you have a higher incidence of problems or not?

CHAIRMAN: The next question and the last at this session.

M. STOPCZYK *(Warsaw, Poland):* A short comment on intra-cavitary signals. The inhibitory potential of demand pacemakers is not only a function of amplitude, but a function of rate of rise as well.

CHAIRMAN: Thank you gentlemen. We have finished the questions and now we will try to answer them starting with Dr. Furman.

S. FURMAN *(New York, U.S.A.):* First, I agree that the rate of rise is absolutely critical and that was the point I made with the rounded signal as opposed to the sharply rising vertical signal.

Second, I think that there will be a much higher incidence of difficulty if there is not an elevated S-T segment. The problem is that, acutely, in a variety of sick patients, you may not see it all the time; you must then reassure yourself that you have achieved the best signal which is possible under the circumstances.

CHAIRMAN: Thank you. Dr. Steinbach.

K. STEINBACH *(Vienna, Austria):* The question Dr. Meibom raises is very important and can easily be answered. You cannot measure and do not have to measure the capacity of the pacemaker output and you will never find it in the specifications of the pacemaker as presented by the companies. But, if you ask the representative, he will tell you the exact capacity: usually, it is 3.5 micro-Farads. Some companies use condensors with higher capacities.

CHAIRMAN: Thank you. Dr. Kozlowski.

J.W. KOZLOWSKI *(Lodz, Poland):* Responding to Dr. Meibom's remark, I had the possibility to see his work in Copenhagen and I agree with him. This team work should be established. There is a lack of arrangements and this is the reason why the technician does not take part in every pacemaker implantation, in Poland. As to reimplantations, cardiologists are doing these, too.

CHAIRMAN: Although I see that there are some more question, we have to close this session. Perhaps some of these questions could be presented to the Round Table on the Pacemaker Clinic.

Thank you for your attention.

I thank the speakers for their cooperation.

Section VII

PACEMAKER ELECTROCARDIOGRAPHY

ECG SURVEY OF VARIOUS PACEMAKER MODES

MAJ LEVANDER-LINDGREN

Let us omit the pioneer, the asynchronous, stubborn mode of pacing and start directly with the more complicated ones, where sensing of spontaneous ECG complexes, mostly QRS, sometimes P-waves, is the prerequisite for adequate function.

Energy wasting, *ventricular synchronized pulse generators* are certainly giving way to energy saving ventricular inhibited pacers. Let us therefore take the opportunity of studying the important sensing, which is clearly indicated with ventricular synchronized pacing, but only indirectly indicated with the ventricular inhibited method.

We will study a series of ECGS from one and the same patient with Mobitz type II A-V block and varying bundle-branch block, treated with a ventricular synchronized pulse generator, at a rate of 60/min. The endocardial electrode is in the apical region of the right ventricle, the pulse generator pocket is abdominal, as in all ECGS shown here. The first, third and fourth ventricular complexes in Figure 1 A are pacemaker induced after blocked A-V transmission. The second ventricular complex is transmitted with LBBB. As the right ventricle is activated early, the synchronized pacing artifact is visible at the very start of QRS. The paced complexes show, as usual, LBBB pattern (1, 2, 3, 4) but the impulse transmission from the electrode is evidently different from that in spontaneous LBBB. The escape interval is a few hundredths of a second longer than the automatic interval, but that is not a true hysteresis.

In Figure 1 B every other impulse is normally transmitted, every other impulse transmitted with LBBB, with early appearance of the synchronized artifact with both types of QRS. That is in contrast with Figure 1 C with RBBB when the artifact appears late in the ventricular complex, as is to be expected with late activation of the right ventricle. This explains, why with inhibited mode of pacing artifacts may appear at escape interval late in a QRS complex: pseudo-fusion beats (5).

In Figure 1 D the patient presented with loss of sensing of spontaneous beats and an asynchronous pacing rate of 52, indicating battery depletion, when the sensing circuit may lose its energy maintenance. The electrode is functioning well and capture is obtained.

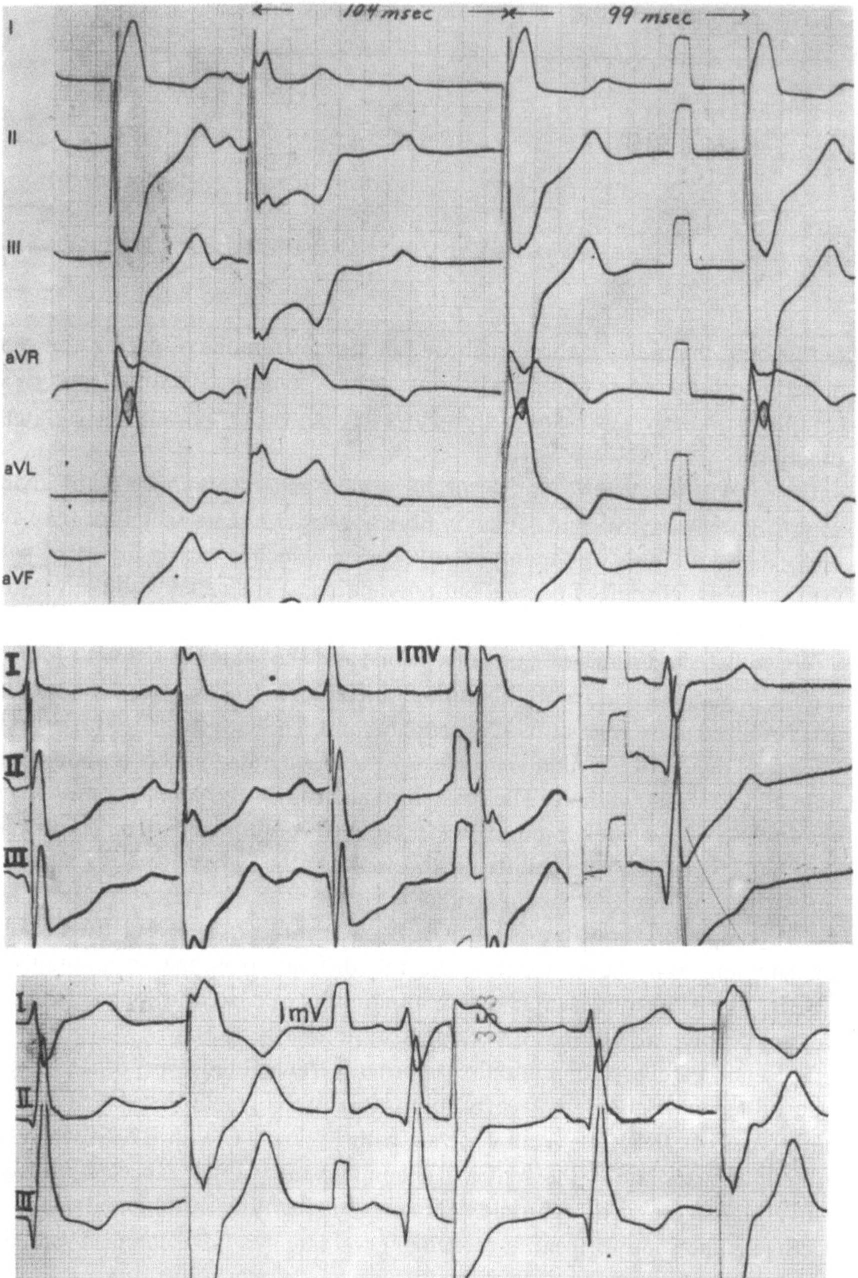

Figure 1. Patient with Mobitz type II block and ventricular synchronized pulse generator, rate 60. A, B and C. The position of the synchronized pacemaker artefact varies with changing intraventricular conduction. D. Battery depletion with decrease in rate and loss of synchronization. Paper speed 50 mm/sec.

Diagnostic problems between triggering by T-waves and premature beats from the electrode area may arise with ventricular synchronized pulse generators as in Figure 2. Thanks to the fact that one of the premature beats started within the refractory period of the pulse generator without synchronizing, the true spontaneous nature of these beats was evident. With ventricular inhibited pulse generators, the spontaneous nature of such premature beats from the electrode area is immediately clear.

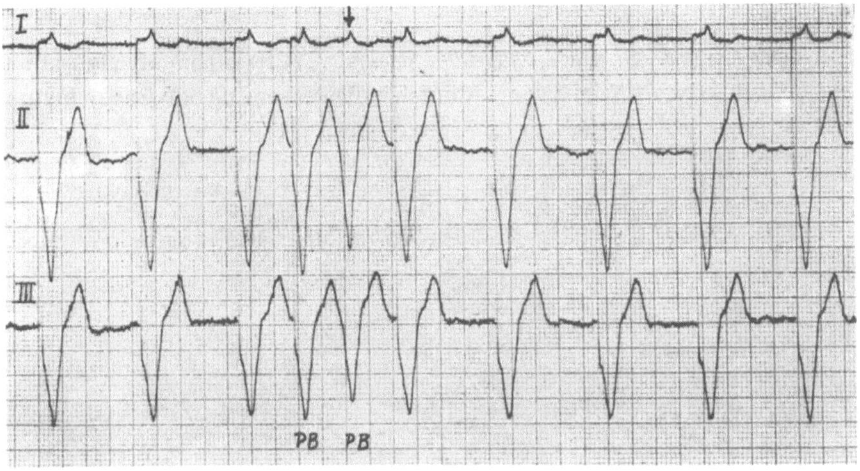

Figure 2. Premature beats (PB) from the electrode area. One of the ectopic beats, indicated by arrow, starts within the refractory period of the ventricular synchronized pulse generator. Paper speed 25 mm/sec.

With *inhibited pulse generators*, the refractory period is as a rule short, often about 350 msec, and the input sensitivity is high, frequently between 1,5 and 2 mV to obtain adequate sensing of spontaneous beats. During an episode of atrial fibrillation a high ventricular rate of about 150 may result in the appearance of some ventricular complexes within the refractory period. This may cause escapes, despite the high ventricular rate.

With long-life pulse generators the problem will probably not be battery depletion but increase of threshold. Threshold measuring on implanted pulse generators will therefore be of the utmost importance. It may be achieved, as in Vitatron pulse generators, by a high frequency receiver circuit which is sharply tuned to 525 kHz. This circuit produces a voltage of reverse polarity to the voltage of the output circuit when the transmitter coil of the pacemaker analyzer is placed over the pulse generator. The pacer is gradually suppressed to values under threshold, which is given in percentage of the total output. The Vario method by Siemens Elema is another approach, by which magnet application converts the pacing mode to asynchronous and stepwise decreases the output down to O, which permits threshold determination. Hysteresis is a method of avoiding unnecessary pacing during physiological slowing down of transmitted sinus rhythm, which may cause symptoms, particularly when there are retrograde P waves. An escape interval of 1200 msec. can be combined with an automatic interval of 1000.

Unnecessary pacing is of course particularly inconvenient when retrograde P waves and even echo-beats appear as may be seen with S-A block. Atrial pacing instead of ventricular pacing is then the method of choice.

In A-V block, *atrial triggered cardiac pacing* (ATCP) is hemodynamically the ideal method of artificial pacing. A notch indicates sensing of P wave, (Figure 3)

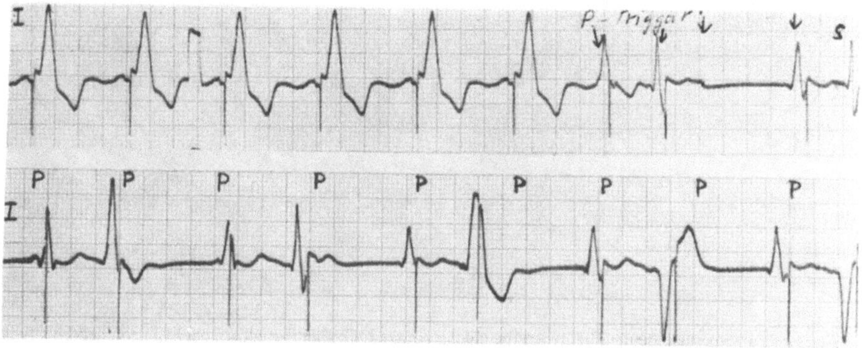

Figure 3. Atrial triggered cardiac pacing interrupted by numerous ventricular premature beats, which trigger the pulse generator. Several P waves appear within the refractory period of the pulse generator. See text. Paper speed 25 mm/sec.

and there is a delay of about 100 msec. till firing of the impulse to the ventricular electrode. There are, however, particular problems associated with ATCP. One of them concerns the refractory period – highest synchronous rate, when the pulse generator starts blocking 2:1. A highest synchronous rate of 150 to 160 will be linked to a short refractory period of 380 to 360 msec, which will make possible stimulation in the vulnerable zone of the T wave. This may happen with atrial ectopic beats or during sinus bradycardia, when the pulse generator starts firing at its basic rate. Some P waves may then appear after the refractory period of a basic beat and trigger the pulse generator, which fires in the vulnerable zone, and may elicit potentially dangerous ventricular ectopic beats.

On the whole, when there is complicating arrhythmia, ATCP may produce a peculiar ECG (6, 7). When first glancing at Figure 3, one does not think of a normally functioning ATCP. The elucidation will be easier, if we start to look at the first part of the ECG with a series of normal sinus rhythm, which ends with a ventricular premature beat. The next two impulses fall within the refractory period of the spontaneous beats. When the following P wave appears, the pulse generator is in its turn refractory. The sinus impulse is probably conducted with a P-R time of 400 msec. A premature beat then reappears which triggers the pulse generator, which thereafter is refractory to the P wave and the series is repeated.

Let us close this review by looking at one of our more recent approaches to cardiac pacing: for treatment of tachycardia, here exemplified by a drug resistant nodal tachycardia. Two myocardial electrodes were implanted on the right auricle, connected to an implanted receiver lead, and activated by a radiofrequency external transmitter. (8). Activating the pulse generator at a rate of 400 during tachycardia restored the sinus rhythm. (Figure 4).

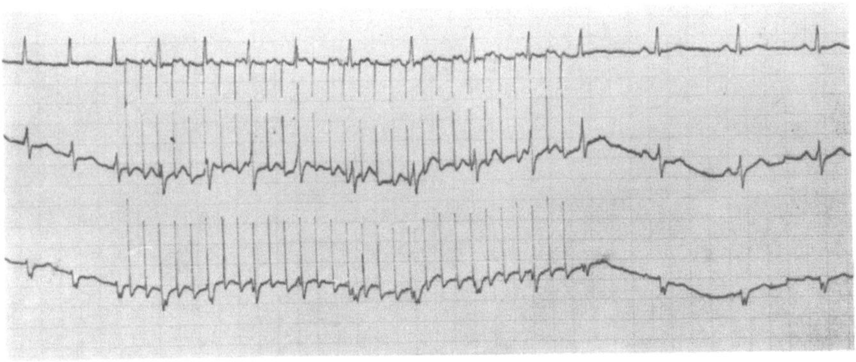

Figure 4. High frequency atrial pacing during nodal reciprocal tachycardia restores sinus rhythm. See text.

References

1. Barold, S. Serge., Modern concepts of cardiac pacing. Heart and Lung. 2, 238 (1973).
2. Castellanos, A., Maytin, Jr. O., Lemberg, L. and Castillo, C., Unusual QRS complexes produced by pacemaker stimuli. Am. Heart J. 77, 732 (1969).
3. Castellanos, A. Jr., Ortix, J.M., Pastis, N. and Castillo, C., The electrocardiogram in patients with pacemakers. Progress in Cardiovascular Dis. 13, 190 (1970).
4. Castellanos, A. Jr., Befeler, B., Myerburg, R.J., Castillo, C.A., Agha, A.S. and Vagueiro, M. C., Functional properties of the ventricular muscle and distal conducting system during right ventricular stimulation. European Cardiol. 1, 41 (1973).
5. Carroll, M., Martin, M. and Kleid, J., Pseudofusion Beats Masquerading as Pacemaker Failure. J. Electrocardiol. 7, 179 (1974).

6. Javier, R. and Samet P., in Samet, P. Cardiac Pacing. P. 115. Electrocardiographic Patterns associated with cardiac pacing. Grune and Stratton, New York 1973.
7. Furman, S. and Escher, D., in Principles and techniques of cardiac pacing. P. 163, 1970. Harper and Row, New York 1970.
8. Kahn, A., Morris, J.J., Citron, P., Patient-Initiated Rapid Atrial Pacing to Manage Supraventricular Tachycardia. Am. J. Cardiol. 38, 200 (1976).

PACEMAKER ELECTROCARDIOGRAPHY – THE IMPORTANCE OF QRS AND T WAVE CONFIGURATION

J. GRAEME SLOMAN, HARRY G. MOND, JITU K. VOHRA AND DAVID HUNT

Summary

The QRS of a pacing rhythm is composed of the stimulus artefact followed by ventricular depolarisation. Depending on the position of the indifferent electrode, the stimulus artefact in unipolar pacing may significantly distort the QRS. A T wave is important in determining if ventricular depolarisation in response to the stimulus artefact has actually occurred.

Right ventricular endocardial pacing produces a left bundle branch block configuration and the frontal plane axis is dependent on the electrode position in the right ventricular cavity. With this type of pacing, a right bundle branch block configuration may result from right ventricular perforation, coronary sinus pacing or, rarely, from pacing in the normal position at the right ventricular apex. Left ventricular epicardial pacing produces a right bundle branch block configuration.

The intracavity electrogram aids in temporary electrode positioning in the right ventricle. The electrogram shows characteristic changes in cases of right ventricular perforation if a continuous recording is performed during electrode withdrawal.

The ventricular pacemaker QRS or depolarisation consists of a stimulus artefact and the subsequent ventricular response.

The stimulus artefact represents the voltage delivered by the pacemaker generator and is seen on the electrocardiograph (ECG) as a perpendicular or voltage deflection of the baseline. The size of this artefact differs according to the ECG lead, but tends to be larger with unipolar compared with bipolar pacing systems. In unipolar pacing, the frontal plane axis of the stimulus artefact is dependent on the position of the indifferent electrode (Fig. 1).

The stimulus artefact may, on occasion, be seen on the ECG without a ventricular response. This may occur with electrode displacement, perforation or threshold problems. If the artefact is large, deflection of the ECG baseline si-

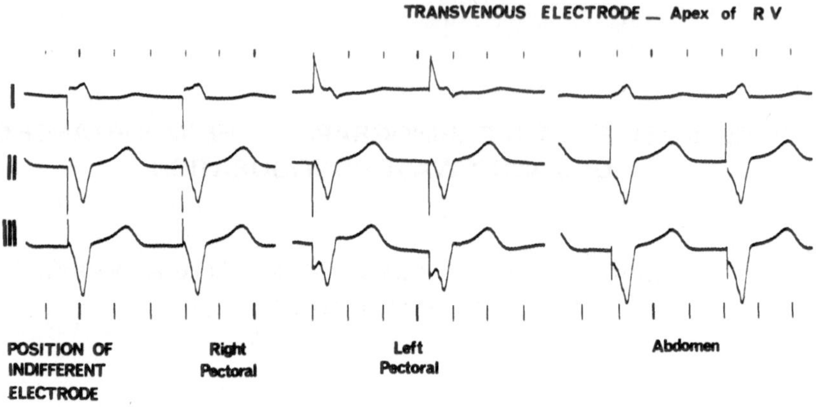

Figure 1. ECG leads 1, 11 and 111 recorded simultaneously, speed 100 mm/sec. Unipolar endocardial pacing was established at five volts with the active electrode at the apex of the right ventricle and the indifferent electrode at three differing positions – right and left pectoral regions and abdomen. The stimulus artefact shows marked vector differences for the three positions. The subsequent QRS complexes show significant distortion by the stimulus artefact. However, only the initial 80 msec of the QRS is distorted. The terminal part of the QRS for each lead is similar, althought its position relative to the baseline may differ.

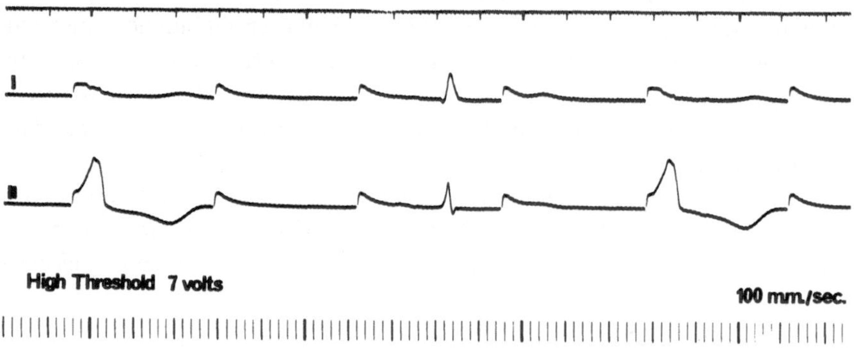

Figure 2. ECG leads 1 and 11 recorded at speed 100 mm/sec. The endocardial electrode has been positioned at the outflow tract of the right ventricle and the pacing threshold was seven volts. Intermittent pacing was established. The pacemaker artefact without ventricular depolarisation (complexes 2, 3, 5 and 7) have shown baseline distortion of the ECG. The first and sixth QRS complexes are paced beats, as they are initiated by a stimulus artefact and are identical to the beats seen at a higher voltage (not shown). The first part of the QRS complex is identical to the early baseline distortion. In lead 11, the QRS has a positive vector as the impulse originates in the right ventricular outflow tract. The fourth complex is a spontaneous QRS resulting from intermittent pacing.

mulating a QRS complex occurs and, therefore, it is important to confirm true ventricular depolarisation by noting a subsequent T wave (Fig. 2).

On inspection of pacing rhythms, the QRS complex may be modified or deformed by the preceding stimulus artefact. This produces a fusion between the true QRS and the baseline deflection. The deformity of the QRS is significant with unipolar high voltage pacing in ECG leads where the stimulus artefact vector is opposite to the QRS vector. In Figure 3, the tip of a temporary bipolar pace-

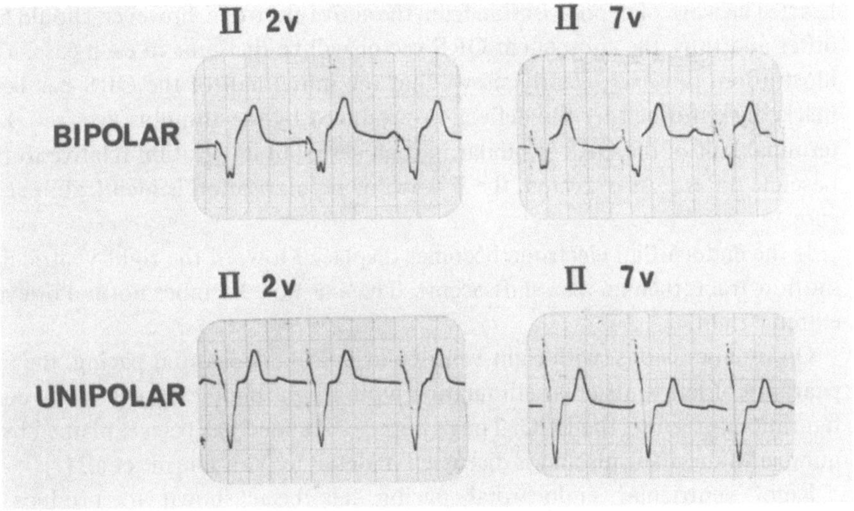

Figure 3. Using a bipolar transvenous electrode positioned at the apex of the right ventricle and a subcutaneous indifferent electrode, both bipolar and unipolar pacing was established at two and seven volts. With both types of pacing there was an increase in the size of the stimulus artefact on increasing the voltage. However, with bipolar pacing, the stimulus artefact vector is similar to the QRS vector and only minor distortion oftthe QRS occurs at high voltages. With unipolar pacing, the vectors are opposite and marked distortion occurs at high voltages.

maker electrode lies at the apex of the right ventricle. Using an external generator and a subcutaneous indifferent electrode plate, cardiac pacing has been established using bipolar and unipolar systems. In both modes, the heart has been paced at two and seven volts. The bipolar artefact is small and its predominant vector negative like the subsequent QRS. Increasing the voltage results in a minor increase in stimulus artefact size and QRS deformity. With unipolar pacing the deformity is minor at two volts. At seven volts, however, the predominant stimulus artefact vector has now become positive and opposite to the QRS vector. There is now a significant QRS deformity.

Vector analysis of the pacemaker QRS reveals typical characteristics when pacing is established from various parts of the heart and a knowledge of the configurations can be very valuable in clinical pacing.

Unipolar endocardial pacing from the apex of the right ventricle results in a characteristic 12 lead ECG. The anterior chest leads show a left bundle branch block configuration and the frontal plane vector is to the extreme left. However, in unipolar pacing this frontal plane axis appears modified by altering the position of the indifferent electrode. In Figure 1, ECG leads 1, 11 and 111 are recorded using three separate indifferent electrode positions. In each case, there has been significant alteration in the stimulus artefact vector as this is dependent on the position of the indifferent electrode relative to the active electrode in the heart. The wave of depolarisation from the active electrode, however, should not differ and thus, the subsequent QRS vector will be the same in each case. The illustration, however, clearly shows that the initial half of the QRS has been markedly deformed by the deflection produced by the stimulus artefact. The terminal half of the QRS is similar in each case, but its position relative to the baseline differs. As expected, the T wave or repolarisation is identical in each case.

If the endocardial electrode becomes displaced toward the right ventricular outflow tract, then an axis shift occurs. The axis now becomes normal or even extreme right.

On rare occasions, with right ventricular apical endocardial pacing, the appearance of left ventricular stimulation with a right bundle branch block configuration is seen on the ECG. The pattern so obtained has been explained by a number of mechanisms and is discussed in detail by Van Durme et al. (1).

Right ventricular endocardial pacing has been shown to produce a right bundle branch block configuration in other situations. Perforation of the anterior right ventricular wall with the tip of the pacemaker electrode in the pericardial cavity will produce a right bundle branch block, provided pacing continues (2). Direct perforation of the intraventricular septum is very rare, but it too will result in right bundle branch block pacing (3).

The other situation which results in a right bundle branch block configuration on the ECG is inadvertent placement of the transvenous electrode in the coronary sinus. This situation should be readily diagnosed with a left lateral chest radiograph. In normal right ventricular apical pacing, the electrode passes anteriorly through the tricuspid valve and is placed against the anterior aspect of the cardiac silhouette. With coronary sinus pacing, however, the electrode is not placed forward, but rather lies on the posterior aspect of the heart in the coronary sinus or cardiac vein. The postero-anterior chest radiograph may not be helpful as the electrode may appear to lie at the apex of the right ventricle. The ECG reveals a right bundle block configuration and the axis is dependent on the positioning of the electrode in the heart. If the electrode lies toward the apex, then the axis is extreme left. If, on the poster-anterior chest radiograph, the electrode is displaced upwards, with the tip directed toward the hilum of the left lung, then the axis is either normal or even to the right.

Epicardial left ventricular pacing has a right bundle branch block configuration. Because these electrodes are implanted at varying positions on the anterior left ventricular surface, the axis will be variable and thus not as significant as with right ventricular endocardial pacing.

The intracavity electrogram is a simple means of recording the electrical potentials from the heart. The technique is useful in placing temporary pacemaker electrodes in the right ventricle when fluoroscopic facilities are not available (4). When the electrode makes contact with the right ventricular endocardium, a "current of injury" pattern characterised by ST elevation and T wave inversion occurs. In contrast, coronary sinus recordings have no such pattern.

As well as being useful for electrode placement, such electrograms are of value for the correct diagnosis of right ventricular perforation. Recordings are performed as the electrode is withdrawn from the epicardial surface (5). Figure 4 is an

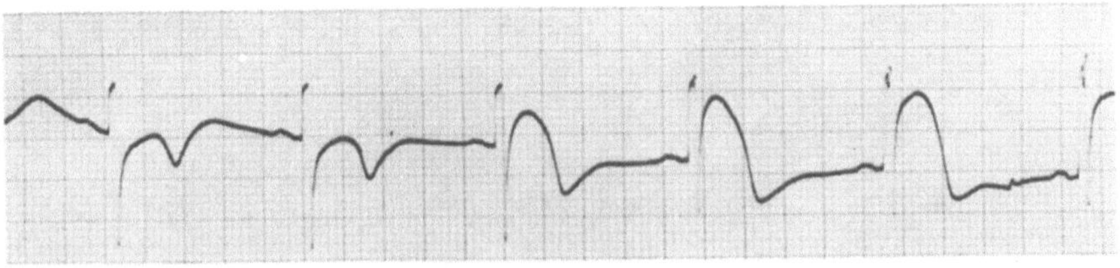

Figure 4. Withdrawal intracardiac electrogram of a perforated unipolar permanent electrode. The initial part of the tracing shows a biphasic QRS with a dominant S wave. On gradual withdrawal of the electrode, the QRS vector becomes markedly positive with an endocardial "current of injury" pattern.

illustration of such a withdrawal. A permanent unipolar electrode had perforated the ventricle at the time of implantation and the threshold of pacing was greater than eight volts. The unipolar intracavity electrogram revealed a biphasic epicardial QRS pattern. With a continuous electrogram recording, the electrode was slowly withdrawn. The QRS vector became markedly positive and an endocardial "current of injury" pattern with ST elevation and T wave inversion noted. The threshold of pacing was now 0.7 volts. This change in electrograph pattern is diagnostic of perforation and thus, this simple procedure should always be performed if myocardial perforation is suspected.

Thus, in conclusion, the interpretation of the pacemaker ECG requires understanding of both the stimulus artefact and the QRS. The stimulus artefact may significantly alter the initial part of the QRS in unipolar pacing. Specific ECG patterns for pacing from various sites have been described. The intracavity electrogram is useful for positioning of temporary electrodes and is diagnostic of electrode perforation if the procedure is performed whilst withdrawing the electrode.

References

1. Van Durme, J.P., Heyndrickx, G., Snoeck, J., Vermeire, P. and Pannier, R., Diagnosis of myocardial perforation by intracardiac electrograms recorded from the indwelling catheter. *J. Electrocardiology* 6, 97 (1973).
2. Barold, S.S. and Gaidula, J.J., Selected electrocardiographic manifestations of cardiac pacing. *Cardiology Digest* 7, 16 (1972).
3. Stillman, M.T. and Richard, A. McD., Perforation of the interventricular septum by transvenous pacemaker catheter. *Amer. J. Cardiol.* 24, 269 (1969).
4. Evans, G.L. and Glasser, S.P., Intracavity electrocardiography as a guide to pacemaker positioning. *JAMA* 216, 483 (1971).
5. Mond, H.G., Stuckey, J.G. and Sloman, G., The diagnosis of right ventricular perforation by an endocardial pacemaker electrode. *Pace* 1, 62 (1978).

ELECTROCARDIOGRAPHIC DIAGNOSIS OF MYOCARDIAL INFARCTION AND CORONARY INSUFFICIENCY IN THE PACEMAKER PATIENT

B. DODINOT, L. KUBLER, E. ALIOT AND A. RIO

For more than 10 years after the worldwide acceptance of ventricular pacing, the electrocardiographic (ecg) diagnosis of myocardial infarction (M.I.) was considered as impossible to make in the paced patients in the absence of spontaneous ventricular complexes, the abnormal ventricular depolarization and the presence of the stimulus masking the usual pattern of M.I.

Cardenas (1) was the first to show that the diagnosis of M.I. was occasionally possible. Several papers were recently published on this subject which was particularly studied by Barold (2, 3, 4) in the United States and Kulbertus (5) in Europe.

The same negative attitude was also adopted relative to the diagnosis of coronary insufficiency since secondary abnormalities of the repolarization were present not only on the paced but also on the spontaneous complexes as described in 1964 by Chatterjee (6).

Most papers published on these subjects deal with temporary pacing or bipolar permanent pacing and refer to cases report.

From 1962 to 1976, 2700 patients had a permanent pacemaker implanted in our institution. More than 1800 are alive and in most instances treated by transvenous unipolar pacing.

The purpose of this paper is to try to find out if the diagnosis of M.I. and coronary insufficiency is effectively possible in the permanently paced patient.

1. Myocardial infarction

Out of 1820 pacemaker patients alive and followed in our clinics, 72 (4%) had a M.I. prior (59) or after (13) implantation.

Spontaneous ventricular activity was present in 68 patients either during passive ecg recording or after pacemaker artificial inhibition. Analysis of these spontaneous complexes made the diagnosis of M.I. possible in 64 cases. No definite conclusion could be drawn in the 4 remaining patients with left bundle block (LBBB) or right ventricular ectopic beats from the aspect of the autonomous complexes.

A. Analysis of the paced QRS

All patterns described as typical of M.I. in the presence of LBBB were searched in our 72 patients on 12 lead electrocardiograms recorded at different intervals.

1. Inferior wall myocardial infarction (31)

In no instances was it possible to see any particular pattern suggesting a M.I. even in the six cases who developed M.I. after their implantation.

2. Anterior wall infarction (38 cases)

Included in this group are 7 patients with associate diaphragmatic M.I. Out of 35 patients treated by unipolar pacemakers, the ST QR pattern described by Castellanos was never found in lead I and VL in all instances and apparently present in V5 V6 in only one patient. It was present in one out of the 3 patients treated by bipolar pacing (fig. 1).

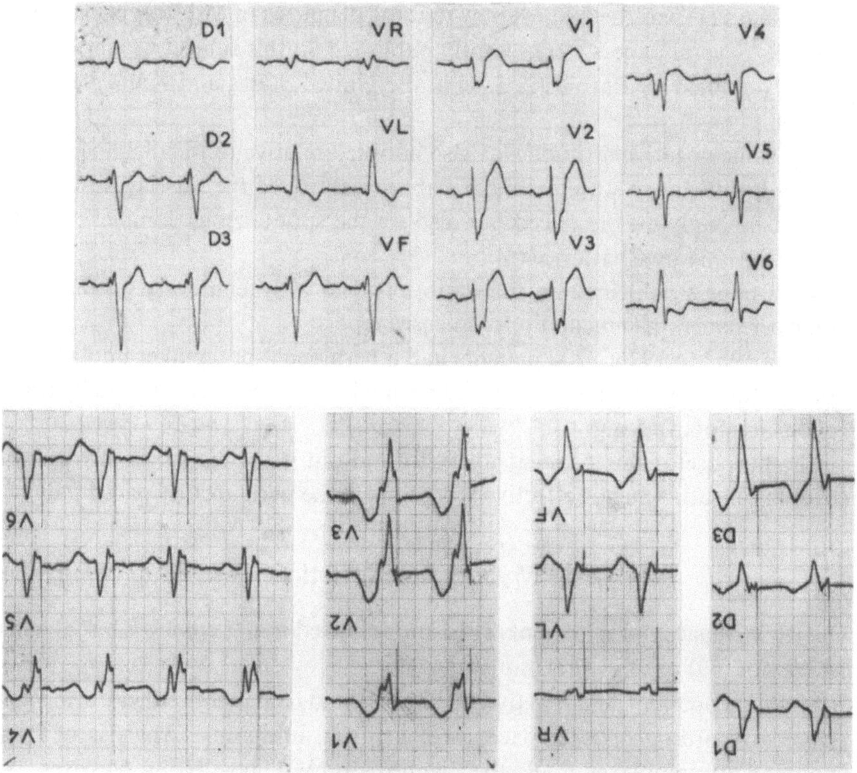

Figure 1.

The most constant aspect evoking an extensive anterior wall infarction was a large and late notch of the S wave (> 0,05 s) in lead V3 V4 and occasionally V5 (fig. 1 and 2). This aspect was described by Cabrera in patients with LBB and anteroseptal myocardial infarction exhibiting Q waves from V1 to V6 but not in localized anteroseptal myocardial infarction. No specific axis deviation was found in patients with myocardial infarction compared to others.

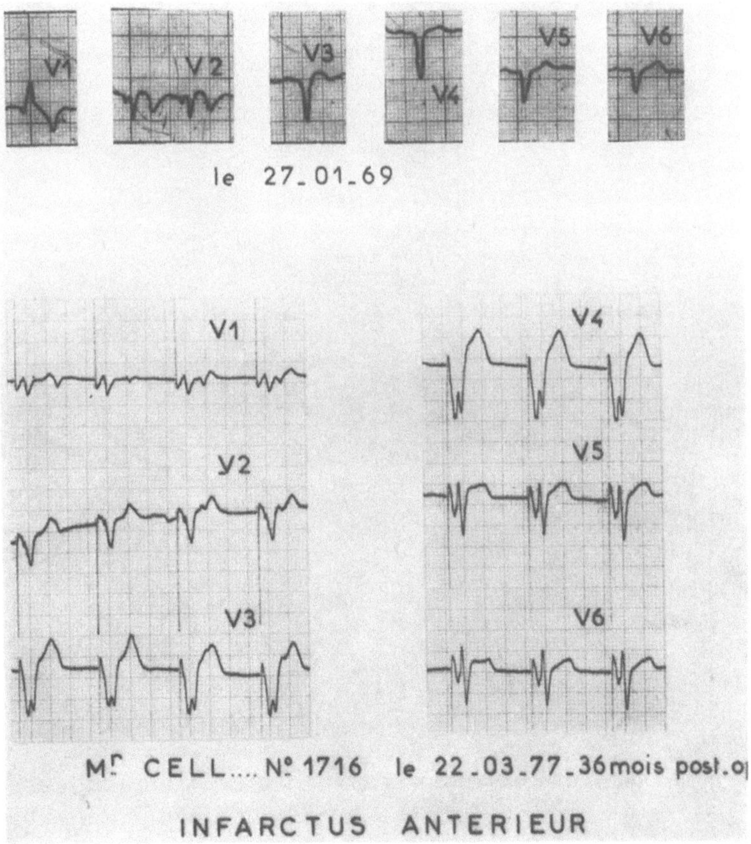

Figure 2.

3. *Non-localized myocardial infarction (3)*

In 3 patients the diagnosis of M.I. was made solely by clinical and biological criteria in the absence of any electrocardiographic abnormalities.

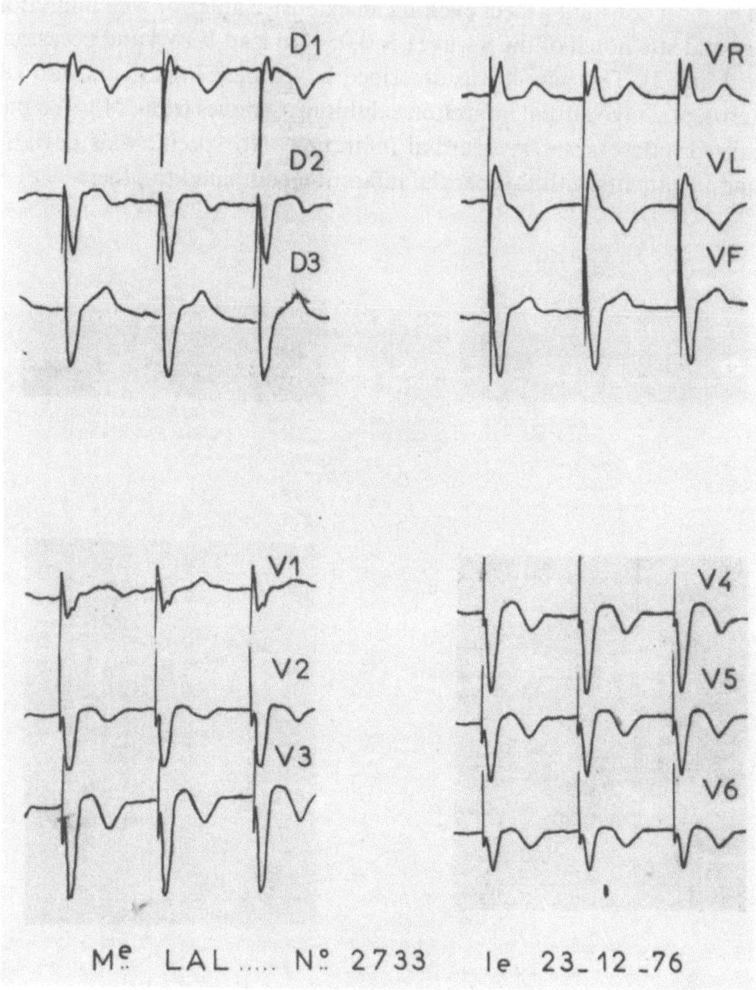

Figure 3a.

B. Repolarization

No statistical difference was found in the repolarization of the paced beats in patients with sequellae of M.I. and others.

In one patient, marked ST T waves elevation in chest leads contrasting with the negative T waves observed in the same leads several days before appeared two hours before death (fig. 3). Autopsy of this patient treated by a unipolar implanted transvenous pacemaker showed a massive anterior wall infarction.

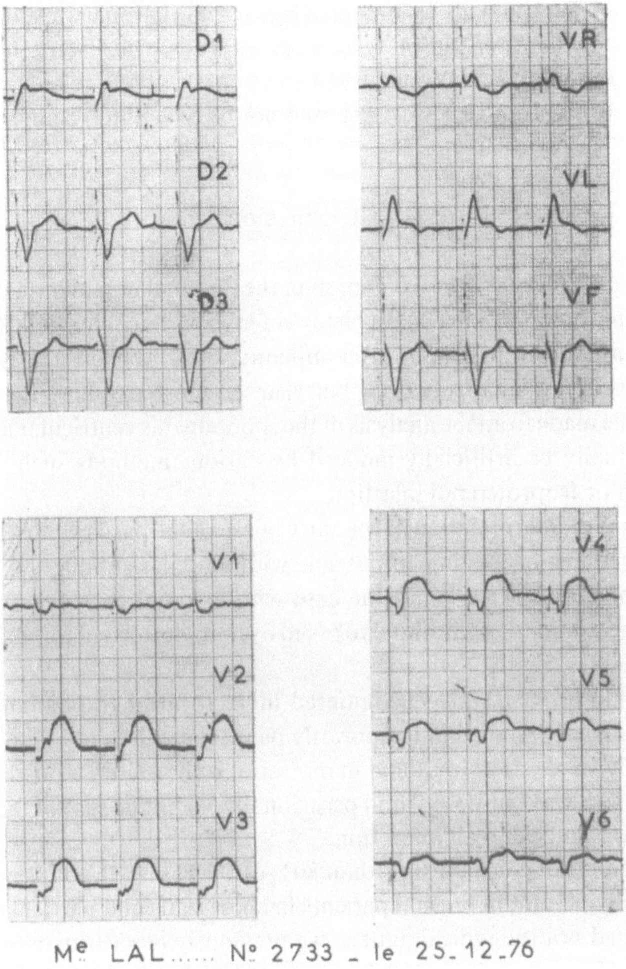

Figure 3b.

2. Coronary insufficiency

Permanent ventricular stimulation induces secondary marked changes of the repolarization of the spontaneous complexes. This is however only evident in the absence of intra-ventricular conduction defects. In the pacemaker patient, the incidence of T waves changes depends upon the relationship between paced and spontaneous beats.

A patient with a constantly inhibited pacemaker will have normal spontaneous T waves which may become inverted if he returns to complete heart block. Too many patients were treated for an acute coronary insufficiency on the basis of massive inversion of T waves in all leads which were in fact the consequence of the cardiac stimulation.

Inversely all negative T waves should not be related to pacing.

Discussion

Myocardial infarction is not common in the pacemaker patient: less than 4% of our patients presently alive had a history of myocardial infarction. The incidence of acute myocardial infarction after implantation is even lower: less than 0,5% in our series, approximatively 0,2% per year. In most instances the diagnosis of M.I. can be made from the analysis of the spontaneous ventricular activity which can eventually be artificially induced by various methods such as chest wall inhibition or Isoproterenol injection.

Attempts of interpretation of the early phase of the paced ventricular depolarization are most of the time impossible with unipolar stimulation and even bipolar stimulation. This is not the case with external pacemakers adjusted at border line stimulation threshold to avoid overshoots related to a high amplitude signal.

The same problems are encountered in vectocardiographic analysis which were particularly studied in temporarily paced patients.

The only valid criterium found in our series is the presence of a large and late notch of the S wave in V3, V4 and occasionally V5, in the case of the presence of an extensive anterior wall infarction.

This sign is not constant (less than 80% of the cases). If notched S waves are occasionally present in normal patients in chest leads and particularly V5, they however had not the typical pattern we previously described: either present in one lead only and particularly V5 or not sufficiently late or large.

Little information can be drawn from the study of the repolarization of the T waves of the paced beats. If occasionally marked changes can be obviously related to an acute coronary insufficiency with or without myocardial infarction as described by Barold and met twice in our series, this appears to be an exception. In the absence of obvious alterations or marked changes recorded between two electrocardiograms made with the same type of recorder, the morphology of these pacemaker induced T waves should not be interpreted.The same careful attitude should be adopted to interpret the repolarization of the spontaneous ventricular complexes which may vary in the same patient depending upon the frequency of the stimulation.

Conclusion

The diagnosis of myocardial infarction and coronary insufficiency in patients treated by cardiac pacemakers is always difficult and occasionally impossible even in the presence of spontaneous ventricular depolarization. Clinical symptoms and biological changes should not be neglected and should be considered as determinant when the electrocardiographic aspect is not convincing. This is one of the paradoxes of modern technology to sometimes oblige the medical profession to rely more on old clinical medicine than on sophisticated tests.

References

1. Cardenas, M.L., Sanz, G., Linares, J.C., Zamora, C., Medrano, G.A., Estandria, A., Diagnostico electrocardiographico de infarto del miocardio en pacientes con estimulacion endocardica del ventriculo derecho por marcapasos. *Arch. Instit. Cardiol. Mexico* 42, 345 (1972).
2. Barold, S.S. and Ong, L.S., Electrocardiographic diagnosis of myocardial infarction in patients with transvenous ventricular pacemakers. In Proceedings of Colloquium on Cardiac Pacing, J. Norman and A. Rickards, eds. *Arnheim, The Netherlands*, 1975.
3. Barold, S. Serge, Ong, Ling, S. Heinle, Robert A., Electrocardiographic Diagnosis of Myocardial Infarction in Patients with transvenous pacemakers. *J. Electrocardiol.* 9; 99 (1976).
4. Barold, S. Serge, Wayne, A.N., Wallace, Ong, Ling, S. and Heinle, Robert A., Primary ST and T Wave abnormalities in the diagnosis of Acute Anterior Myocardial Infarction during permanent ventricular pacing. *J. Electrocardiol.* 9, 387 (1976).
5. Kulbertus, G.E. and Deleval Ruiten, F., Vectorcardiographic study of QRS in patients with transvenous pacemakers and myocardial infarction. *J. Electrocardiol.* 7, 27 (1974).
6. Chatterjee, K., Harris, A., Davies, G., Leatham, A., Electrocardiographic changes subsequent to artificial ventricular depolarization. *Br. Heart J.* 31, 770 (1969).
7. Castellanos, A., Zoble, R., Procacci, P.M., Myerburg, R.J., Berkovits, B.V., ST-qR pattern: New sign for diagnosis of anterior myocardial infarction during right ventricular pacing. *Br. Heart J.* 35, 1161 (1973).
8. Cabrera, E., Friedland, C., La Onda de Activacion ventricular en el bloqueo de rama izquierda con infarto miocardico (un nuevo signo electrocardiografico); *Arch. Inst. Mexico* 23, 441 (1953).

THE IRREGULAR PACEMAKER: MECHANISMS AND CLINICAL SIGNIFICANCE

A. Wirtzfeld, Ch. Himmler and H.W. Präuer

An implanted cardiac pacemaker usually stimulates the heart in an extremely regular fashion and any irregularity documented in the electrocardiogram must be recognized and analyzed for its mechanism and clinical significance. It is certainly impossible within fifteen minutes to give a complete discourse on the numerous mechanisms which may lead to an irregular pacemaker discharge and I will rather confine myself to the discussion of a few clinical examples of irregularly discharging pulse generators.

Fig. 1 represents the ECG of a patient with a totally irregular R-wave inhibited demand pacemaker. The intervals between the stimuli vary from 920 to 1380 ms.

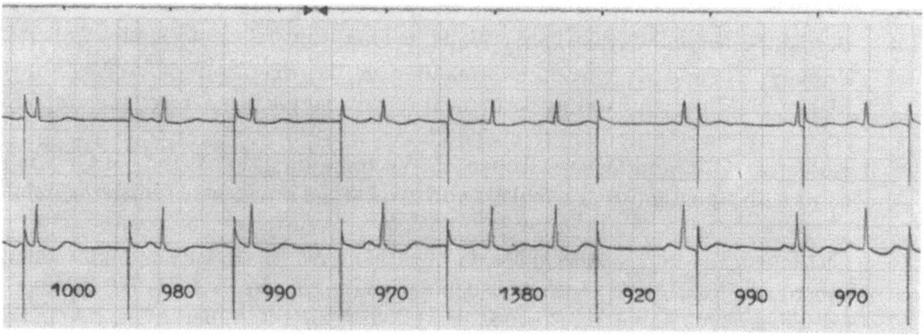

Figure 1. Irregular pacemaker discharge and complete exit- and entrance block in a defective R-wave inhibited pulse generator.

The pacemaker discharge remained irregular even when the magnet for reversion to asynchronous pacing was applied and the pulse generator could no longer be inactivated by chest wall stimulation. In addition, there is complete exit block as the stimuli are not followed by ventricular depolarizations.

The reason for this malfunction was an electronic defect in the pulse generator's circuit and this diagnosis was confirmed by the manufacturer. Erratic pacing is a very uncommon manifestation of a pacemaker defect indeed, and – in our experience – this diagnosis is often made too liberally before other more common mechanisms leading to pacing irregularities have been excluded. Of course, such a pacemaker has to be exchanged immediately.

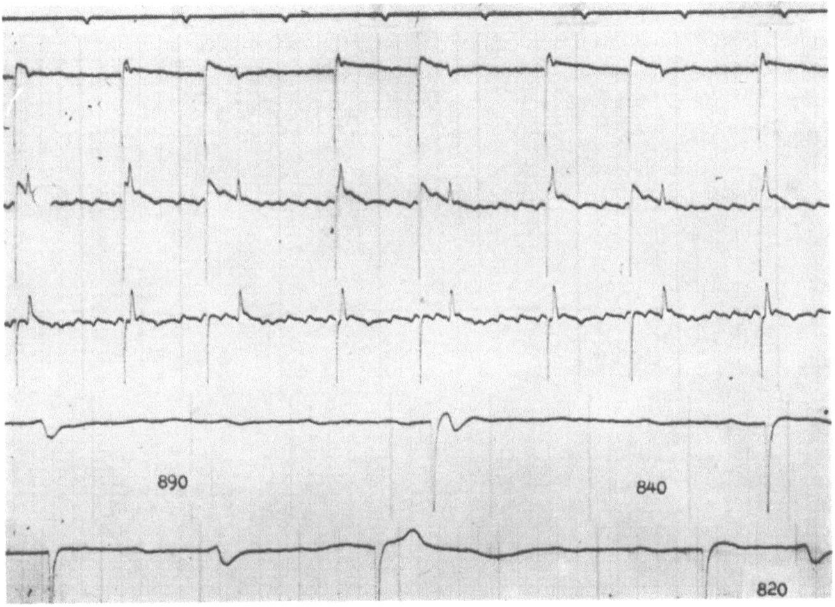

Figure 2. Pacemaker exit block due to a rise in myocardial threshold in a normally functioning R-wave inhibited pulse generator leading to irregular pacemaker discharge.
a) Lead I, II and III (25 mm/sec).
b) Lead I (100 mm/sec).
c) Lead I (100 mm/sec) after applying the test magnet.

Fig. 2 represents an ECG which superficially resembles the previous one. Again the pacemaker discharge is irregular and the heart does not respond to the electric stimuli. A more careful examination of the tracing, however, reveals that the discharge rate is not completely erratic as in fig. 1 but that the intervals between some of the spontaneously occurring beats and the next pacemaker discharge are identical amounting to 890 ms which equals the escape interval of this pacemaker model. Besides, the short intervals between two consecutive pacemaker discharges are identical amounting to the normal pace interval of 840 ms. Application of the magnet reveals a normal fixed-rate interval of 820 ms. These observations indicate that the sensing as well as the discharge mechanism of this pulse generator are intact; those QRS complexes which failed to recycle the pacemaker fall within the pacer's refractory period and so could not be detected.

The diagnosis of the pacemaker malfunction in this case, therefore, is complete exit block due to a rise in myocardial threshold and repositioning of the stimulating lead rather than exchanging the pulse generator will be the appropriate treatment.

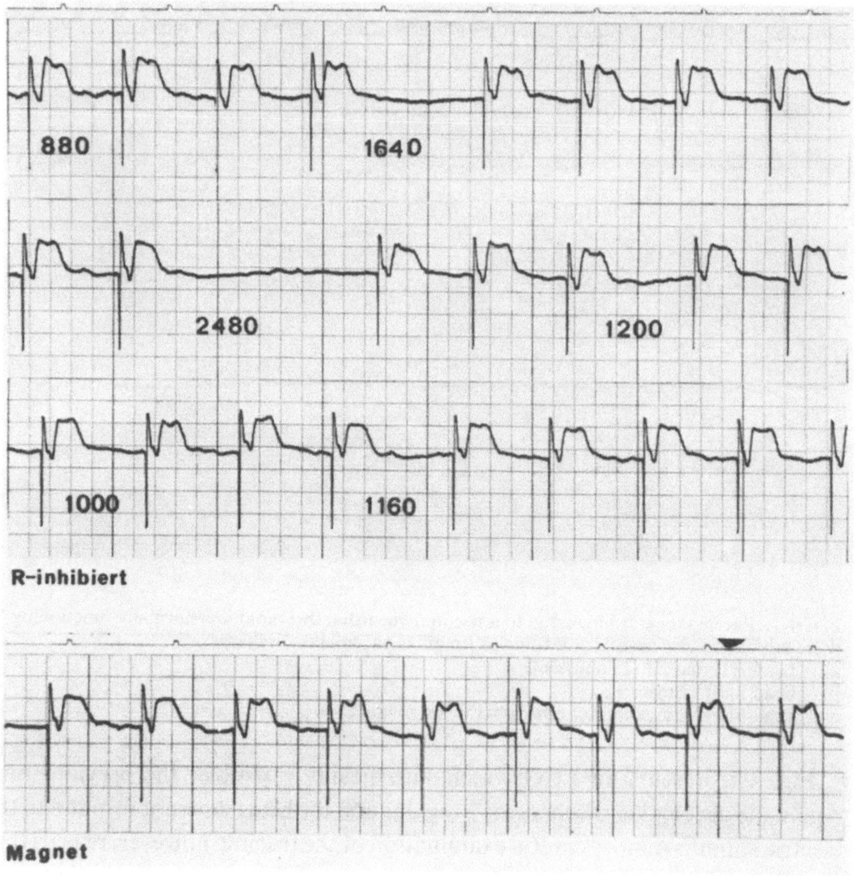

Figure 3. Irregular pacing due to intermittent pacemaker inhibition by false signals originating from a fractured electrode lead.
a) Continuous rhythm strip in the R-wave inhibited mode.
b) Regular pacing after application of the magnet.

Fig. 3 shows another example of a grossly irregular pacemaker discharge. But this time there is no exit block, all the electrostimuli are followed by ventricular depolarizations. Besides, on close inspection of the tracing one realizes that unlike the example in fig. 1 many pacing intervals are identical corresponding to the normal automatic interval of this pacemaker of 880 ms. These periods of regular pacing are interrupted by longer pauses of asystole which are not a multiple of the basic automatic interval. This pattern should alert us to the possibility that false signals intermittently inhibit the pacer's demand circuit and we can confirm this assumption by converting the pulse generator to fixed rate pacing by applying the test magnet resulting in uninterrupted regular pacing.

The source for the false signals in this patient was a fractured electrode lead which by intermittent resistance changes produced voltages sufficiently high to saturate the input amplifier and to simulate spontaneous cardiac activity.

Quite a similar ECG pattern of chaotic pacing may occasionally be encountered in patients with unipolar demand pacemakers when they activate the skeletal muscles close to the implantation site of the pulse generator. In these cases myopotentials originating from the activated muscles may inhibit the demand circuit. The example shown in fig. 4 represents an unusually marked disturbance in pacemaker function by skeletal muscle activity during movement of the right arm necessitating the exchange of the ventricular inhibited generator to a fixed rate unit.

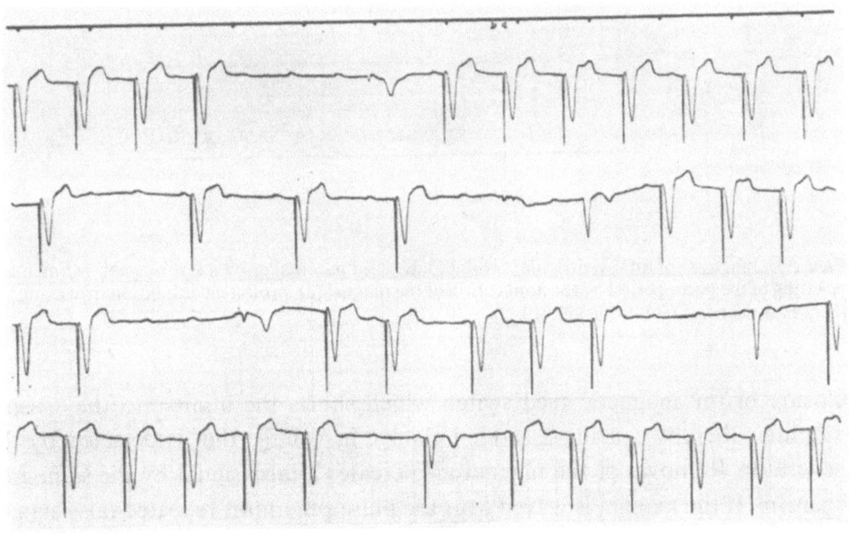

Figure 4. Irregular pacing due to muscle potential interference. Continuous rhythm strip lead III during movement of the right arm.

The differential diagnosis between myopotential interference and false signals originating in a broken lead or a loose pacemaker-electrode connection may sometimes be difficult. But in the latter case irregular pacing can usually be provoked by active as well as passive movements whereas myopotential interference requires a strong active muscle contraction. Besides, a broken lead can usually be diagnosed by photoanalysis.

False signals may also originate from various other sources including those coming from outside the body. For example, moving a test magnet towards a demand pulse generator creates a false signal which will temporarily inhibit a demand pacemaker and reset the pacing period (fig. 5). The signal is produced by

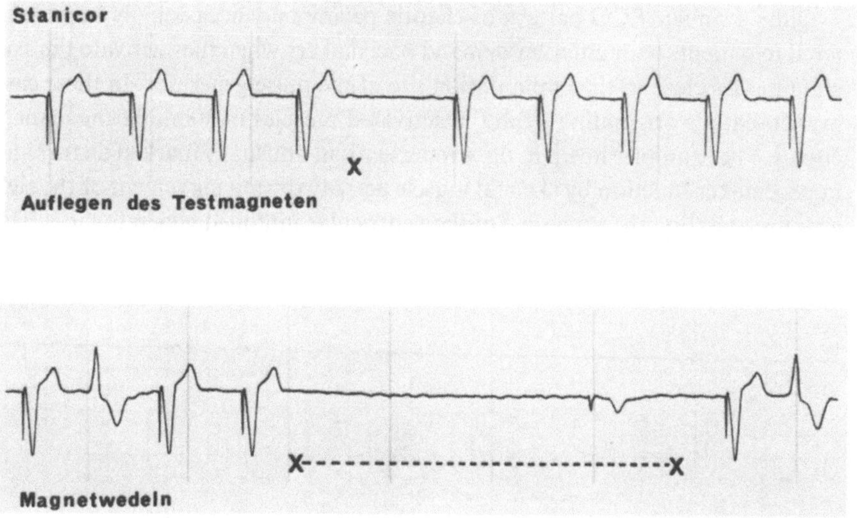

Figure 5. Inactivation of a ventricular inhibited demand pacemaker by a test magnet. Momentary resetting of the pacer period by the application of the magnet (a), prolonged inhibition by waving the magnet over the implantation site (b).

closure of the magnetic reed switch which shorts the input into the sensing amplifier thereby causing a sudden change in voltage that is detected by the generator. Removal of the magnet also creates a false signal by the same mechanism. If the magnet is waved over the pulse generator, repeated false signals may be produced and the pacemaker may respond by longer periods of inhibition. R-wave synchronous pacemakers will respond to false signals by acceleration of the pacing rate (fig. 6).

Another source of electrical interference producing irregular pacing of an implanted on demand pacemaker recently occurred at our Coronary Care Unit (fig. 7). In this unit motor operated hospital beds are used, and we noticed that every time the patient activated the bed's electric hydraulic mechanism the monitor ECG was superimposed by AC interference which quite obviously in-

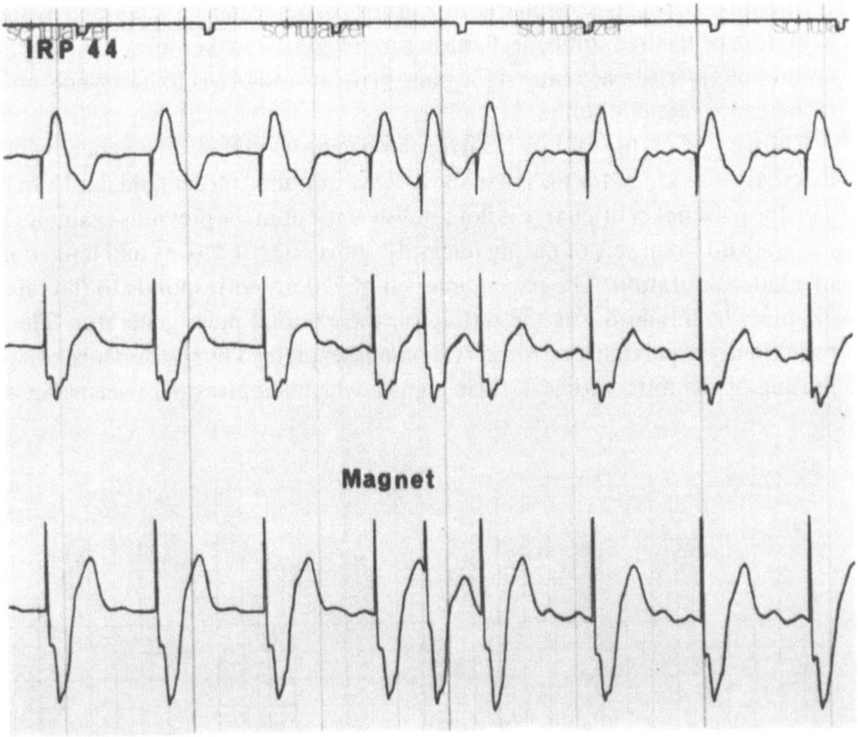

Figure 6. Triggering of extrastimuli in a ventricular-synchronous standby-pacemaker by moving a test magnet.

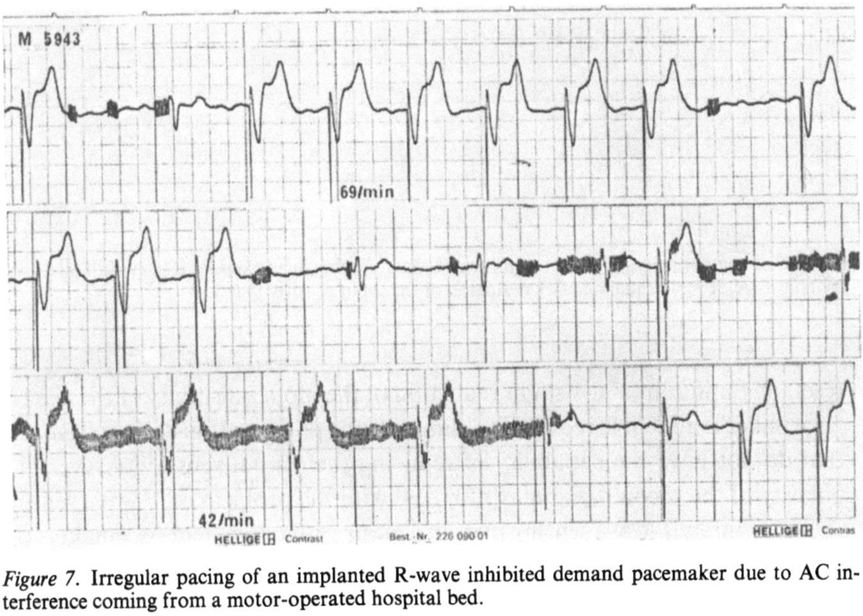

Figure 7. Irregular pacing of an implanted R-wave inhibited demand pacemaker due to AC interference coming from a motor-operated hospital bed.

fluenced the pacemaker discharge rate. Bursts of interference, generated by short actuation of the hydraulic mechanism provoked pacemaker inhibition whereas continuous interference caused the pulse generator to revert to its asynchronous interference rate of 42/min.

The next ECG (fig. 8) showing irregular pacing was taken on a patient with an external pulse generator pacing in the R-wave inhibited on demand mode. In this case the pacemaker discharge is not totally erratic as in the previous examples but there are different sets of pacing intervals: short ones of 770 ms and longer ones of 1320 ms duration. The pacing interval of 770 ms corresponds to the rate of 78/min which indeed was the setting on the external pulse generator. The intermittently occurring longer intervals can be explained by the presence of oversensing of the intracardiac T-wave signals which suppress the pacemaker and

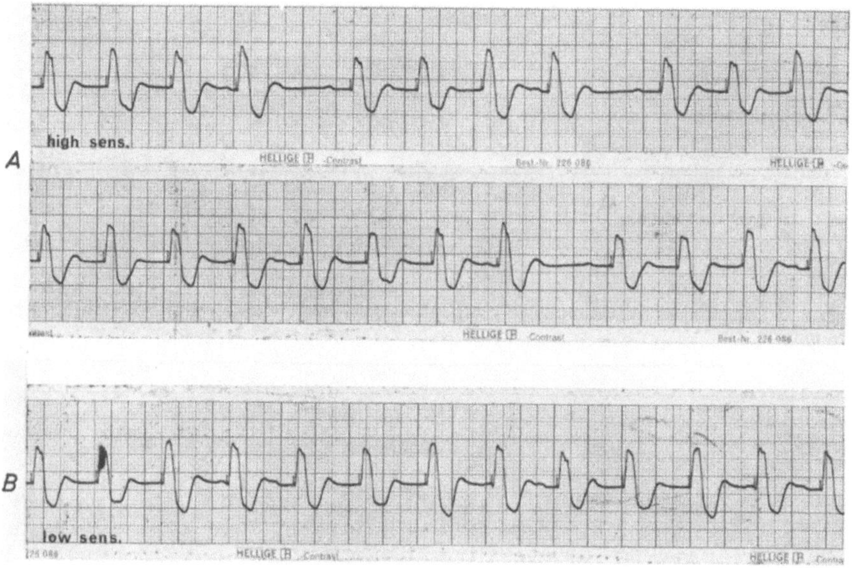

Figure 8. Irregular pacing due to intermittent T-wave sensing in an external R-wave inhibited pulse generator (A). Regular pacing after reduction of the input sensitivity (B).

reset the timing circuit. A slight reduction of the input sensitivity of the external pacemaker is all that is required to eliminate the problem (fig. 8). In pacemakers that do not have the capability of reducing their input sensitivity reversal of polarity of the bipolar lead may also deal with the problem of T-wave sensing.

Occasionally T-wave sensing may also occur with permanent pacemakers (fig. 9). During spontaneous on demand pacing the pacing interval temporarily in-

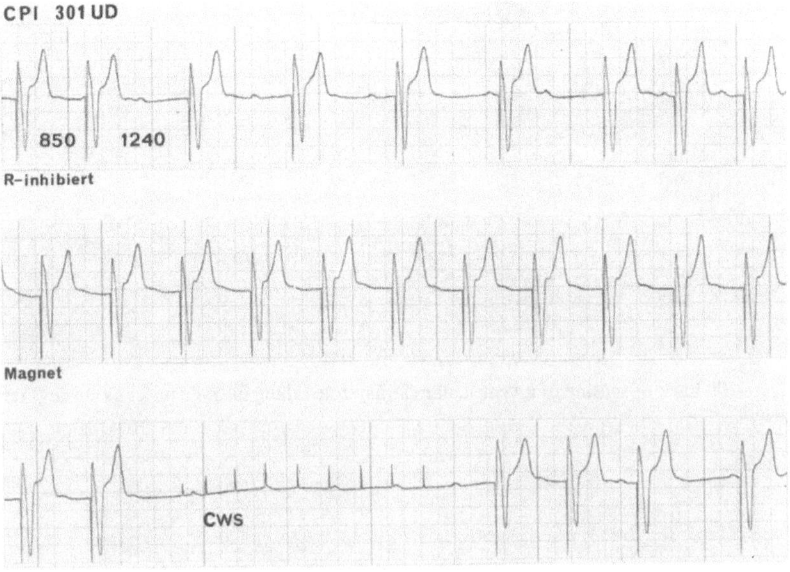

Figure 9. Intermittent T-wave sensing in an implanted R-wave inhibited pulse generator (a). Normal reversion to regular fixed rate pacing by applying the magnet (b). Inhibition of the pacemaker by chest wall stimulation (c).

creases from its normal 850 ms to 1240 ms which represents a drop in pacing rate from 70 to 48/min. The presence of oversensing can easily be confirmed by conversion to fixed rate pacing by applying the test magnet (middle tracing). The bottom tracing demonstrates the pacer's normal demand mechanism by inactivating the pacemaker by external chest wall stimulation.

The phenomenon of intermittent T-wave sensing may sometimes disappear a few days after insertion of the electrode but in other cases the pulse generator has to be changed to a less sensitive model or to a model with different input filter characteristics.

Not only the various manifestations of oversensing but also the phenomenon of undersensing may lead to an inappropriate and irregular pacemaker discharge. In fig. 10, showing the ECG from a patient with an implanted Omnistanicor pacemaker programmed at a rate of 60/min the ventricular extrasystole occurring after the third spontaneous beat does not reset the timing circuit. The reason for it not being detected is quite obvious in this case: The PVC falls within the pacer's (sensing) refractory period which in an Omnicor pacemaker set at 60/min amounts to 375 ms. The tracing therefore represents a normal pacemaker function and no corrective measures are warranted.

Fig. 11 represents an example of true undersensing leading to an intermittent

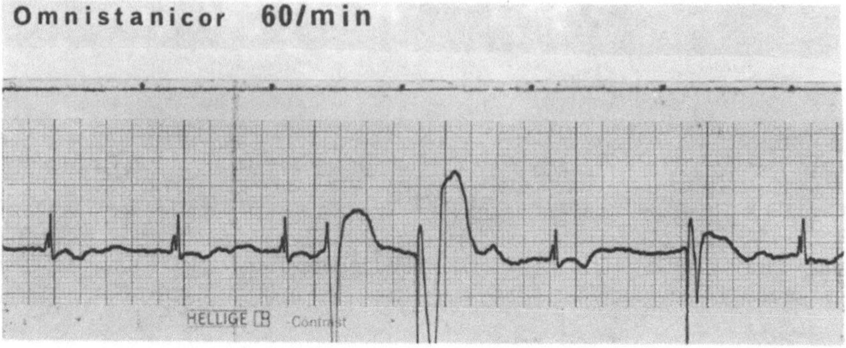

Figure 10. Lack of sensing of a ventricular extrasystole falling into the pacer's (sensing) refractory period.

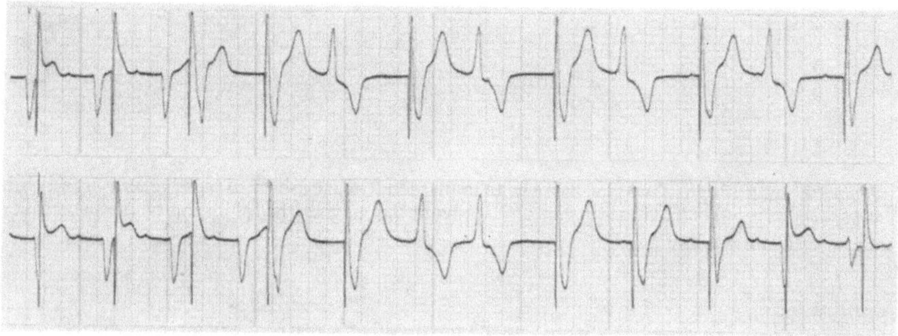

Figure 11. Undersensing leading to intermittent entrance block.

entrance block. In this case the pulse generator's refractory period is certainly not responsible for the lack of sensing, as the undetected ventricular depolarizations occur rather late during the pacing cycle. The strange finding in this tracing is that evidently only those QRS-complexes are sensed by the pacemaker which in the lead shown have a positive deflection whereas the negative complexes are not able to inhibit the pacemaker.

The reason for this finding is not too obvious; but it must be assumed that the negative QRS complexes generate too little voltage at the electrode implant site and the pacemaker does not receive an adequate signal. One has to realize that there is no relationship between the voltage picked up by conventional EKG leads and the intraventricular electrogram and that from a high deflection in a given lead one cannot predict sufficient intracardiac voltage.

The treatment in this case, of course, would be repositioning of the stimulating lead and it would be advisable not only to measure the stimulating threshold but also the amplitude of the various intracardiac electrograms.

The last ECG (fig. 12) on a first glance appears to be a common example of a pacemaker parasystole due to complete entrance block. But there is one peak to peak interval of 1160 ms which is considerably longer than the automatic pacing interval of this pulse generator of 860 ms. What mechanism may be responsible for this irregularity? If we assume a sensing of the fifth QRS complex why wasn't it capable to reset the pacemaker completely and to initiate a full escape interval?

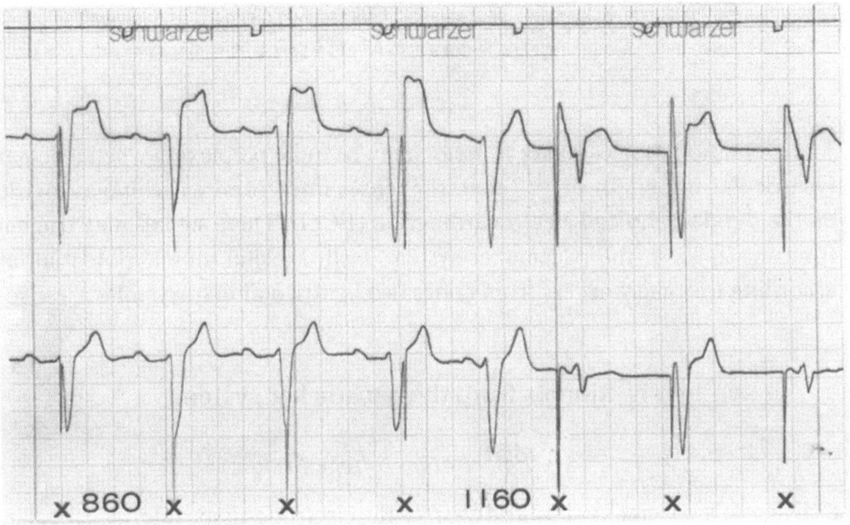

Figure 12. Partial sensing because of marginal voltage of the intracardiac R-wave signal.

This tracing probably represents an example of the phenomenon of partial sensing. The intracardiac signals are marginal in amplitude (or frequency content!); some of them are too small to be detected at all whereas others just reaching threshold cause incomplete discharge of the timing capacitor with a corresponding shorter escape interval.

With these few examples of clinical electrocardiography we tried to illustrate the differential diagnosis of the irregular pacemaker, which admittedly may sometimes produce rather confusing ECG patterns. In view of the numerous potential mechanisms which may be involved, a detailed knowledge of the mode of operation of the various types of pacemakers including their individual technical data is essential, and every case must be assessed thoroughly in order to find the appropriate treatment.

COMPLEX DEMAND PACEMAKER ARRHYTHMIAS: THE DIFFERENTIAL DIAGNOSIS OF PACEMAKER PAUSES

S. SERGE BAROLD, LING S. ONG, MICHAEL FALKOFF AND ROBERT A. HEINLE

The evaluation of pacemaker function may be quite perplexing when a demand (ventricular-inhibited) pulse generator senses intracorporeal voltages invisible on the standard 12-lead electrocardiogram (ECG). These signals may originate from the T-wave, the pacemaker system itself, skeletal muscle potential, and according to some workers from concealed ventricular extrasystoles.

1. Signals from the pacemaker system

A. Polarization voltage (1-3)

Delivery of a pacemaker impulse charges the electrode-tissue interface to a large DC potential (polarization voltage) which will subsequently dissipate over a relatively long period. The decay of this waveform represents a time-changing voltage that may be sensed when the pulse generator comes out of its (paced) refractory period. Thus, a relatively short refractory period associated with a prolonged and sharp decay of the pacemaker "afterpotential" may allow a pulse generator to sense its own discharge, recycle and alter its firing rate (double-reset phenomenon) (1, 2). This may mimic T-wave sensing and should be suspected whenever the interval between two consecutive pacemaker spikes (SS interval) lengthens to a value approximately equal to the sum of one automatic interval and the delivery (paced) refractory period of the pulse generator. Better design has greatly reduced the incidence of this problem but a recent report from Japan serves as a reminder that this problem may still occur with contemporary pulse generators. Taniguchi et al. (4) observed the double-reset phenomenon (false triggering) with two types of implantable demand pacemakers and reproduced the abnormality in dogs with epicardial electrodes under the following circumstances: 1) superficial placement of one pacing electrode (in either a unipolar or bipolar system); the problem disappeared as soon as the electrodes were more deeply implanted in the myocardium. 2) Placement of bipolar electrodes very close to each other.

B. False signals (electrical transients)

Abrupt changes in resistance within a pacing system produce corresponding voltage changes between the anode and the cathode and may generate relatively large signals capable of being sensed by a demand pulse generator (3, 5, 6). Two basic mechanisms are involved (3): (i) interruption of the polarization voltage after the pacemaker pulse and, (ii) disturbance of the much smaller permanent DC voltage across the electrode in the absence of pacemaker stimuli. Sudden changes in resistance generate false signals responsible for the sensing problems seen with the brief derangement of the pacemaker circuit by intermittent loose connections, short circuits, and wire fractures with otherwise well apposed ends. A loose connection between electrode and pulse generator is probably the commonest cause of false signals during temporary pacing. The interaction of two pacing catheters within the heart may also generate false signals when the functional and inactive electrodes lie side by side and make intermittent contact (7).

False signals often create difficult diagnostic problems because they are invisible on the standard 12-lead ECG. Recycling of a pacemaker from false signals sometimes resembles T-wave (or polarization voltage) sensing (8). This differential diagnosis is important because T-wave sensing can lead only to pacemaker bradycardia and is therefore relatively harmless. In contrast, oversensing of false signals may be the earliest indication of a potentially catastrophic situation when an intermittent wire fracture becomes permanent.

The following points should be considered in the diagnosis of false signals.

(i) False signals tend to occur at random and often much later than the timing of the T-wave.

(ii) Very long ECG strips will often reveal relatively long, irregular and constantly changing pauses without pacemaker stimuli or spontaneous beats (Figure 1 B-D).

(iii) The testing magnet may help in the diagnosis because its application eliminates all arrhythmias related to oversensing (except in some pacemaker models, e.g. Starr-Edwards units retain their demand function). Application of the magnet will convert the irregular and constantly changing SS intervals to a mathematically precise value which may be double, triple or an exact multiple of the basic SS or automatic interval (3) (Figure 1 E, F). The demonstration of pacemaker pauses (SS intervals) that are exact multiples of the automatic interval during fixed-rate pacing (with the magnet) is virtually diagnostic of an intermittent wire fracture (or electrode problem) and reflects the correct and undisturbed timing of a normally functioning pulse generator delivering its impulse into a transiently disrupted circuit (3, 9). Mathematically precise (exact multiple) prolongation of the SS interval with the magnet may permit the early diagnosis of an intermittent wire fracture and indeed this finding may be the only

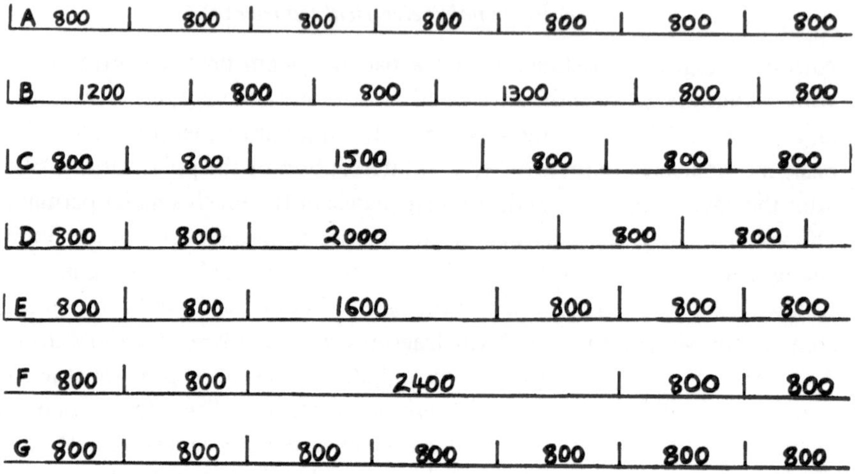

Figure 1. Diagrammatic representation of various demand pacemaker arrhythmias. *A*) Firing of demand pacemaker with an automatic interval of 800 msec. *B & C*) Show irregular prolongation of the SS intervals consistent with either sensing of the "T wave" or false signals. *D*) Sudden prolongation of the SS interval to 2000 msec. This obviously rules out sensing of the T waves or polarization voltage and the pattern suggests a defective electrode. Irregular prolongation of the SS interval may be partly or totally due to sensing of false signals. Upon application of the magnet an intermittently defective electrode system (i.e. fracture) causes precise doubling (*E*) or tripling (*F*) of the automatic interval. If an intermittent fracture presents as a pure sensing problem as in (*B*) application of the magnet may cause regular pacing as in strip (*G*).

diagnostic clue when the spontaneous rhythm is faster than the preset rate of the pacemaker, a situation where false signals will remain undetectable and irregular prolongation of the SS interval will obviously not occur (9).

An intermittent wire fracture may occasionally present as a pure sensing problem if its timing always allows the fractured ends to be in contact whenever the pacemaker delivers its impulse. The defective portion of the pacemaker catheter may induce rhythmic recycling of a demand pacemaker if mechanical systole consistently creates a false signal by making and breaking the circuit (3, 8). Such an abnormality may be electrocardiographically indistinguishable from T-wave sensing because of its timing and regularity (Figure 1B) and indeed regular pacing will occur with conversion to fixed-rate pacing (Figure 1G). Consequently the diagnosis of an intermittent electrode problem cannot be positively ruled out if conversion to fixed-rate pacing eliminates abnormalities of the SS interval. This point is important because some authors have stated that in the presence of an irregular pacemaker rhythm, restoration of regular pacing with the magnet provides sufficient evidence to rule out an intermittent wire fracture (10).

(iv) Wire fractures or loose connections may produce false signals and irregular SS intervals only in relation to certain body movements such as changes from the supine to sitting or standing position, arm raising, etc. (11, 12). In the latter situation if the pulse generator is unipolar, the problem may mimic sensing of skeletal muscle potentials especially if regular fixed-rate pacing occurs after application of the magnet.

(v) The presence of false signals (electrical transients) should be demonstrated by intracardiac recordings if the diagnosis remains in doubt. The timing of an intermittent electrode problem may give rise to normal measurements of electrode impedance if there is electrical continuity whenever the pulse generator fires. Consequently the demonstration (or absence) of interfering electrical transients by intracardiac recordings becomes imperative for diagnosis.

2. Diagnostic techniques for demonstrating false signals or electrical transients

A. Recordings of the intracardiac electrogram during spontaneous rhythm

Intermittent wire fractures often cause obvious interference of the baseline but may also give rise to less conspicuous electrical transients measuring only a few millivolts (9, 13). In the absence of pacemaker stimuli, changes in the small permanent DC voltage across the electrode produces these signals. Obviously when the electrode ends separate during pacing, sudden changes of the much higher residual polarization voltage will generate considerably larger signals. The absence of electrical transients during recording of the electrogram of spontaneous beats makes the diagnosis of an intermittent fracture unlikely but does not completely rule it out as pointed out by Waxman et al. (8) who showed that occasionally only the superimposed pacemaker voltage waveform during pacing (at threshold or subthreshold values) may bring out the culpable electrical transients. Therefore if the electrogram of spontaneous depolarization remains normal and a fracture is strongly suspected steps b) and c) should be undertaken.

B. Recordings of intracardiac electrograms during pacing

When a patient has a poor spontaneous rhythm, recordings must be made during pacing. With a bipolar system, unipolarization allows recording from each electrode in turn; one electrode is used for pacing, the other one for recording the electrogram. For example, if a bipolar electrode has an intermittent fracture in its proximal electrode, unipolarization with the distal electrode as the cathode should yield absolutely regular pacing as the defective electrode now resides outside the pacing circuit. Recording of the intracardiac electrogram of paced beats from the (free) proximal electrode may be obtained easily on an ordinary electrocardiograph and should clearly show electrical transients if sufficiently long strips are taken. Conversely when the defective proximal electrode becomes the cathode during unipolar pacing prolongation of the SS interval should recur if the fracture is confined to the proximal electrode and intracardiac recordings from the inactive distal electrode will reveal no electrical disturbances. The recording of electrical transients from both electrodes suggests fractures of both electrodes or an additional internal short circuit.

C. Direct recordings of pacemaker waveform during pacing

The above techniques obviously cannot demonstrate electrical transients in a pacemaker-dependent patient with a unipolar electrode. In this situation the diagnosis requires simultaneous recordings of the pacemaker waveform *directly* from the pacemaker terminals and the surface ECG. During pacing, recordings from the pacemaker terminals tend to saturate ECG preamplifiers and an ordinary electrocardiograph may be unsuitable. Waxman et al. (8) recorded satisfactory pacemaker waveform by placing a 10,000 ohm resistor in series with the electrode to attenuate the signal to avoid preamplifier saturation. We have, however, successfully recorded pacemaker waveforms directly without the need of a resistance in series by using appropriate sensitivity and filter settings on a standard physiological recorder (Electronics for Medicine). The pacemaker waveform must be recorded *simultaneously* with the surface ECG and when an intermittent fracture occurs, prolongation of the SS interval should coincide with the sudden disruption of the pacemaker waveform producing a large signal (Figure 2). This technique is very useful in the investigations of elusive pacemaker problems because it records the presence and precise timing of electrical transients making it simple to determine whether they recycle the pacemaker.

3. Concealed ventricular extrasystoles (14)

Massumi et al. (15) described an unusual demand pacemaker arrhythmia explained in terms of sensing of concealed ventricular extrasystoles (ventricular depolarization confined to the His-Purkinje system invisible on the standard 12-lead ECG). The advent of His bundle recordings has clearly demonstrated the existence of such concealed extrasystoles (14) but the intriguing possibility that a demand pacemaker may detect such localized depolarization must remain speculative in the absence of direct recordings from the pacing catheter to prove that such "beats" can indeed generate sufficient voltage to be sensed. Unfortunately direct intracardiac recordings were not available to substantiate

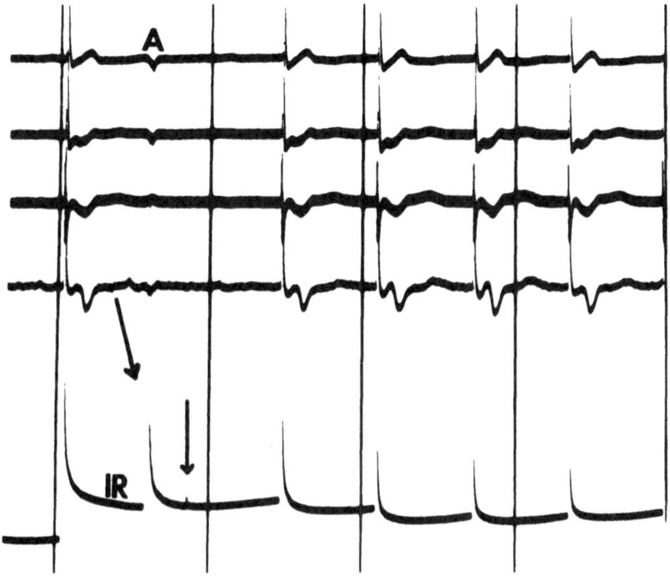

Figure 2. Irregular prolongation of the SS interval due to an intermittent wire fracture causing false signals. Diagnosis by intracardiac recording (IR) of the pacemaker waveform. Several electrocardiographic leads are seen on top. There is a sudden break in the intracardiac voltage (first arrow) due to momentary separation of the fractured ends. The second arrow points to another false signal which actually initiates the last escape interval terminating with the next pacemaker spike. Note the variability of amplitude and morphology of the false signals and how relatively small disturbances could be missed with improper settings of the physiological recorder. A) Refers to an artefact occasionally seen on the surface ECG with intermittent wire fractures during *unipolar* pacing. A sudden and large change of the electrical field inside the heart may cause corresponding small artefacts on the surface electrocardiogram of unipolar systems. These electrode artefacts are usually tiny, but distinct, on the surface electrocardiogram, but may be invisible on the standard electrocardiograph because of attenuation.

the report of Massumi et al. (15). In this respect any unusual sensed signal recorded directly from a pacing electrode should always be considered as extracardiac (false signals, etc.) in origin until proven otherwise. The possibility that a demand pacemaker might sense a concealed ventricular extrasystole will always remain intellectually stimulating and may eventually be proven but from the practical standpoint one must always exclude the following causes whenever the SS interval lengthens intermittently.

4. Differential diagnosis of pacemaker pauses (prolongation of the SS interval)

1. Invisible ventricular extrasystoles (in contrast to concealed).
   Invisible *isoelectric* ventricular extrasystoles in certain leads usually become

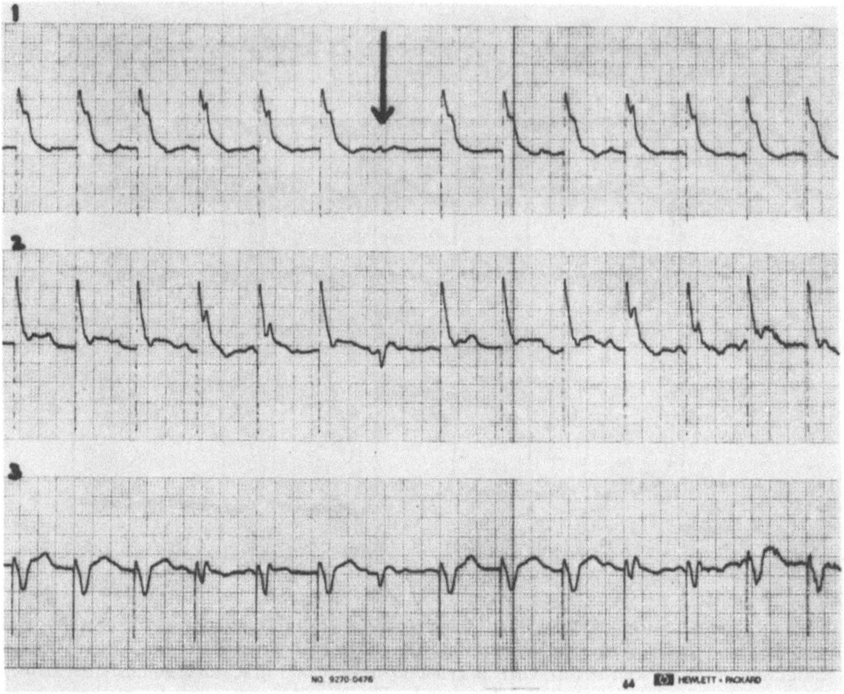

Figure 3. Simultaneous recordings of leads 1, 2 and 3 showing a sensed ventricular extrasystole clearly seen in leads 2 and 3, but not in lead 1 (invisible extrasystole). This electrocardiogram illustrates the importance of obtaining recordings with three simultaneous leads.

obvious in other leads. Electrocardiographic recording of three simultaneous leads (used routinely in our clinic) is essential to avoid this pitfall. (Figure 3).

2. *Sensing of the polarization voltage* or "afterpotential" (double reset).
3. *False signals* from various sources.
4. *Musculoskeletal potentials.*

Inhibition of demand pacemakers by musculoskeletal potentials has been reported to occur only with unipolar pacing systems (16). Mymin et al. (17) however described one case of apparent suppression of a bipolar unit by myopotentials (presumably originating near the implantation site) but gave no details about the mechanism of interference. Their observation is difficult to understand because the geometry of the sensing electrode in a bipolar system and perhaps their observation represents an example of pseudointerference (baseline blurring) or sensing of false signals from a loose connection or wire fracture. In this respect an insulation leak close to skeletal muscle could conceivably detect myopotentials and suppress a bipolar pulse generator (12).

Peter et al. (10) recently described transient inhibition of a unipolar demand pacemaker during deep respiration and suggested without direct proof that the pacemaker was being suppressed by myopotentials originating from the muscles of respiration. We recently clearly documented transient inhibition of a bipolar demand pacemaker by diaphragmatic potentials. This unusual phenomenon became apparent only with active contraction of the diaphragm such as deep respiration, straining, Valsalva maneuver, coughing, sneezing and laughing (18). The patient had no spontaneous rhythm and we made the diagnosis during pacing by recording the pacemaker waveform directly from the two pacing terminals simultaneously with the surface ECG (Figure 4). There were no sudden

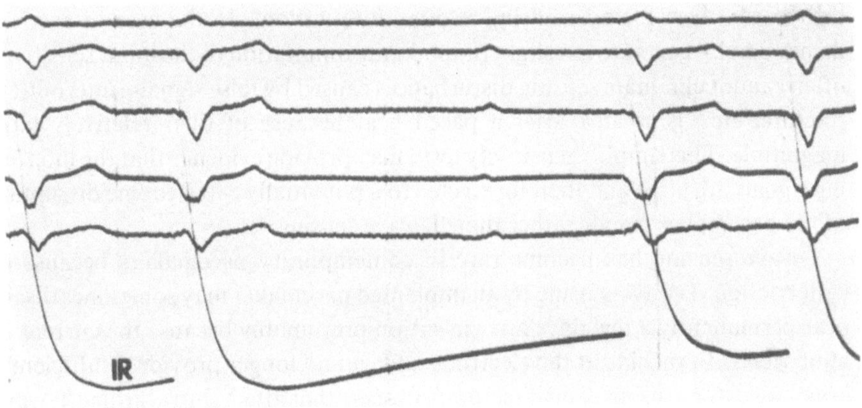

Figure 4. Sensing of diaphragmatic muscle potentials by a bipolar demand pacemaker. Irregular prolongation of the SS interval was present on deep respiration, coughing, sneezing, the Valsalva maneuver and laughing. Intracardiac recordings of the pacemaker waveform during periods of inhibition failed to show the characteristic disturbances seen with false signals. This recording illustrates the importance of documenting the absence of false signals as part of the problem-solving approach in unusual situations. Subsequent magnified recordings of the pacemaker waveform on a storage oscilloscope showed myopotential disturbances up to 2 mV in magnitude (18).

and large disruptions of the pacemaker waveform characteristic of a transient electrode problem and diaphragmatic myopotential voltages of about 2 mV. were recorded intermittently (18).

5. T-wave sensing

This problem is relatively rare and is usually seen after paced rather than spontaneous beats probably because the polarization voltage contributes a larger signal and therefore tends to generate a larger "T-wave" signal (19). Indeed, cases of T-wave sensing of paced ventricular beats may actually represent the detection of total voltage from the pacemaker afterpotential and the relatively small, if any, contribution from the T-wave. The diagnosis of T-wave sensing should always be one of exclusion and we agree with the admonition of Waxman et al. (8) that many cases of so-called T-wave sensing may represent a partial wire fracture producing signal artefacts corresponding with the timing of the T-wave.

When T-wave sensing is seen during temporary pacing slight reduction of the sensitivity control of the external pacemaker usually eliminates the problem because the unwanted signal is often barely above the sensitivity of the pulse generator. Conversion to a unipolar system or reversing the polarity of the electrodes may occasionally be useful. Compensation for T-wave sensing by increasing the pacing rate is potentially dangerous and may lead to pacemaker tachycardia because oversensing is often intermittent. In the case of external demand pulse generators a slight or moderate diminution of the input sensitivity often cannot eliminate sensing disturbances caused by false signals (intermittent fracture, etc.) generated after a paced beat because of their relatively large magnitude. This simple "sensitivity test" may provide evidence that the interfering signals are large and therefore a clue to a potentially catastrophic disruption of the pacemaker circuit rather than T-wave sensing.

T-wave sensing has become rare in contemporary pacemakers because of better design. T-wave sensing by an implanted pacemaker may sometimes disappear permanently a few days after insertion presumably because the current of injury tends to subside at the electrode and can no longer provide a sufficiently large signal for sensing. Conversely any process that affects intracardiac T-wave voltage such as ischemia, electrolyte imbalance, trauma, etc. could conceivably cause late T-wave sensing. Some workers have successfully used Quinidine to eliminate apparent T-wave sensing of paced ventricular beats (20, 21). Quinidine probably acts by altering the intracardiac T-wave signal in terms of voltage or dv/dt or both. Indeed a similar mechanism could easily explain the finding of Massumi et al. (15) who attributed the disappearance of their unusual pacemaker arrhythmia to the elimination of concealed ventricular extrasystoles by antiarrhythmic therapy.

6. Other causes of pacemaker pauses

Sensing of P-waves always enters the differential diagnosis of pacemaker pauses but this complication is fortunately very rare (6). Partial recycling from a borderline signal (3) is no longer a design feature of contemporary pacemakers but may still be seen with existing Medtronic units 5944 and 5945. Application and removal of the magnet from some normally functioning pulse generator may create a pause related to signals generated in their reed switch mechanism. Static electricity (triboelectric phenomena) may play a role in unexplained sensing problems (6). Brief inhibition of the 5880 and 5880A external Medtronic pulse generators often occurs by simply touching the metal front panel. Finally, true pulse generator malfunction should always be considered in the evaluation of pacemaker pauses and this diagnosis is often one of exclusion (Figure 5).

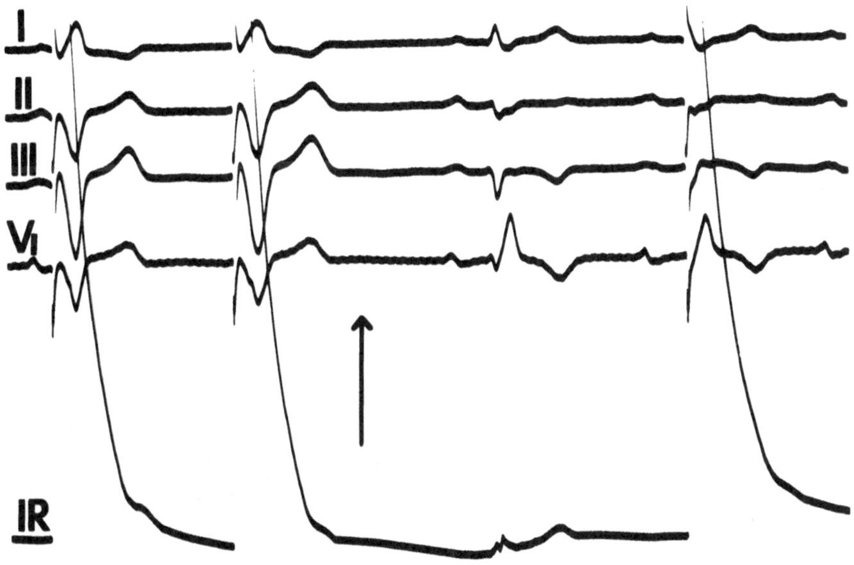

Figure 5. Apparent sensing of the T wave by unipolar demand pacemaker. Application of the magnet eliminated the sensing problem. Unipolar ventricular electrograms from the tip electrode showed no abnormality and no false signals. Intracardiac recordings (IR) of the pacemaker waveform during pacing again showed the absence of false signals. The appearance of late "T wave sensing" at 26 months suggested component failure. Indeed analysis of the pulse generator by the manufacturers revealed a leaking capacitor.

7. Conclusions

1. The differential diagnosis of pacemaker pauses may occasionally be difficult. As a general rule a chaotic pattern during demand pacing should always suggest the presence of false signals. This possibility should always enter into the differential diagnosis of oversensing from true pacemaker failure to avoid the unnecessary replacement of a normally functioning pulse generator in the presence of a defective electrode system.

2. An intermittent wire fracture may occasionally present as a pure sensing problem and in this situation normal and regular pacing may occur during conversion to fixed-rate pacing.

3. In elusive cases an intermittent electrode problem must be positively excluded by the direct recording of the waveform from the pulse generator terminals together with the surface ECG. The demonstration of false signals (or their absence) avoids making a diagnosis with only circumstantial evidence. This approach may lead to the correct diagnosis of special sensing problems in situations where the clinical findings suggest an intermittent electrode problem (Figure 4, 5).

4. Unipolar or bipolar demand pacing systems may occasionally sense diaphragmatic myopotentials. This is probably rare but the true extent of this problem remains to be defined.

5. The concept of a demand pacemaker sensing concealed ventricular extrasystoles though accepted by many (22, 23) must remain speculative in the light of our present knowledge.

6. The diagnosis of T-wave sensing should always be one of exclusion. The warnings of Waxman et al. (8) are worthy of repetition. These workers believed that many cases of so-called T-wave sensing described in the literature probably represented an intermittent wire fracture.

Intermittent electrode problems may occasionally present with subtle manifestations and the diagnosis may be exceedingly difficult. These problems will undoubtedly become more frequent as the longevity of pulse generators continues to increase and the population of patients with aging electrodes continues to grow. Appreciation of these potentially misleading problems and accurate knowledge of pacemaker specifications are essential for the proper interpretation of demand pacemaker function.

References

1. Barold, S.S., Caroll, M., Double reset of demand pacemakers. *Amer. Heart J.*, 84, 276 (1972).
2. Keller, J.W., Gosselin, A.J., Nathan, D.A., Stults, R.H., Bhavati, S., Lister, J., Rhythm anomalies in contemporary demand pacing. *Amer. J. Cardiol.*, 29, 572 (1972).
3. Barold, S.S., Keller, J.S., Sensing Problems with demand pacemakers in cardiac pacing. Edited by Samet P. New York. *Grune and Stratton*, p. 385, 1973.
4. Taniguchi, K., Takaoka, T., Fujiwara, H., Tabuchi, K., Takeuchi, J., Clinical experiences and experimental studies of false sensing with demand pacemakers. In Cardiac Pacing, Watanabe Y, Editor, Excerpta Medica, Amsterdam, 1977, p. 333.
5. Lasseter K.C., Buchanan, J.W., Yoshonis, K.F., A mechanism of "false" inhibition of demand pacemakers. *Circulation* 42, 1093 (1970).
6. Barold, S.S., Gaidula, J.J., Evaluation of normal and abnormal sensing functions of demand pacemakers. *Amer. J. Cardiol.* 28, 201 (1971).

7. Widmann, W.D., Mangolia, S., Lubow, L.A., Dolan, F.M., Suppression of demand pacemakers by inactive pacemaker electrodes. *Circulation*, 45, 319 (1972).
8. Waxman, M.B., Berman, N.D., Sanz, G., Downar, E., Mendler, P., Taylor, K.W.G., Demand pacemaker malfunction due to abnormal sensing. *Circulation* 50, 389 (1974).
9. Coumel, P., Mugica, J., Barold, S.S., Demand pacemaker arrhythmias caused by intermittent incomplete electrode fracture. Diagnosis with Testing Magnet. *Amer. J. Cardiol.* 36, 105 (1975).
10. Peter, T., Harper, R., Sloman, G., Inhibition of demand pacemakers caused by potentials associated with inspiration. *Brit. Heart J.* 38, 211 (1976).
11. Hillis, J.S., Arm raising: An unusual cause of intermittent pacemaker malfunction. *J. Indiana Med. Ass.* 65, 114 (1972).
12. Widlansky, S., Zipes, D.P., Suppression of a ventricular-inhibited bipolar pacemaker by skeletal muscle activity. *J. Electrocardiol.* 7, 371 (1974).
13. Furman, S., Escher, D.J.W., Lister, J., Schwedel, J.B., A comprehensive scheme for management of pacemaker malfunction. *Ann. Surg.* 63, 611 (1966).
14. Rosen, K.M., Rahimtoola, S.H., Gunnar, R.M., Pseudo A-V block secondary to premature non-propagated His bundle depolarizations. Documentation by His bundle electrocardiography. *Circulation.* 42, 367 (1970).
15. Massumi, R.A., Mason, D.T., Amsterdam, E.A. et al., Apparent malfunction of demand pacemaker caused by non-propagated (concealed) ventricular extrasystoles. *Chest* 61, 426 (1972).
16. Wirtzfeld, A., Lampadius, M., Ruprecht, E.O., Unterdrückung von Demand-Schrittmachern durch Muskelpotentiale. *Deutsch. Med. Wschr.* 97, 61 (1972).
17. Mymin, D., Cuddy, T.E., Sinha, S.N., Winter, D.A., Inhibition of demand pacemakers by skeletal muscle potentials. *JAMA.* 223, 527 (1973).
18. Barold, S.S., Ong, L.S., Falkoff, M.D., Heinle, R.A., Inhibition of bipolar demand pacemaker by diaphragmatic myopotentials. *Circulation.* (In press).
19. Jacobson, L.B., T-wave sensing during temporary demand pacing. *West. J. Med.* 123, 314 (1975).
20. Wiehmeyer, J., Korrektur einer T-Wellen-induzierten Schrittmacherbradykardie durch Chinidin. *Dtsch. med. Wschr.* 100, 1172 (1975).
21. Barold, S.S., Inapparent signals to demand pacemakers. *Chest.* 63, 467 (1973).
22. Langendorf, R., Editorial expression of Ref. 15. *Chest.* 61, 431 (1972).
23. Escher, D.J.W., Types of pacemakers and their complications. *Circulation.* 47, 1119 (1973).
24. Rubenfire, M., Timmis, H., Freed, P. et al., Electromechanical suppression of a demand pacemaker associated with electrode perforation. *J. Electrocardiology.* 6, (4), 367 (1973).

ELECTROCARDIOGRAPHIC PATTERNS IN SICK SINUS SYNDROME

R. SUTTON, P. BARRETT AND R. EMANUEL

The first year's experience of a new London pacemaker clinic shows a high incidence of sick sinus syndrome – 17 or 33% of 51 new patients. The diagnosis was made in 15 patients by documenting sinoatrial block with delayed escape mechanism either on routine electrocardiography or on 24 hour Holter monitoring (1). 2 patients showed persistent sinus bradycardia at less than 60 beats per minute and abnormal sinus node behaviour with intravenous atropine and isoprenaline (1) and after rapid atrial pacing (2). Clinically 14 of these patients presented with syncope as the primary symptom and 3 with dyspnoea. Of the important additional symptoms of sick sinus syndrome 5 had paroxysmal tachycardias and 3 had angina pectoris. Ventricular pacing is generally the chosen mode of therapy in patients with sick sinus syndrome. It is noteworthy that in only 12 of 14 syncopal patients were the attacks abolished by ventricular pacing. Both of the other patients were subsequently converted to atrial pacing with abolition of the attacks, the patients confirming dependance on atrial systole. Its persistent lack in ventricular pacing appeared to be due to retrograde atrial activation via the atrio-ventricular node. 2 of 3 dyspnoeic patients were given relief by ventricular pacing. The other patient required digitalis and diuretics. In contrast paroxysmal tachycardias were not well suppressed by pacing alone and 4 of 5 required drug therapy also. Angina pectoris required drug therapy in all patients.

6 (35%) patients had evidence on routine electrocardiogram, 24 hour Holter monitoring or His bundle electrography of His-Purkinje system disease (3). Patients with complete atrio-ventricular block have not been included. One patient showed atrial paralysis which is thought to be a variant of sick sinus syndrome (4). It is often familial (5, 6, 7) and is probably so in this case; although only 2 first degree relations have been examined both have abnormal P waves. For the purpose of expanding the available information on atrial paralysis 3 additional cases studied by us at the National Heart Hospital, London have been included in this presentation. Electrocardiographically 2 patients are illustrated (Patients 2 and 3 in Tables 1 and 2). Figure 1 shows a 12 lead electrocardiogram (Patient 2) with an idionodal rhythm at 58 per minute. There is an absence of sinus node activity and no evidence of retrograde atrial conduction. The mean

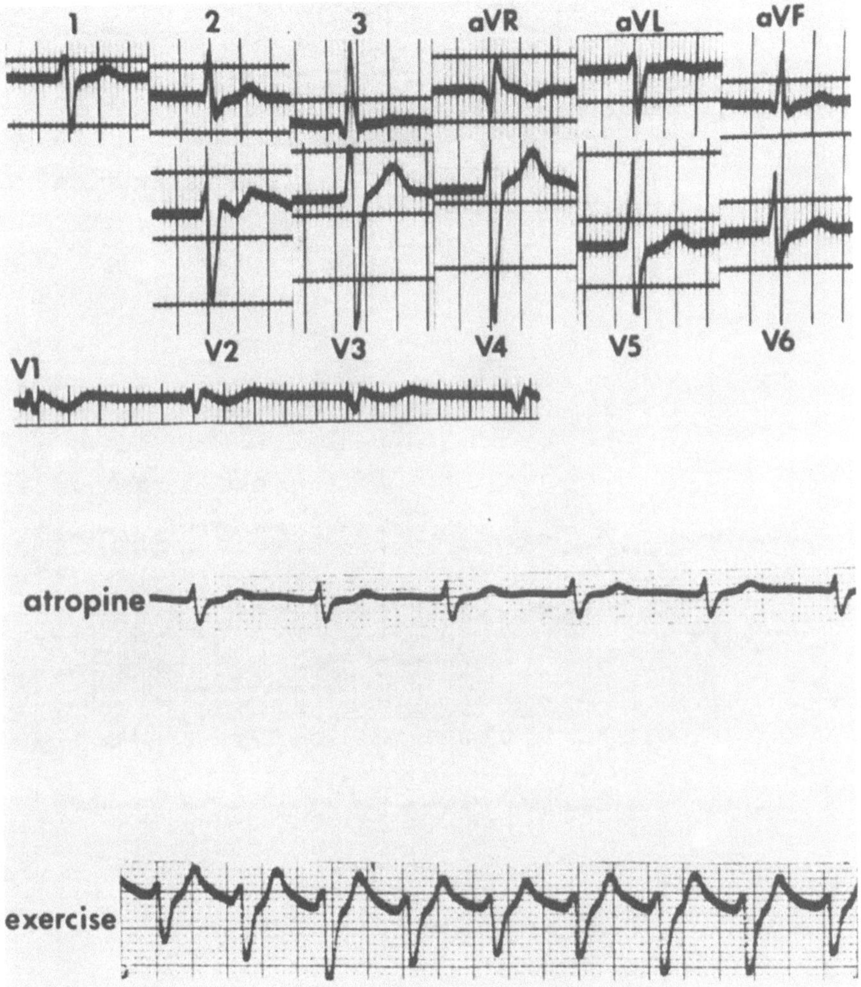

Figure 1. A 12 lead electrocardiogram and rhythm strips showing effects of atropine and exercise in Patient 2 with atrial paralysis. For description of the findings see text.

frontal QRS axis is +120° and in the absence of right ventricular hypertrophy this indicates left posterior hemiblock. The lower panels show the effect of atropine 1.2 mg. intravenously and exercise recorded on a monitor lead accelerating the idionodal rhythm. Again no atrial activity antegrade or retrograde is seen. The upper panel of Figure 2 shows a 12 lead electrocardiogram recorded recently (Patient 3). No atrial activity is seen. Left anterior hemiblock is present. The middle panel shows a 12 lead electrocardiogram recorded 17 years pre-

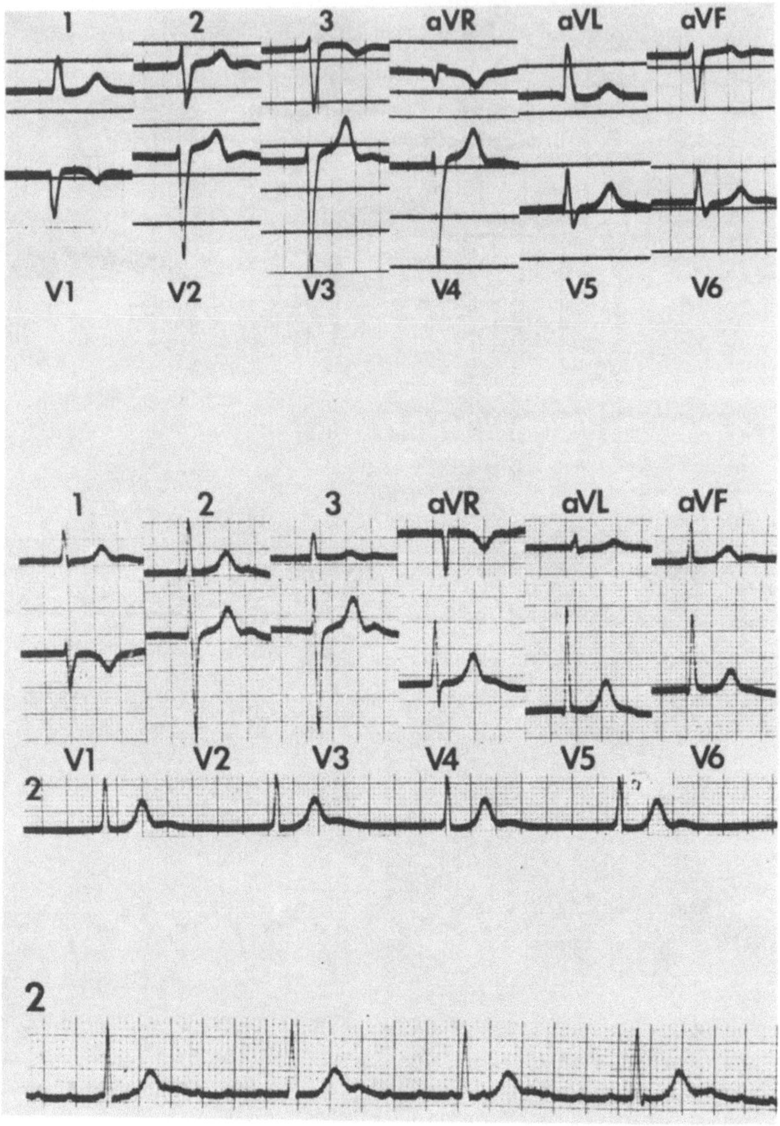

Figure 2. A 12 lead electrocardiogram (upper panel on Patient 3 with atrial paralysis. The middle panel shows a 12 lead electrocardiogram on the same patient taken 17 years previously. The lower panel shows a rhythm strip taken one week after the recording in the middle panel. For description of the findings see text.

viously. The rhythm is similar but left anterior hemiblock is absent. The lower panel shows evidence of atrial flutter recorded on a monitor lead one week after the tracing in the middle panel. The lack of atrial activity could result from sinus arrest, third degree sinoatrial block or sinus rhythm with sinoventricular conduction along internodal pathways without activation of surrounding atrial myocardium. No atrial ectopic activity or retrograde atrial activation was noted. Evidence of His-Purkinje system disease is present, also evidence of progression of this and atrial disease is seen. At times, irregularity of the idionodal rhythm was seen but no pattern could be identified; regularity was always achieved by any chronotropic mechanism suggesting the possibility of a varying second degree atrio-ventricular nodal block at rest.

Table 1. Clinical features of atrial paralysis

Patient	*1.*	*2.*	*3.*	*4.*
Age (Yrs)	33	35	42	67
History (Yrs)	28	28	2	0
Syncope	+	+	+	0
Dyspnoea	+	+	0	+
Familial	+	+	No rels.	+
HR (bpm)	29	44	40	32
BP (mmHg)	120/90	130/80	130/70	200/80
LVH	+	+	+	+
S_1 variation	0	0	0	0
S_3	+	+	+	+
S_4	0	0	0	0

Table 1 illustrates the clinical features of the 4 patients. The age range is wide suggesting a very chronic disease. When the length of history is available the chronicity of the disease is emphasised. Patients 1 and 2 are brothers and first presented 28 years ago. Long follow-up was also obtained in Patient 3. The leading symptoms were syncope and dyspnoea. Amongst relations of patients 1 and 2 sinus node and His-Purkinje abnormalities were found in two other generations. Patient 3 was brought up in an orphanage and nothing is known of his relations. Patient 4's relations have been mentioned above. On physical examination no evidence of atrial activity could be detected but clinical manifestations of ventricular volume overloading were apparent in all.

Investigative data (Table 2) revealed cardiac enlargement in the patients (1 and 4) with slowest heart rates. Patient 1 with the slowest resting heart rate showed the most severe volume loading of the left ventricle reflected in both echocardiographic dimension and angiographic volume. Left ventricular function was normal in all in whom it was studied but patient 1 showed definite increase in left ventricular mass. Right ventricular biopsy in 3 patients all showed simple hypertrophic changes. In none was there any suggestion of amyloid disease previously reported as a cause of atrial paralysis (5, 6). Atrial biopsies were not performed. The electrophysiological studies showed atria which were refractory to high output stimulation in 3 of 4 patients. His-Purkinje disease was

Table 2. Investigative data in atrial paralysis

Patient	*1.*	*2.*	*3.*	*4.*
CXR – HT +	+	0	0	+
– PVH	0	0	0	0
Echo – LVESD (cm)	4.1	3.5	4.6	–
– LVEDD (cm)	6.6	5.7	7.0	–
– LAD	3.8	3.1	3.8	–
Other features	N	N	N	–
Haemodyn: "a"	0	0	0	0
Other features	N	N	N	N
Electrophys:				
RAE "a"	0	0	0	0
RA Stim.	0	0	0	+
H-V (msec)	70	65	70	35
RV Stim.	N	N	N	N
RV Biopsy	VH	VH	VH	–
LVV ES (Ml)	174	55	–	–
ED (Ml)	501	228	–	–
EF (%)	66	76	70	–
Peak VCF (circ/sec)	2.06	2.48	–	–
LV Mass g/KgBW	4.05	2.50	–	–
Cor. Angio.	N	N	N	–

present in 3 of 4 patients also. This has been noted previously (7). The right ventricles behaved normally with electrical stimulation. Haemodynamics were normal in all cases except for the lack of atrial activity. The definition of atrial paralysis given in man first by Bloomfield and Sinclair-Smith (8) may be expanded to:

(1) Absence of P waves in any lead of the electrocardiogram
(2) Absence of any haemodynamic evidence of atrial activity
(3) Absence of atrial activity on right atrial electrogram
(4) Refractoriness of the atria to all but high output stimulation
(5) Normal ventricular stimulation
(6) High incidence of His-Purkinje disease
(7) Normal ventricular function

When all the possible electrocardiographic variants of sick sinus syndrome are taken into consideration it is possible to put forward a new pacing policy for the condition. When syncope is the dominant symptom requiring treatment and the cardiac output fall between resting sinus rhythm and ventricular pacing at 70 per minute is less than 25% and no retrograde atrio-ventricular conduction can be demonstrated, the choice is ventricular demand pacing. Also for atrial paralysis the choice is ventricular demand pacing. However, in syncopal patients where the cardiac output fall between sinus rhythm and ventricular pacing is greater than 25% and there is retrograde atrial activation and furthermore the His-Purkinje system is unequivocally normal on routine electrocardiogram, Holter monitoring and His Bundle electrography as progression of His-Purkinje disease is well recognised (9) atrial demand pacing is the method of choice. When the His-Purkinje system is abnormal atrio-ventricular sequential pacing is required. When syncope is not present experience so far suggests that ventricular demand pacing is adequate.

In conclusion, sick sinus syndrome has become a common indication for permanent cardiac pacing; additional His-Purkinje system disease is common in sick sinus syndrome. Attention should be given to the haemodynamics and electrophysiology in the choice of pacing system. Paroxysmal tachycardias and angina pectoris in association with sick sinus syndrome usually require drugs in addition to pacing for a good clinical result. Atrial paralysis is probably an uncommon familial variant of the sick sinus syndrome which is frequently associated with His-Purkinje system disease. Long-standing bradycardia in atrial paralysis is associated with ventricular volume overload and ventricular hypertrophy but not with ventricular disease and ventricular function is normal.

References

1. Ferrer, M.I., The Sick Sinus Syndrome. *Circulation* 47, 635 (1973).
2. Mandel, W., Hayakawa, H., Danzig, R., Marcus, H.S., Evaluation of sino-atrial function in man by overdrive suppression. *Circulation* 44, 59 (1971).
3. Rosen, K.M., Loeb, H.S., Sinno, M.Z., Rahimtoola, S.H., Gunnar, R.M., Cardiac conduction in patients with symptomatic sinus node disease. *Circulation* 43, 836 (1971).
4. Harris, C.L., Baldwin, B.J., Permanent atrial paralysis. *J. Electrocardiology* 9, 81 (1976).
5. Allensworth, D.C., Rice, G.J., Lowe, G.W., Persistent atrial standstill in a family with myocardial disease. *Amer. J. Med.* 47, 775 (1969).
6. Harrison, W.H., Derrick, J.C., Atrial Standstill: A review and presentation of two new cases of familial and unusual nature with reference to epicardial pacing in one. *Angiology* 20, 610 (1969).
7. Williams, D.O., Jones, E.L., Nagle, R.E., Smith, B.S., Familial atrial cardiomyopathy with heart block. *Quat. J. Med.* 61, 491 (1972).
8. Bloomfield, D.A., Sinclair-Smith, B.C., Persistent atrial standstill. *Amer. J. Med.* 39, 335 (1965).
9. Narula, O.S., Atrio-ventricular conduction defects in patients with sinus bradycardia. Analysis by His Bundle recordings. *Circulation* 44, 1096 (1971).

DISCUSSION VII. PACEMAKER ELECTROCARDIOGRAPHY

CHAIRMAN: J. NIEVEEN *(Groningen, The Netherlands)*

J.W. HARTHORNE *(Boston, U.S.A.)*: I have just an observation regarding Dr. Sloman's demonstration of the presence of an electrode in the coronary sinus at autopsy. We, too, have had this same experience. I would submit – and I think Dr. Sloman would agree – that, as long as the pacemaker functions it does not particularly matter where the electrode ends up being found. We, too, have found chronic perforations of the ventricular lead system lying in the pericardial space and we found electrodes in the coronary sinus in functioning pacemakers. We had one patient with chronic ischemic cardiomyopathy, with a very large right ventricle in whom we could not achieve stable position and purposely perforated the right ventricle using a stiff stylet and probed the epicardial surface of the left ventricle until we found a satisfactory threshold. That patient paced reliably for the subsequent seven years of his life.

We have had one further patient, recently, who was an elderly lady with a prosthetic valve in the tricuspid position, who had a persistent A-V block following tricuspid and mitral valve replacement. It was possible, by negotiating an electrode into the coronary sinus and down the posterior ventricular vein to create succesful ventricular pacing. The lead position in the coronary sinus and the great cardiac vein can be identified on a lateral chest X-ray as being directed posteriorly. Usually, the threshold is too high for effective ventricular stimulation. If the electrode can be negotiated down the posterior interventricular vein, one often finds a satisfactory ventricular stimulation threshold, the only risk being of also having diaphragmatic stimulation.

J.G. SLOMAN *(Melbourne, Australia)*: Certainly, I agree with the comments. The point I was making, was that we must know what we are doing. I showed the slide to point out that in 1963 we really had no appreciation of this potential problem, we did not look at the electrocardiogram properly and we did not screen the patient properly. But, as Dr. Harthorne said, the function of the pacemaker, luckily for the patient, was quite satisfactory.

S. BERENS *(Santa Monica, U.S.A.)*: I would just like to make a few comments about the intracardiac electrogram. We have routinely used it for the last 5 years and have come to really depend on it for evaluation of the electrode position and to see how deep we are into the myocardium i.e. have we perforated it or not? We also use it to analyze if we are in an epicardial position like in the coronary sinus. The QRS configuration will really tell you if you are too deep or if you are epicardial or not. The only problem with that is that the classic small R deep S wave pattern of the intraventricular right ventricular cavitary position, is only present at the apex. If you are on the floor of the ventricle, or on the septum, you will not have the classical pattern.

Perhaps Dr. Barold might want to expand on those comments. I know he published something on that subject. Is not the classic pattern of small R deep S only delectable when you are right at the apex?

S.S. BAROLD *(Rochester, U.S.A.):* I think, in about 98% of the cases, this is exactly what you see: a small "R" followed by a deep "S." In about 2 or 3% of the cases, we have seen an R-wave taller than the S-wave. When you see this type of unusual pattern, you are never sure where you are until the patient comes to the autopsy table and we do have some cases where it has been shown that the catheter was at the apex of the right ventricle. So it can happen, but I think it is rare.

S. BERENS *(Santa Monica, U.S.A.):* I think if you explore the right ventricle, you can record various patterns. I want to bring up the point that you may be in a perfectly unsatisfactory position, not quite at the apex, when you do not record that classic pattern.

S.S. BAROLD *(Rochester, U.S.A.):* Yes. I think an electrocardiogram at the right ventricular apex may have an equiphasic pattern, the R-wave being equal to the S-wave. Occasionally, the R-wave may be taller than the S-wave. If the threshold is good, we will leave the catheter there. But it is important that, if the R-wave is very tall and ST segment elevation is very high, you may not be at the proper site and perhaps in the wall. In this situation you should withdraw the catheter while recording the electrogram.

CHAIRMAN: Dr. Sutton would like to make some comments?

R. SUTTON *(London, England):* With regard to the ST elevation of the complex, I think it is very important to take the idio-ventricular complex. If you have the patient on a temporary pacemaker and you cannot get him off, then do not use the electrogram for evaluation. In some cases even the conducted complex can conceal a perforation pattern.

CHAIRMAN: Other comments from the table?

S. DALLA VOLTA *(Padova, Italy):* I would like to make a short comment on Dr. Sutton's presentation on the sick sinus syndrome and the relief of angina by pacing. We have seen, that, if you reduce the stimulation frequency to about 56, 58 or 60, you will have much better results. In two of five cases, we have seen the disappearance of angina only with stimulation. I must tell you that our cases were different, in the sense that while in your three cases the coronary angiogram was normal, in our cases out of seven cases five had abnormal non-critical lesions of coronary arteries.

CHAIRMAN: We have to close this interesting discussion now. Thank you all for your contributions.

Section VIII

TACHYCARDIA AND PACING

DIAGNOSTIC PACING IN TACHYCARDIA

HEIN J.J. WELLENS

As shown in table 1 several aspects of tachycardia can be studied by combining programmed electrical stimulation of the heart with simultaneous recording of extremity and precordial ECG leads and intracavitary electrograms (1).

Table 1. Use of pacing in tachycardia

1.	Study of the mechanism of tachycardia	
2.	Localisation of site of origin and pathway of tachycardia	
		drugs
3.	Selection of proper therapy	pacemaker
		surgical interruption of tachycardia circuit

1. Mechanism of tachycardia

In the distinction between abnormal automaticity or re-entry as the mechanism of the arrhythmia, reproduceable initiation and termination of tachycardia by premature stimuli given within a well defined and reproduceable zone of timing intervals (the tachycardia zone) has been accepted as suggestive for a re-entrant mechanism. While tachycardia based upon re-entry can be terminated by pacing at rates above the frequency of the tachycardia ("overdrive pacing") tachycardia due to abnormal enhanced automaticity can at best be only temporarily suppressed or slowed.

It is important however to realize that inability to demonstrate initiation and termination of tachycardia by timed stimuli or "overdrive pacing" does not rule out in a given patient the possibility of a re-entrant mechanism.

Factors like: a) rate of tachycardia b) site of origin of tachycardia c) distance between site of origin of tachycardia and site of stimulation and d) the electrophysiological properties of the tissues in between these two sites all affect the outcome of the stimulation study. This should be kept in mind in interpreting the data given in table 2.

This table shows the mechanism of different types of tachycardia as found

Table 2. Mechanism of tachycardia in relation to site of origin

		Pts	*Focus*	*Re-entry*
Atrial Tachy		27	+	+
Atrial Flutter		38	+	
	Intra nodal	59		+
AV Junctional Tachy	Conc. Acc. P.	20		+
	Pathw. unknown	3		+
	Digitalis	3	+	
Wolff-Parkinson-White		139		+
Other Forms of Pre-excitation		10		+
Ventricular Tachy		64	+	+

Abbreviations: Tachy = Tachycardia; Conc. Acc. P. = Concealed Accessory Pathway; Pts = Patients.

during a programmed stimulation study using the criteria for differentiation between re-entry and enhanced automaticity given above.

In all patients classified as "re-entry" the tachycardia could reproduceably be initiated and terminated during the study. Patients in whom this could not be accomplished were labelled "focal." The actual mechanism of tachycardia in this group is less clear. We can for reasons given above not rule out the possibility that in some of the patients from this group the mechanism of tachycardia was based upon re-entry rather than abnormal automaticity. A possible example of difficulties in differentiating between mechanisms are patients with atrial flutter in whom a re-entry mechanism in a small area cannot be excluded (1). Both patients with atrial and ventricular tachycardia (2) showed striking differences in mechanism of tachycardia.

2. Localisation of site of origin and pathway of tachycardia

Determination of the site of origin of a tachycardia is of diagnostic, prognostic and therapeutic importance. By simultaneously recording the activation process during tachycardia from several different intracardiac sites, it has become possible not only to determine the site of origin of tachycardia, but also to answer the question whether an accessory atrio-ventricular pathway is incorporated in the tachycardia circuit.

In 139 patients with the Wolff-Parkinson-White syndrome consecutively studied by programmed electrical stimulation and multiple intracardiac recordings, the accessory pathway was incorporated in the tachycardia circuit in 87 patients. In 8 patients the tachycardia was confined to the AV node, in 3 patients to the atrium and in one patient to the ventricle only. In 15 patients the exact site of their tachycardia could not be determined (3).

It has become increasingly clear that a number of patients originally diagnosed as suffering from AV nodal tachycardia, are actually using during tachycardia an accessory atrio-ventricular pathway conducting in ventriculo-atrial direction only (4).

In our own series 20 out of 85 consecutively studied patients suffering from AV junctional tachycardia never showing any evidence of AV conduction over an accessory pathway, used an accessory pathway in ventriculo-atrial direction during tachycardia. These observations may have consequences as far as choice of anti-arrhythmic drug is concerned and also when surgical interruption of the tachycardia circuit or chronic pacemaker implantation is considered.

3. The effect of drugs

In patients in whom tachycardia can reproduceably be initiated and terminated by programmed electrical stimulation of the heart, repetition of the same stimulation program from the same stimulation site following drug administration, gives the opportunity to study the effect of drugs on mechanism of tachycardia. This has been done in patients with the Wolff-Parkinson-White syndrome (5), AV nodal tachycardia (6, 7) and ventricular tachycardia (8). During these studies it has become clear:

1) that the effect on AV and VA conduction over the AV node – His pathway and accessory atrio-ventricular connections may be quite different (9),

2) that in patients with re-entrant tachycardia the interplay between conduction velocity and refractoriness in the re-entry circuit may be affected by drug administration in such a way that initiation and perpetuation of tachycardia is actually facilitated by drug administration (9),

3) that the effect of acute intravenous drug administration may be quite different from the effect during chronic oral use (10).

If these studies following acute and chronic drug administration fail to demonstrate control of tachycardia, the outcome of the stimulation study will be helpful in selecting either surgical therapy or implantation of a specially designed pacemaker.

References

1. Wellens, H.J.J., Electrical stimulation of the heart in the study and treatment of tachycardias. *Baltimore, University Park Press.* 1971.
2. Wellens, H.J.J., Düren, D.R., Lie, K.I., Observations on mechanisms of ventricular tachycardia in man. *Circulation* 54, 237 (1976).

3. Wellens, H.J.J., Modes of initiation of circus movement tachycardia in 139 patients with the Wolff-Parkinson-White syndrome studied by programmed electrical stimulation. In: Re-entrant arrhythmias. H. Kulbertus (Ed.). M.T.P. *Lancaster*. p. 153. (1977).
4. Wellens, H.J.J., Durrer, D., The role of an accessory atrioventricular pathway in reciprocal tachycardia. Observations in patients with and without the Wolff-Parkinson-White syndrome. *Circulation* 52, 58-72 (1975).
5. Wellens, H.J.J., Contribution of cardiac pacing to our understanding of the W.P.W. syndrome. *Brit. Heart J.* 37, 231 (1975).
6. Wellens, H.J.J., Liem, K.L., Düren, D.R., Lie, K.I., Effect of digitalis in patients with paroxysmal A-V nodal tachycardia. *Circulation* 52, 779-788 (1975).
7. Wellens, H.J.J., Tan, K., Lie, K.I., Düren, D.R., Dohmen, H., Effect of verapamil in re-entrant A-V nodal tachycardia. *Brit. Heart J.* (in press).
8. Wellens, H.J.J., Lie, K.I., Düren, D.R., Dohmen, D., Effect of procainamide, propranolol and verapamil on mechanism of recurrent ventricular tachycardia. *Amer. J. Cardiol.* (in press).
9. Wellens, H.J.J., The electrophysiological properties of the accessory pathway in the Wolff-Parkinson-White syndrome. In: The conduction system of the heart. H.J.J. Wellens (Ed.). *Lea and Febiger*. p. 567, p. 567 (1976).
10. Wellens, H.J.J., Bär, F., Dohmen, H., Düren, D.R., Durrer, D., Effect of amiodarone in the Wolff-Parkinson-White syndrome. *Am. J. Cardiol.* 38, 189 (1976).

PACING IN SUPRAVENTRICULAR TACHYCARDIA

THOMAS A. PRESTON

Cardiac pacing is a feasible and largely successful method of treatment of supraventricular tachycardias (SVT) of all types excepting atrial fibrillation, and even this one exception has on occasion been successfully treated partially by pacing. In general, pacing is effective in one of three manners: (1) pacing may be employed to prevent onset of SVT; (2) pacing may be successful in terminating a SVT which is already in progress; (3) pacing may be used to control (but not terminate) a SVT so that it is clinically manageable, with or without ancillary use of drugs.

There are also three methods of pacing for SVT: (1) interruption; (2) overdrive; (3) rapid atrial stimulation (R.A.S.). Interruption pacing is the delivery of stimuli which depolarize a portion of a re-entry circuit, thereby making that part of the circuit refractory, and interrupting the re-entry arrhythmia. This form of pacing is therefore used to terminate a tachycardia. It is well known that in a classic re-entry SVT, a single properly-timed stimulus can either initiate or terminate the arrhythmia, but frequently two or more stimuli are necessary to interrupt and terminate a SVT. When multiple stimuli are required, it is thought that the first stimulus "peels back" the surrounding area, and it is a subsequent stimulus which interrupts the pathway (1). Sometimes bursts of multiple stimuli are necessary to interrupt a SVT, (2) and, when careful timing of single or double stimuli is not possible, continuous slow pacing can produce a random stimulus that interrupts a re-entry pathway (3, 4).

Overdrive pacing is frequently effective in prevention of SVT by suppression of premature beats which otherwise would lead to repeated bouts of SVT. This is particularly useful therapy in treating arrhythmias associated with acute problems, such as acute myocardial infarction. Overdrive pacing for prevention is often effective at pacing rates considerably slower than that of the SVT being prevented. The combination of anti-arrhythmic drugs plus overdrive pacing at a rate slightly in excess of the sinus rate is very effective in prevention of SVT. Occasionally a SVT can not be interrupted, and overdrive pacing at a rate in excess of that of the SVT is necessary in order to suppress the tachycardia, often with termination of the SVT when the pacing rate is subsequently reduced or stopped.

Rapid atrial stimulation (usually at rates above 250 per min.) is effective in termination of SVT. Short bursts of RAS, either programmed or random, can interrupt re-entry SVT, and the use of scanning with bursts of RAS has proven effective (2). RAS can also be applied as a form of overdrive which captures the atria, suppressing the SVT in the process. In cases in which suppression is possible but the SVT recurs when R.A.S. is stopped, continuous R.A.S. is frequently very effective in producing atrial fibrillation, or an atrial fibrillation equivalent, which usually results in a real reduction in the ventricular rate, as compared to the ventricular rate with the S.V.T. Thus, the application of continuous R.A.S. can provide control of a serious S.V.T., especially in conjunction with suitable cardiac drugs (5).

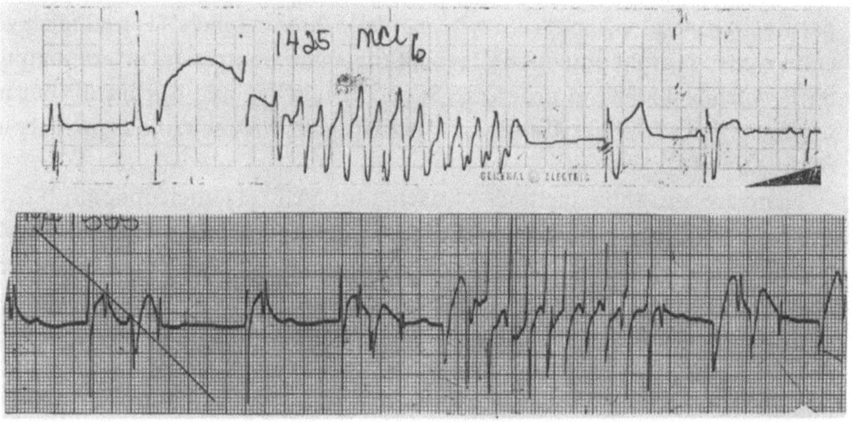

Figure 1. Above. Modified chest lead 6 shows a paroxysm of tachycardia. Ventricular pacing did not suppress the arrhythmia.
Below. Intra-atrial lead demonstrates that the arrhythmia is atrial flutter.

The technical methods of pacing in treatment of S.V.T. can be a determinant of the success of this mode of therapy. Right atrial pacing is possible by placement of a catheter electrode in the area of the S-A node, curved against one of the atrial walls, or hooked into the right atrial appendage. Left atrial stimulation is possible through catheter positioning in the coronary sinus, and either right or left atrial pacing can be achieved with epicardial electrodes. Success of pacing may be possible in one atrium but not the other (14), in one ventricle but not the other (6), and with atrial pacing but not ventricular, or vice versa (7).

Patients with sick sinus syndrome and the bradycardia-tachycardia syndrome are often treated with ventricular demand pacers and suppressant drugs. In cases in which the tachycardia is not well controlled, it is possible to use ventricular demand pacing to control periods of bradycardia or arrest, and other pacing methods to control S.V.T. Paroxysmal S.V.T. usually can be terminated by interruption pacing, using single, double, or multiple stimuli, bursts of stimuli, or continuous pacing. This rhythm, if refractory to medical management, is particularly well treated by pacing, including the use of ingenious scanning pacers which scan the cardiac cycle with single or multiple stimuli (8), or which gradually increase the pacing rate until the tachycardia is terminated (9). It is important to remember that S.V.T. can be terminated sometimes by ventricular pacing (3), as well as by atrial pacing (10).

Non-paroxysmal S.V.T. frequently can not be terminated, although this should be attempted first. Failing termination of this arrhythmia, R.A.S. can produce atrial fibrillation or its equivalent, which in almost every instance suppresses the S.V.T. and maintains the ventricular response rate in a therapeutically desirable range (1, 5, 11). We recently treated a patient with non-paroxysmal S.V.T. and a ventricular rate of 180/min, using R.A.S. at a rate of 500/min. Although the S.V.T. always returned when the R.A.S. was stopped, during R.A.S. the ventricular rate slowed to 110, due to an equivalent atrial fibrillation produced by the R.A.S. This treatment was used continuously for 2½ days, following which the S.V.T. terminated and the patient recovered.

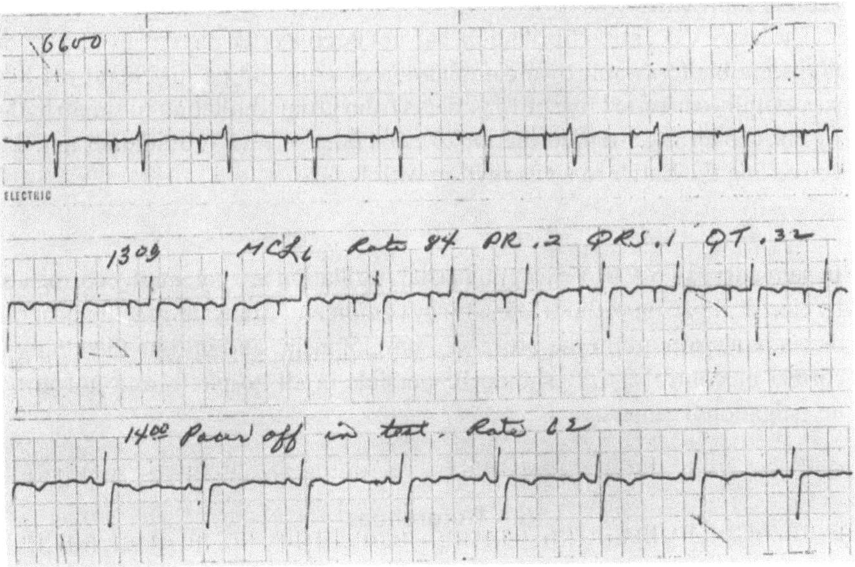

Figure 2. Same patient as figure 1. Right atrial pacing at rate of 75 per minute prevents the supraventricular tachycardia.

Atrial flutter, if not successfully controlled medically, can usually be terminated or controlled by atrial pacing. Although flutter does not convert to sinus rhythm or sustained atrial fibrillation in every attempt by pacing, (1) for intermediate periods (hours to days) it can be suppressed by temporary R.A.S. This is particularly useful and easy to accomplish with post-operative patients who have atrial wires (4). The production of atrial fibrillation almost always results in a ventricular rate which is slower than that with atrial flutter. Conversion of atrial flutter to sinus rhythm, either directly or through an intermediate stage of atrial fibrillation, is successful using R.A.S. in about 70% of cases (1). Success is enhanced by patience in probing (stimulating) at different sites (low in the right atrium is usually best), stimulating at different rates (300-600), and using prolonged over-drive pacing of the atria. On some occasions it is necessary to pace the atrium (R.A.S.) for 10 minutes or longer before atrial flutter is suppressed and does not return upon cessation of pacing. Success is most directly related to capture of the atrium, which is perceived by a change in the ventricular response.

I wish to report one patient in whom atrial flutter was converted only by pacing both atria simultaneously. R.A.S. of the right atrium, at various sites, and of the left atrium alone, did not produce conversion. After ten seconds of R.A.S. of both atria simultaneously, the heart reverted to sinus rhythm. This suggests some functional independence between the atria, and the need to suppress both atria in some cases.

The last S.V.T., atrial fibrillation, can not be converted directly by pacing, but is susceptible to assault by a combination of drug and pacing therapy. I have successfully converted five of 15 patients from atrial fibrillation to sinus rhythm by first converting atrial fibrillation to atrial flutter with I.V. quinidine, and then converting the flutter to sinus rhythm with R.A.S.

In summary, all S.V.T.'s excepting atrial fibrillation are potentially correctable by electrical pacing without using fancy equipment. Many new methods of cardiac stimulation are in the process of development, and in time the ability to correct or control S.V.T. should be possible in all hospitals, and not just at investigational centers.

References

1. Barold, S.S., Therapeutic uses of cardiac pacing in tachyarrhythmias. In Narula, O.S., His bundle electrocardiography and clinical electrophysiology. *F.A. Davis, Philadelphia*, p. 407-435, (1975).

2. Fisher, J.D., Mehra, R. Furman, S. et al., Serial electrophysiologic-pharmacologic testing for control of recurrent tachyarrhythmias in 38 patients. *Amer. J. Cardiol.* 39, 307 (1977).
3. Ryan, G.E., Easley, R.M., Zaroff, L.I. et al., Paradoxical use of a demand pacemaker in treatment of supraventricular tachycardia due to the Wolff-Parkinson-White syndrome. *Circulation* 38, 1037 (1968).
4. Preston, T.A. and Kirsh, M.M., Permanent pacing of the left atrium for treatment of WPW tachycardia. *Circulation* 42, 1073 (1970).
5. Lister, J.W., Gosselin, A.J., Nathan, D.A. and Barold, S.S., Rapid atrial stimulation in the treatment of supraventricular tachycardia. *Chest.* 63, 995 (1973).
6. Arthur, A. and Basta, L.L., Termination of recurrent supraventricular tachycardia by right ventricular endocardial pacing, but not by left ventricular epicardial pacing. *J. Electrocardiol.* 6, 345 (1973).
7. Haft, J.I., Treatment of arrhythmias by intracardiac electrical stimulation. *Prog. Cardiovasc. Dis.* 16, 539 (1974).
8. Spurrell, R.A. and Sowton, E., The management of paroxysmal supraventricular tachycardia using a scanning pacemaker system. *Organizing Committee, Vth International Symposium on Cardiac Pacing, Tokyo*, p. 41, (1976).
9. Mandel, W.J., Lacks, M.M., Yamaguchi, I., et al., Recurrent reciprocating tachycardias in the Wolff-Parkinson-White syndrome. Control by the use of a scanning pacemaker. *Chest* 69, 769 (1976).
10. Kahn, A., Morris, J.J. and Citron, P., Patient-initiated rapid atrial pacing to manage supraventricular tachycardia. *Amer. J. Cardiol.* 38, 200 (1976).
11. Waldo, A.L., MacLean, W.A., Karp, R.B. et al., Continuous rapid atrial pacing to control recurrent or sustained supraventricular tachycardias following open heart surgery. *Circulation* 54, 245 (1976).

RISKS OF DELAYED POTENTIALS IN PACEMAKER PATIENTS PRONE TO VENTRICULAR TACHYCARDIA*

G. FONTAINE, R. FRANK, J.C. PETITOT AND Y. GROSGOGEAT

Introduction

The widespread use of demand pacemakers has opened up a new field in clinical electrophysiology. One of the problems encountered with demand pacemakers concerns the characteristic feature of these devices, the sensing function which permits correct inhibition (or triggering) when the patient's spontaneous rate overrides the automatic escape rate of the pacemaker (2).

For a given pacemaker the sensing function is related to the electrogram recorded by the cardiac electrode. Excluding cases of poor electrode-myocardium contact, several circumstances may alter pacemaker sensing performances such as when the endocardial electrogram is disturbed by altered electrophysiological properties of fibres surrounding the elecrodes (18).

It has been reported that myocardial infarction may diminish the endocardial signal in such a way that the magnitude of the recorded potential is insufficient to inhibit the pacemaker (3). A similar effect has been also reported after administration of anti-arrhythmic therapy (15, 16). In these cases, the loss of sensing is the result of the abnormal activation. Conversely, oversensing is also a possibility (26, 25, 30). Our department has recently demonstrated the presence of doubled potentials recorded during epicardial mappings of patients with chronic V.T. (13).

This abnormal activation is usually completely invisible on the surface ECG and substantiates the concept of concealed extrasystoles put forward long ago by Schamroth (27) by deduction from ECG studies. Up to now there had been no direct proof of this concept in a clinical situation (22).

This paper demonstrates some examples of abnormal potentials observed during electrophysiological explorations in man and goes on to discuss the possible rhythmological consequences for pacemaker patients.

* Supported in part by: L'Association de Recherche et d'Entraide Cardiologique et Angéiologique (A.R.E.C.A.). La Caisse Régionale d'Assurances Maladie de Paris (C.R.A.M.P.).

Doubled potentials

a) Materials and methods

Doubled potentials were recorded, during epicardial mapping with a tripolar electrode similar to WALDO's triple bipolar system (19). This investigation, a routine procedure in patients with chronic recurrent V.T. uncontrolled by anti-arrhythmic therapy, is performed to locate the site of origin of the V.T. (28, 12).

We have treated 26 of these patients surgically: In nine out of twelve cases of V.T. not related to coronary artery disease, the initiation and termination of tachycardia by electrical stimulation suggested a reentrant mechanism. During epicardial mapping, all of these cases showed doubled potentials, the morphology and area of origin (mostly right ventricle) of which, varied from patient to patient. Areas of dilatation with thinning of the right ventricular wall observed either on right ventricular angiography or at operation seemed typical features in these patients (14).

Delayed endocardial potentials have recently been recorded by our group during electrophysiological exploration with the bipolar USCI C-51 catheter positioned near the abnormal area localised by right ventricular angiography.

Delayed potentials have also been recorded in two out of 14 cases of reentrant V.T. after myocardial infarction which were treated surgically. Most of these cases showed either a ventricular aneurysm, an akinetic area or a global increase in cardiac volume on angiography. The morphology of the doubled potentials observed over the left ventricle in these cases did not differ substantially from the first group (10).

b) Description

A bipolar derivation with electrodes 1mm apart positioned on the epicardium will record a single rapid deflection of 5mV over healthy right ventricle and of between 15-20mV over healthy left ventricle (Fig. 1-b). This potential occurs during the QRS complex of the ECG and is called the "synchronous potential" (14).

If this bipolar system is placed over an area of delayed potentials a second deflection may be recorded after the synchronous potential coupled with the preceding complex at a constant time interval (Fig. 1-a and c). The second potential may sometimes be situated inside the QRS complex (Fig. 1a). – In other areas or other patients, it may be recorded during the ST segment (Fig. 1c) or near the peak of the T wave. The most delayed potential we have recorded occurred 340ms after the onset of QRS complex.

The morphology of the doubled potentials was very varied. In several cases,

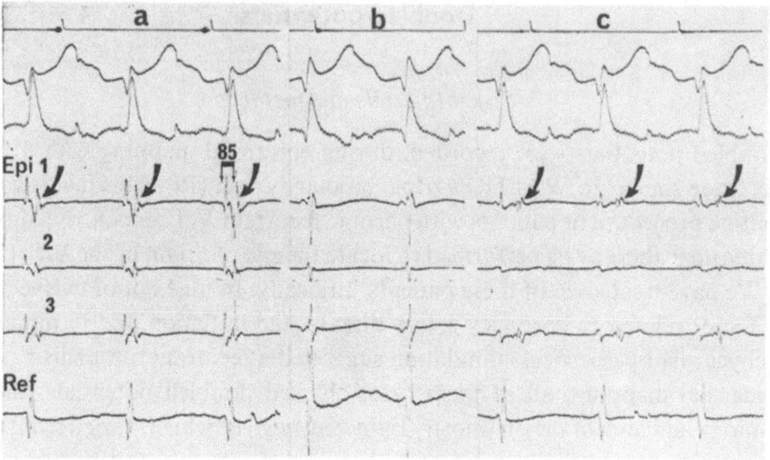

Figure 1. Potentials recorded during epicardial mapping with a tripolar system (giving 3 bipolar derivations, Epi 1, 2, 3).

REF: A fixed reference electrode.

The tracings were recorded during atrial pacing which notches the second part of the T wave on the two surface leads II and III.

In B, the point explored shows normal activation with a single deflection occurring inside the QRS complex (synchronous potential).

In A and C, the phenomenon of doubled potentials is observed. A second potential (arrowed) occurring 85ms after the start of the synchronous potential in A, and, in C, after a longer delay after the end of ventricular depolarisation, is recorded.

the synchronous potential was of relatively small amplitude and had low frequency content, the delayed potential being of larger amplitude and higher frequency. The converse has also been observed. Fragmentation of ventricular depolarisation, making it possible to distinguish the second potential from the synchronous potential, both of very diminished amplitudes, has also been recorded.

Doubled potentials have been recorded in sinus rhythm and during ventricular tachycardia usually in the same zones. In this case (during V.T.) their morphology differed and periodic modification in their order of appearance suggesting the presence of intra-myocardial conduction defects was observed. A more detailed study of these potentials is needed (11).

c) Interpretation

The synchronous potential corresponds to the normal activation sequence. The separate second potential is though to signify a delay of the propagation of activation in adjacent areas of abnormal myocardium which show in some cases dilatation and macroscopic thinning of the ventricular wall (12). These zones show much fibrous change and are thought to delay the conduction so that the activation occurs in an uneven manner.

In a hypothetical example of a bundle of fibres in site A and another in site B, separated by an area of fibrosis (Fig. 2), one could imagine an activation pathway travelling in site A far away from the exploratory electrode giving rise to weak potentials of low frequency. Then, possibly after a phenomenon of slow conduction or reflection, the activation could depolarise the fibres in site B giving rise to a stronger deflection of higher frequency.

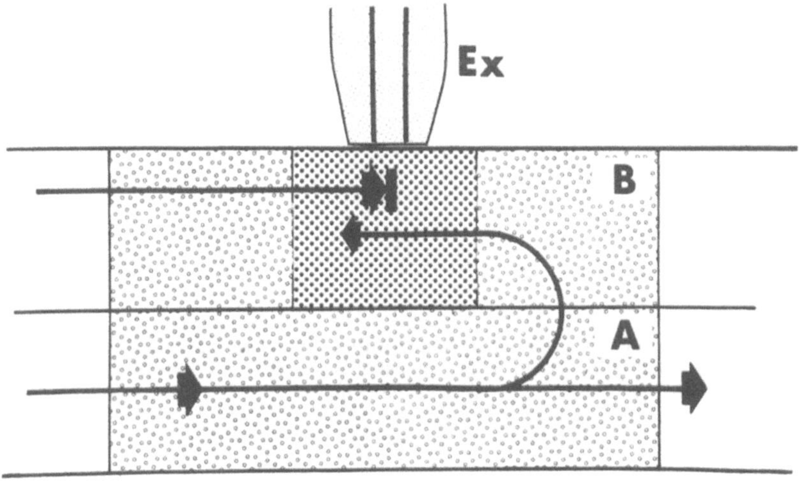

Figure 2. A possible explanation of how a doubled potential recorded with an exploratory bipolar lead (EX) might arise by a phenomenon of reflection (see text).

Theoretically, the outcome of these potentials would depend on a number of factors which vary from one area to another:

– They could be conducted into an impasse blocked by the refractory period of surrounding healthy fibres.

– They could exceed the refractory period of adjacent healthy fibres, but be too weak to excite neighbouring healthy fibres.

– They could be so delayed as to exceed the refractory period of the healthy fibres and be in a position to reactivate them and initiate a reentrant phenomenon (14).

The results of epicardial mapping do not provide absolute proof but the variations of the coupling intervals and of the morphology of the delayed potentials arriving at the peak of the T wave strongly suggest this mechanism, and in some cases, lead to the propagation of a ventricular extrasystole (8).

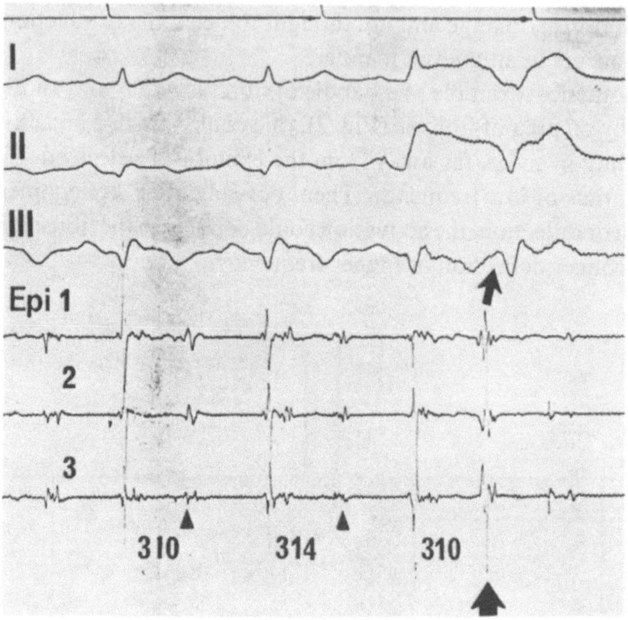

Figure 3. The recording of a doubled potential with a tripolar lead positioned at the edge of a posterior myocardial infarction. A second potential is seen 310 or 314ms after the start of the synchronous potential. The last one (arrowed) gives rise to a propagated ventricular extrasystole (Fontaine et al. Ref. 8). The last arrowed delayed potential is of greater amplitude than the synchronous potential and would have been large enough to inhibit a pacemaker.

The sequence recorded by the surface ECG during preceding cardiac cycles may only show normal ventricular depolarisation dependent on sinus rhythm.

The dynamic electrophysiology of these potentials is virtually unknown at present but we may surmise that abrupt changes of the cardiac cycle, be they intrinsic or extrinsic, disturb this unstable equilibrium (23). When the underlying disorder is sufficiently serious the delayed potential could give rise to ventricular extrasystoles and in favourable conditions for reentry, to a sustained V.T.

In the same manner, a further disturbance spontaneous or provoked which would modify the conduction properties of either normal or abnormal fibres, could lead to:

– Reversion to sinus rhythm.

– V.T. by a different pathway with a different morphology and rhythm from the original tachycardia.

– Degeneration of V.T. to ventricular fibrillation if the desynchronisation of the myocardium is serious enough to give rise to multiple reentry phenomena.

Pacemaker patients

In the following circumstances a pacemaker may be implanted in a patient prone to V.T.:

Pacemakers may be used to stop attacks of V.T. by bursts of rapid ventricular stimulation. This was made possible by knowledge acquired from electrophysiological studies (29). This function may be triggered by the patient placing a magnet over the pacemaker (6) or by radiofrequency stimulation of an implanted receiver. In these cases the pacemaker functions at a rapid fixed rate, and so there is no risk of interference from delayed potentials.

Permanent pacing by endocavitary catheter either by a fixed rate slightly faster than the normal sinus rhythm (7) or by premature ventricular stimulation triggered by ventricular extrasystoles (17, 19) has been used to prevent attacks of V.T. Permanent atrial pacing at a fixed rate faster than the sinus rhythm has also been used (24, 20).

Atrial or ventricular permanent pacing may occasionally be used during cardiac surgery for aneurysmectomy when sinus arrhythmia, bradycardia or atrial arrhythmias cause unfavourable haemodynamic situations (30).

The occurrence of ventricular extrasystoles pre- or postoperatively suppressed by permanent pacing and the use of large doses of anti-arrhythmic drugs which may depress the heart rate to unacceptable limits, are also indications for temporary and in some cases, permanent pacing.

Finally the average age of patients who have a pacemaker implanted being over 60, a substantial number of them are susceptible to attacks of V.T. as a complication of acute or chronic myocardial ischaemia (4).

Consequences

In patients in the last four groups, the proximity of the pacing catheter to regions liable to give rise to delayed potentials could in theory lead to abnormal inhibition of the demand pacemaker as it exits from its post-inhibition refractory period. This oversensing could lead to prolonged diastole which is known to increase the unevenness of repolarisation and favorise the occurrence of ventricular extrasystoles or arrhythmias. Oversensing may be suspected when an ECG shows:

– A slower pacing rhythm than automatic rhythm as suggested by ventricular sensing during atrial demand pacing (21, 9).

– An irregular triggering which may resemble an electronic circuit fault or an intermittent rupture of a pacing wire (5).

Up to the present, we have not observed these abnormalities in demand pacemaker patients with idiopathic V.T. or myocardial infarctions complicated by

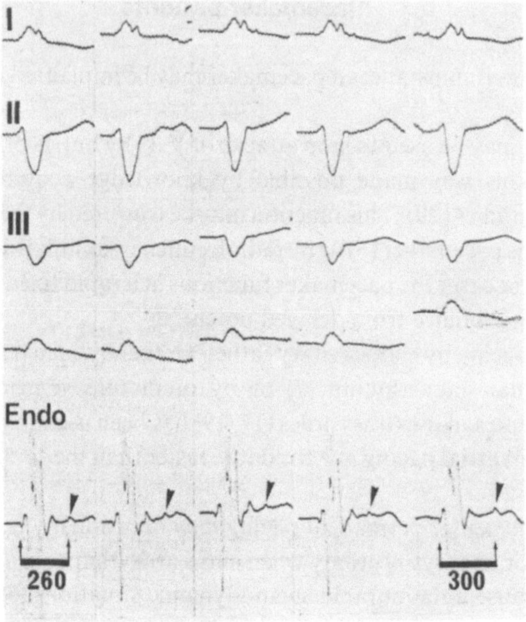

Figure 4. Endocardiac potentials recorded with a monopolar catheter during the replacement of a pacemaker of a patient with a large anteroseptal infarction. The filters were fully opened so as to eliminate the possibility of recording abnormal potentials arising from the filtering during the repolarisation phase. The synchronous potential is observed to be very polyphasic and lasting 0,16 s. The delayed potential arrowed has a varying coupling interval of between 260 and 300ms with reference to the start of the synchronous potential. Its amplitude is too small to be able to inhibit a pacemaker.

arrhythmias. Nevertheless during pacemaker replacement abnormally delayed or fragmented potentials have been recorded in two patients:

– In the first case, a delayed potential coupled with the synchronous potential was recorded, but was of too small amplitude to have been sensed by the pacemaker (Fig. 4).

– In the other patient (Fig. 5), a very fragmented high frequency potential was recorded. This patient had a pacemaker with unipolar right ventricular endocardial electrodes implanted after cardiac surgery for excision of an aneurysm. If more delayed potentials had occurred, abnormal inhibition presenting as an abnormal triggering of the pacemaker would perhaps have been observed.

– Delayed atrial (Fig. 6) and ventricular potentials were also recently observed during clinical electrophysiological studies but their magnitude was not sufficient to inhibit a demand pacemaker.

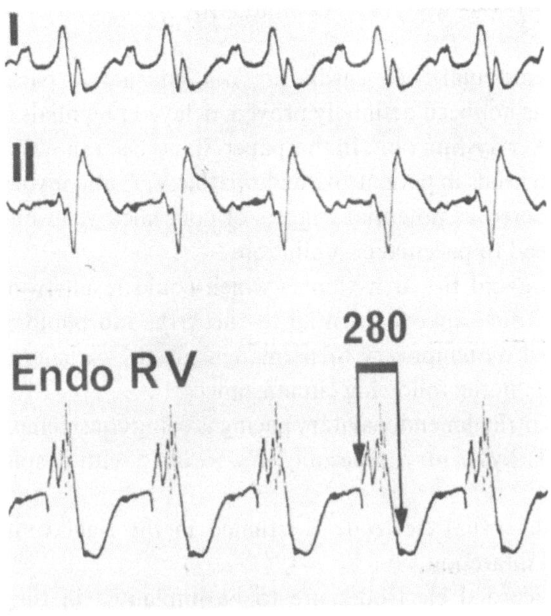

Figure 5. Endocavitary potentials recorded with a monopolar endocavitary catheter in a patient with an antero-septal infarction. The endocavitary potential is very fragmented and lasts nearly 280ms (recorded after opening the filters to have the largest bandpass).

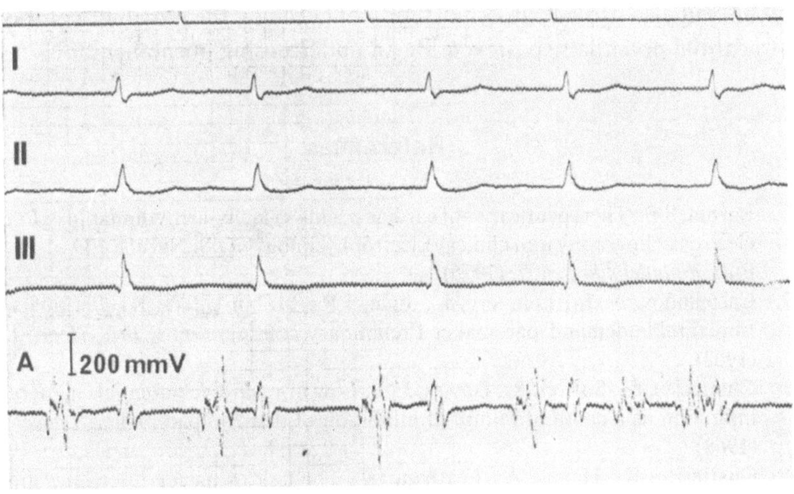

Figure 6. Recording of a polyphasic atrial potential during an electrophysiological investigation of a patient complaining of repeated syncope, and in whom the atrio-ventricular conduction was normal. The potential was recorded with a bipolar USCI C-51 catheter positioned at the midzone of the external wall of the right atrium. In this position, the amplitude of the recorded potential would have been too small to have recycled an atrial demand pacemaker.

Conclusion

Attacks of ventricular tachycardia are not unusual in pacemaker patients. Although it has not been definitely proved, delayed potentials could theorically cause pacemaker dysfunction. In this paper, it has been shown that the presence of delayed potentials in patients with idiopathic V.T. and myocardial ischaemia may be considered as potential triggers of concealed ventricular extrasystoles which could lead to pacemaker inhibition.

In order to avoid the arrhythmias which could result from this abnormal activation, it would appear essential to check the morphology of the electrograms recorded by temporary or permanent pacing catheters in patients susceptible to V.T. in the following circumstances:

– If right ventricular endocavitary pacing is being considered in a patient with idiopathic V.T. by reentry, especially if associated with dysplasia of the right ventricle.

– If an endocardial electrode is situated in the right ventricle in case of postero-septal infarction.

– If the epicardial electrodes are to be implanted in the left ventricular myocardium of patients with chronic myocardial ischaemia. In this latter case, the macroscopic appearance of the heart is no assurance that the electrodes are not overlying a subendocardial ischaemic area of myocardium capable of giving rise to abnormal potentials.

This will also provide an opportunity of checking the possibility of too weak intracardial potentials so preventing an undersensing phenomenon.

References

1. Barold, S.S., Therapeutic uses of cardiac pacing in tachy-arrhythmias in "His bundle electrocardiography and clinical Electrophysiology" O.S. Narula, ED., F.A. Davis Pub. *Philadelphia* p. 407, (1975).
2. Castellanos, A. Jr., Lemberg, L., Jude, J.R., Mobin-Uddin, K., Berkovits, B.V., Implantable demand pacemaker Preliminary considerations. *Brit. Heart J.* 1, 29 (1968).
3. Chatterjee, K., Sutton, R., Davies, J.G., Low intracardiac potentials in myocardial infarction as a cause of failure of inhibition of demand pacemaker. *Lancet* 1, 511 (1968).
4. Chatterjee, K., Harris, A., Leatham, A., The risk of pacing after infarction and current recommendation. *Lancet* 2, 1061 (1969).
5. Coumel, P.H., Mugica, J., Barold, S.S., Demand pacemaker arrhythmias caused by intermittent incomplete electrode fracture Diagnosis with testing magnet. *Amer. J. Cardiol.* 36, 105 (1975).

6. Fisher, J.D., Furman, S., Mehra, R., Ectopic ventricular tachycardia treated with bursts of pacing at 300 per minute from an implanted ventricular pacer. *Circulation* 51, 52, 182 (1975).
7. Fontaine, G., Le rôle du médecin traitant dans la surveillance des porteurs de pacemakers. *La vie médicale* 23-24, 2031 (1976).
8. Fontaine, G., Surgical treatment of resistant ventricular tachycardia (22 cases). *Work-shop on sudden death*, Gent 1976.
9. Fontaine, G., Beneton, H., Frank, R., Guiraudon, G., Grosgogeat, Y., Facquet, J., Prévention de la tachycardie ventriculaire après infarctus du myocarde par pacemaker intracorporel. *Arch. Mal. Coeur* 68, 961 (1975).
10. Fontaine, G., Guiraudon, G., Frank, R., Le syndrome de post-excitation I – en rythme sinusal. *En préparation* 1977.
11. Fontaine, G., Guiraudon, G., Frank, R., Le syndrome de post-excitation II – en tachycardie ventriculaire. *En préparation* 1977.
12. Fontaine, G., Guiraudon, G., Frank, R., Gebraux, A., Cousteau, J.P., Barillon, H., Gay, J., Cabrol, C., Facquet, J., La cartographie épicardique et le traitement chirurgical par simple ventriculotomie de certaines tachycardies ventriculaires rebelles par réentrée. *Arch. Mal. Coeur* 68, 113 (1975).
13. Fontaine, G., Guiraudon, G., Frank, R., Vedel, J., Coutte, R., Dragodanne, C., Epicardial mapping and surgical treatment in 6 cases of resistant ventricular tachycardia not related to coronary artery disease. In – The conduction system of the heart – H.J.J. Wellens, K.I. Lie, M.J. Janse ed., H.E. Stenfert Kroese B.V., Pub. Leiden p. 545, (1976).
14. Fontaine, G., Guiraudon, G., Frank, R., Vedel, J., Grosgogeat, Y., Cabrol, C., Facquet, J., Stimulation studies and epicardial mapping in ventricular tachycardia: study of mechanisms and selection for surgery. In – Reentrant arrhythmias – *Kulbertus Ed. MTP Pub.* Lancaster 1977.
15. Gaspar, H.C.G., De Caprio, Y., Escher, D.J.W., Furman, S., Influence of lidocaine and propranolol on temporary pacer sensing. *Circulation* 51-52, Sup. II, 187 (1975).
16. Gay, R.J., Brown, D.F., Pacemaker failure due to procainamide toxicity. *Amer. J. Cardiol.* 34, 728 (1974).
17. Guize, L., Zacouto, B., Meilhac, B., Le Pailleur, C., Di Matteo, J., Stimulations endocardiaques orthorythmiques. Intérêt diagnostique et thérapeutique. *Nouv. Presse Med.* 3, 2083 (1974).
18. Gurdiel, O., Paris, A., Aleman, C., Penso, M., Gordo, J., Harris, A., Low right ventricular endocardial potentials in chronic Chagas' disease. *Brit. Heart J.* 36, 1239-1243 (1974).
19. Kaiser, G.A., Waldo, A.L., Bowman, F.O., Hoffman, B.F., Malm, J.R., The use of ventricular electrograms in operation for coronary artery disease and its complications. *Ann. Thor. Surg.* 10, 153 (1970).
20. Kastor, J.A., De Sanctis, R.W., Harthorne, J.W., Schwartz, G.H., Transvenous atrial pacing in the treatment of refractory ventricular irritability. *Ann. Int. Med.* 66, 939 (1967).
21. Kramer, D.H., Moss, A.J., Permanent pervenous atrial pacing from the coronary vein. *Circulation* 42, 427 (1970).
22. Massumi, R.A., Masn, D.T., Apparent malfunction of demand pacemaker caused by nonpropagated ventricular extrasystoles. *Chest* 61, 426-431 (1972).

23. Mendes, C., Grihzit, C.L., Moe, G.K., Influence of cycle length upon refractory period of auricles, ventricles and A-V node in the frog. *Am. J. Cardiol.* 184, 287 (1956).
24. Moss, A.J., Rivers, R.J., Griffith, L.S.C., Carmel, J.A., Millard, E.B. Transvenous left atrial pacing for the control of recurrent ventricular fibrillation. *N. Engl. Med. J.* 278, 928 (1968).
25. Mymin, D., Cuddy, T.E., Synha, S.N., Inhibition of demand pacemaker by skeletal muscle potentials. *Circulation* 46, Sup. 11, 208 (1972).
26. Peter, T., Harper, R., Sloman, G., Inhibition of demand pacemakers caused by potentials associated with inspiration. *Brit. Heart J.* 38, 211 (1976).
27. Schamroth, L., The disorders of cardiac rhythm. *Blackwell Pub.* Oxford and Edinburgh 1971.
28. Spurrell, R.A.J., Sowton, E., Deuchar, D.C., Ventricular tachycardia in 4 patients evaluated by programmed electrical stimulations of the heart and treated in 2 patients by surgical division of anterior radiation of left bundle branch. *Brit. Heart J.* 35, 1014 (1973).
29. Wellens, H.J.J., Schuilenburg, R.M., Durrer, D., Electrical stimulation of the heart in patients with ventricular tachycardia. *Circulation* 46, 216 (1972).
30. Woodson, R.D., Friesen, W.G., Starr, A., Use of atrial pacing in cardiac surgical patients. *Amer. J. Cardiol.* 21, 120 (1968).

A SPECIAL APPROACH IN THE MANAGEMENT OF RE-ENTRY TACHYCARDIAS

R.A.J. Spurrell

In recent years programmed electrical stimulation of the heart and intracardiac recording techniques have demonstrated that a re-entry mechanism is the basis for many paroxysmal supraventricular tachycardias and that the site of re-entry is commonly within the AV node (1). In patients who have re-entry tachycardias of this type it is usually possible to terminate the tachycardia by correctly timed single or double atrial or ventricular premature beats (2).

Various pacing techniques have been used in the treatment of re-entry tachycardias. Conventional demand pacemakers which can be converted to a fixed rate mode by the application of a magnet over the pacemaker site have been used in a way such that the pacemaker is converted to its fixed rate mode during a tachycardia and pacing stimuli then occur at a rate slower than that of the tachycardia. Eventually a pacing stimulus will occur at such a time in the cardiac cycle that it produces a suitably timed premature beat which terminates the tachycardia (3, 4).

Other techniques have also been used such as rapid atrial pacing (5) and triggered high frequency bursts of stimuli into the atria (6) to produce appropriately timed atrial premature beats.

An ideal pacing system for the automatic termination of re-entry tachycardias would be one which senses intracardiac electrical potentials, is activated when a tachycardia occurs and then fires one or two stimuli to produce one or two premature beats which are triggered by the intracardiac electrogram to occur at the correct time in the cardiac cycle to terminate the tachycardia. However it has been found that the point in the cardiac cycle where a premature beat can be consistently relied on to terminate a tachycardia varies in different attacks in the same patient (2), and so a preset coupling time for the premature stimuli cannot be relied on to consistently terminate an attack in any one patient.

In conjunction with Devices Instruments Ltd.* the author has developed a pacing system (Devices 4273) which overcomes this problem.

An electrode catheter for sensing and stimulating is positioned in an appropriate chamber, preferably the right ventricle. This catheter is connected to the

* Devices Instruments Ltd., Welwyn Garden City, Hertfordshire, England.

pacemaker. Intracardiac potentials are sensed and when the cardiac cycle length is sensed at a shorter interval than a preset level, i.e. following the onset of a tachycardia then the output circuit of the pacemaker is activated. This induces a premature stimulus with a preset coupling time following the intraventricular endocardial potential. This coupling time is such that the first stimulus occurs within the refractory period of the ventricle. One second later a further stimulus is induced but the coupling time is lengthened by 5 msecs. About every second a further stimulus occurs but each one is delayed by a further 5 msecs. In this way 100 msecs. of the cardiac cycle is scanned at which time the pacemaker recycles and starts the scan again. Once a stimulus has been induced outside the refractory period of the ventricle then ventricular premature beats are induced. As the scan progresses eventually a suitably timed ventricular premature beat will occur which terminates the tachycardia and the pacemaker then switches itself off. In those patients who require two correctly timed premature beats for tachycardia termination this system can be used such that the scan occurs with two premature stimuli scanning, there being a fixed coupling time between the two stimuli. This system can therefore be used with single or double premature stimuli and for ventricular or atrial stimulation, bearing in mind the problems of long-term atrial stimulation.

Figure 1 is a recording obtained from a patient with a re-entry supraventricular tachycardia demonstrating the termination of a paroxysm using the scanning pacing system. The first thirteen beats are part of the tachycardia. The scanning pacemaker is activated and the first pacing stimulus can be seen occurring at 185 msecs. after the preceding QRS complex. This stimulus occurs within the refractory period of the ventricle and so no ventricular premature beat is seen. The next two stimuli occur with delays of 190 and 195 msecs. respectively and both occur within the refractory period of the ventricle. The fourth pacing stimulus has scanned out to 200 msecs., this occurs outside the refractory period of the ventricle, a ventricular premature beat (VPB) is induced which occurs at the right time in the cardiac cycle to terminate the tachycardia. The last two beats are the first two beats of sinus rhythm and the output circuit of the pacemaker is now inactive.

Two patients (one using a single premature stimulus scan and the other a double premature stimulus scan) have been successfully treated using a semi-implanted system on a long-term basis. Monitoring has demonstrated that their spontaneous paroxysmal re-entry supraventricular tachycardia has always been terminated in less than twenty seconds.

At the present time an implantable scanning system which can be programmed external is under development. The principles of function of this system will differ from that described above in that the scan will start late in the cardiac cycle and the premature stimuli will occur with progressively shorter coupling times.

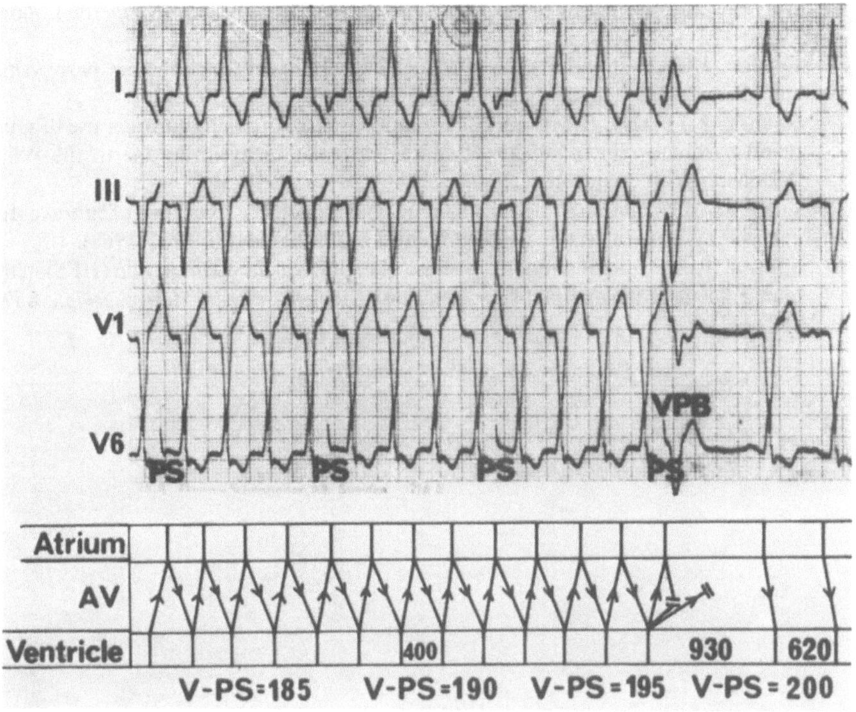

Figure 1. Recording showing the termination of a re-entry supraventricular tachycardia using the scanning pacing system.

I, III, V_1, V_6	– surface electrocardiographic leads
VPB	– ventricular premature beat
PS	– pacing stimulus
AV	– atrioventricular junction
V-PS	– time in milliseconds from the onset of the QRS complex to the pacing stimulus artefact.

In this way it is hoped to improve the safety of the system by avoiding, when possible, the firing of a pacing stimulus in the early vulnerable part of the cardiac cycle.

References

1. Durrer, D., Schuilenburg, R.M. and Wellens, H.J.J., The role of the atrioventricular junction in the genesis of arrhythmias in the human heart. *Proc. Kon. Ned. Akad. Wet.* 72, 515 (1969).
2. Spurrell, R.A.J., The study and management of tachycardias using intracardiac elec-

trograms and programmed electrical stimulation of the heart. *MD thesis*, London 1972.

3. Kitchen, J.G. and Goldreyer, B.N., Demand pacemaker for refractory paroxysmal supraventricular tachycardia. *New Eng. J. Med.*, 287, 596 (1972).
4. Ryan, G.F., Easley, R.M., Zaroff, L.I. and Goldstein, S., Paradoxical use of a demand pacemaker in treatment of supraventricular tachycardia due to the Wolff Parkinson White syndrome. *Circulation*, 38, 1037 (1963).
5. Lister, J.W., Cohen, L.S., Bernstein, W.H. and Samet, P., Treatment of supraventricular tachycardia by rapid atrial stimulation. *Circulation*, 38, 1044 (1968).
6. Spurrell, R.A.J. and Sowton, E., The use of high frequency stimulation (HFS) in the management of paroxysmal supraventricular tachycardia. *J. Electrocardiol.*, 8 (3), 287 (1975).

DISCUSSION VIII. TACHYCARDIA AND PACING

CHAIRMAN: H.J.J. WELLENS *(Maastricht, The Netherlands)*

CHAIRMAN: To warm things up a little bit, I would like to ask the audience a question.

I want to know how many of you are actually using programmed electrical stimulation in the investigation of patients with tachycardia. Would those who are doing this raise their hands?

So that would mean that approximately 20 people out of this audience of about 400 persons are using this method.

This will probably increase now that specially designed programmed stimulators are becoming commercially available.

I would like to address my first question to Dr. Fontaine. I have recently moved from Amsterdam to Maastricht. Maastricht is a new university in the south of Holland. One of the first patients we studied there was a patient with idiopathic ventricular tachycardia. In this particular patient with a right-sided ventricular tachycardia, we were able to record within the cavity a late potential. We could demonstrate that, during programmed stimulation of the right ventricle, the delayed potential moved to a later and later position with a critical position at initiation of re-entry. I would like to know, Dr. Fontaine, whether you observed this phenomenon also, either endo-cavitary or during epicardial mapping studies.

G. FONTAINE *(Paris, France):* Up to now, we observed both, in two separate cases. If you do mapping of sinus rhythm at the time of surgery, you can find a localized area of delayed potentials. With the exploring probe in this area of delayed potential, you try to initiate tachycardia by a premature stimulus or by a rapid burst of stimuli. We were able to find in these patients when the extra stimulus was given, that the delayed potential showed further delay sometimes resulting in ventricular tachycardia. We also got the same results from one case during the intracavitary investigation.

CHAIRMAN: Thank you very much, Dr. Fontaine. Would you like to comment on this particular point, Dr. Spurrell.

R.A.J. SPURRELL *(London, England):* We have seen these late potentials, but not during preoperative studies. We have seen these in two patients with ventricular tachycardia during operative investigation of the patients prior to the surgical interruption of a re-entry pathway. During study of the maps that we obtained during sinus rhythm and with premature stimulation, we were not able to record late potentials in the area where we subsequently recorded that the tachycardia was initiated.

CHAIRMAN: There is a question from Dr. Narula.

O.S. NARULA *(Chicago, U.S.A.):* The question is directed to Dr. Preston. I was just fascinated by the slides on your first patient, where you showed what looked like a VT, but the catheter showed a SVT. I was puzzled that from the slide the ventricular rate seemed to be about 250, whereas the patient had a normal PR, no WPW; how could that patient be conducting 250 beats a minute through the A-V node, was it really SVT? Or could it be a VT with a retrograde conduction of 250 atrial impulses?

T.A. PRESTON *(Seattle, U.S.A.):* This was a patient with acute myocardial infarction and it fascinated us, to accept that this was supra-ventricular. You could see in fact that there are periods of this supra-ventricular tachycardia and that there is antegrade A-V conduction. We never had a conduction of 300 or 250, except for a few instances. I believe also that the patient was, because of hypotension, getting a sympathomimetic amine agent at the time, which enhances A-V nodal conduction.

O.S. NARULA *(Chicago, U.S.A.):* It seems hardly likely that a man with a normal PR would conduct 300 impulses, does it not?

T.A. PRESTON *(Seattle, U.S.A.):* Sure. But have you not seen that before? Patients with essentially normal QRS conducting flutter one-to-one. Especially in the presence of sympathomimetic amines?

O.S. NARULA *(Chicago, U.S.A.):* But the PR interval during atrial pacing, which you showed subsequently, is relatively long.

T.A. PRESTON *(Seattle, U.S.A.):* That was later on. The drugs have changed.

O.S. NARULA *(Chicago, U.S.A.):* I believe there are no simultaneous recordings, are there?

T.A. PRESTON *(Seattle, U.S.A.):* That is right, there are not.

O.S. NARULA *(Chicago, U.S.A.):* But could you be sure this impulse is going from the atrium to the ventricle, or could it have been the ventricle conducting to the atrium? Was it truly SVT and not a VT?

T.A. Preston *(Seattle, U.S.A.):* What we can say is that it involved the atrium and that is the important point in terms of treatment with atrial pacing. We also know that with atrial pacing, this arrhythmia, which was recurring 15 times per hour, was totally suppressed.

Chairman: Thank you, Dr. Preston and Dr. Narula. Who else has a question?

M.H. Ellestad *(Irvine, U.S.A.):* I would like to ask Dr. Spurrell if this technique that he uses has to be localized in the appropriate chamber. In other words, can you terminate with this method a ventricular rhythm with a ventricular or with an atrial electrode and vice versa?

R.A.J. Spurrell *(London, England):* This system can be used for either atrial or ventricular stimulation. Of course, particularly with paroxysmal functional tachycardia, in which we think the re-entry mechanism is within the A-V node, it is not uncommon to find that the tachycardia can be terminated either with atrial stimulation or with ventricular stimulation, but not necessarily both. But when you are treating tachycardia it is extremely important to get your electrode positioned as close to the re-entry circuit as you possibly can. We have used this particular technique by stimulation of both chambers. Obviously, we prefer ventricular stimulation with the electrode technology being as it is at the moment, and if we are having to deal with a patient who needs atrial stimulation then we are really committed to sewing the electrodes on directly.

M.H. Ellestad *(Irvine, U.S.A.):* So, almost invariably then, for ventricular rhythm, you have to use ventricular stimulation.

R.A.J. Spurrell *(London, England);* We have not actually used this in a chronic situation in ventricular tachycardia as yet, but we have used it in the acute situation.

Chairman: It is possible to terminate a ventricular tachycardia by an atrial premature beat, assuming that the rate of the ventricular tachycardia is such that you can get through the A-V node, early enough in the ventricle, to get into the re-entry circuit to break the tachycardia. Out of 64 patients with ventricular tachycardia, we were able to terminate ventricular tachycardia, in three, by an atrial premature beat. So it is possible, but it is very rare because you need to have a rather slow rate of your ventricular tachycardia in order to get into that circuit.

M.H. Ellestad *(Irvine, U.S.A.):* In almost every case, then the premature atrial stimulus is blocked in the A-V node.

Chairman: That is right. Dr. Dodinot...

B. Dodinot *(Nancy, France):* I would like to ask Dr. Spurrell a question.

What kind of cases does he select for stopping tachycardia? Are they having very frequent runs of tachycardia, when you apply your scanning system, or are they having them only once a week or twice a month?

R.A.J. Spurrell *(London, England):* Inevitably, because this is still a developing technique we have had to choose patients that are getting intractable disrhythmias with a high frequency, that is getting attacks frequently and that are becoming drug resistant. I think if we get into a stage where we can offer a very reliable implantable system which will function in this manner, then it will open up a very much larger number of patients, who are perhaps not entirely satisfactorily controlled on oral therapy. But at the moment we have only implanted these systems in patients who really have intractable arrhythmias.

Chairman: I would like to make a comment in this regard. If you look at the ability to terminate tachycardias by timed stimuli, there are certain general rules which I think are important to keep in mind.

First of all, it is very unusual to terminate a tachycardia with a rate of above 160 p.m. by one single premature beat. It is only possible under two circumstances: WPW syndrome and a concealed accessory pathway which is incorporated in the tachycardia circuit. In fact, in my experience, when you have a supraventricular tachycardia with a rate of above 160 p.m. and you can terminate it by a single premature beat, all these patients have either overt or concealed accessory pathways. It is an important thing to know, because this finding is highly suggestive for the presence of accessory pathways. So, if you are talking in terms of termination of tachycardia by a single or more than one premature beat, I think this figure – 160 – is a very important one to keep in mind.

R.A.J. Spurrell *(London, England):* I think we would agree entirely with that. I think this really raises the importance of developing systems of this sort. Because patients with tachycardias under 160 are frequently controllable by other means, anyway and they tend to be less symptomatic. They are the sort that if you really have to implant some form of pacing system, the straightforward underdrive pacemaker is suitable. But if they are the very highly symptomatic patients with rates in excess of 160, at the moment we have considerable difficulty in providing adequate electronic therapy for this group and it is this group that requires a system that can induce more than one premature beat.

Chairman: I am afraid this is going to be the last question.

Dr. Joseph *(England):* A question for Dr. Preston. His success in terminating atrial flutter with rapid atrial stimulation seems contrary to other reported experience and also to my own experience. I wonder if he could give some advice, perhaps in terms not only of site of stimulation, but also frequency and energy content.

T.A. PRESTON *(Seattle, U.S.A.)*: The figure of 70% I gave actually was quoted also by Dr. Barold and one can find success rates anywhere from around 10%, I think – in one paper by Rosen – up to almost 90%. I do think it is a function of how meticulous and persistent one is in attempting this. In the great majority of cases, in my experience all I can say is that one can either get the patient directly back to sinus rhythm or, more frequently, to atrial fibrillation. I have seen very few patients in whom you cannot push that patient into atrial fibrillation temporarily, if one paces for ten minutes with rapid atrial stimulation. Some may go back to flutter, but a large number of them will then go back to sinus rhythm.

One must probe around for various pacing sites, low in the atrium. Close to the A-V node is, I believe, probably the best place. As I said, in one patient we were successful only in pacing both atria. So if one could capture both atria, the success rate would be higher. I think there is no magic formula for doing this.

DR. JOSEPH *(England)*: What about frequency and energy?

T.A. PRESTON *(Seattle, U.S.A.)*: The frequency must be greater than the atrial flutter rate, but not much greater. What is important is to be sure that you are actually capturing the atrium. In most unsuccessful attempts, there has been no capture of the atrium. Therefore, obviously, you are going to be unsuccessful. This requires probing around, using high stimulation levels, so that you really do capture the atrium. I believe that if you capture the atrium, that you will have a success rate of at least 70%.

CHAIRMAN: I would like to make a comment in this regard. It is much easier – and this has been the experience of Waldo in Birmingham (U.S.A.) to terminate atrial flutter of the classic sort as to its appearance, than the flutter that does not have this appearance.

Another thing. In my experience, stimulation low in the atrium is much more effective in terminating the classic type of flutter than stimulating high in the atrium. I would certainly endorse what Dr. Preston just said: it is essential to have indeed evidence that you have captured the atrium, then you really have – especially in the saw-tooth type flutter – a very high, almost 100% success rate in terminating atrial flutter.

Now, just one more minute for Dr. Narula.

O.S. NARULA *(Chicago, U.S.A.)*: I wanted to back up both your comments about the success rate of atrial flutter with rapid atrial stimulation. I am very aware of Dr. Rosen's report and before I moved to Chicago, I thought that the Chicago patient population was different so maybe Dr. Rosen had a different experience. Now I use the same County Hospital with the same type of patient material and I have found a very high success rate in all the twenty cases we have done consecutively. I think the basic issue is to capture the atrium, explore different sites, use a higher frequency. We would even go up to 1200 – stimuli per minute. One last comment – which is not related to temporary rapid atrial stimulation, but is related to permanent implantation of rapid atrial stimulation – I wanted to add was: people are using these types of pacemakers and they have a place for it. But I want to warn you that these patients must be selected properly. We must choose people for permanent implantation among the ones who have a relatively healthy atrium and not a fibrosed and a dilated atrium. Patients with a severely diseased fibrous atrium, although they initially might benefit, did not need a rapid atrial stimulator two years later.

CHAIRMAN: Thank you Dr. Narula for your last comment that closes this section.

Section IX

PACEMAKER FOLLOW-UP METHODS

PACEMAKER FOLLOW-UP METHODS

MICHAEL S. LAMPADIUS

The next two sections of the colloquium deal with different methods of pacemaker follow-up. Though these sections are divided into two parts, mainly the follow-up of a pacemaker as a single unit and on the other hand the management of the workload of a pacemaker clinic by computer application, both sections should be combined to a complex system. It will not be possible to regard the pacemaker as an independent technical product, but rather the patient, his pacemaker and the statistical behavior of the whole pacemaker series as a system.

By regarding the topics of the individual papers that will be presented on the next pages it is very astonishing to discover, that none of these papers is mentioning the interrelation of pacemaker and patient. Perhaps, especially after the preceding papers, this is so evident that there is no more uncertainty about exit- or entrance blocks, relative or absolute refractory periods, noise sampling intervals, T-wave sensing and A-V delays. This is due to the fact, that we have learned to interpret a pacemaker ECG and are familiar with the existing pacemakers. But this will change when pacemakers become more complex as it is pointed out in some of the preceding papers.

To give a quick review about the band width of the check-up possibilities the following paragraphs should be discussed.

First	The patient together with his pacemaker
Second	The pacemaker as a single unit
Third	The pacemaker as a series product

When talking about the patient and his pacemaker it must be kept in mind, that depending on the structure of a local health system many pacemaker clinics serve as an outpatient department. That means that the patient will be examined completely not only from the standpoint of his pacemaker, but also with a general internal medical examination. Even in countries where the overall education of the general practioners is on a relative high level, there are hospitals that are performing a complete internal check-up on their patients because they think, that otherwise good care for their patients will not be guaranteed. But this problem is more of a social political issue and this paper will discuss the pacemaker itself.

By examining the pacemaker as a single unit we in part can rely on our experience that we have gathered within the last decade. In most pacemaker clinics a check-up routine has been developed. First of all the functioning of the pacemaker will be evaluated. That means the pacemaker's ability to capture the heart, the ability of the heart to inhibit the demand pacemaker and a proper programmability if it is a programmable unit. This check-up is performed with a simple ECG strip chart recorder and perhaps by means of a magnet to convert the inhibited pulse generator into a fixed mode. And a good deal of common sense of course.

An equally important, but much more difficult procedure is the prognosis of the remaining functional time of the implanted unit. By experience with the Mallory batteries (a mercury primary element) which were used for years exclusively, we learned that it is very difficult, if not impossible, to predict safely an impending pacemaker failure due to energy starvation. Almost all pacemakers now have a repetition rate that is coupled to the power supply voltage. A declining voltage may easily be detected on the strip chart recorder or a digital counter. Nevertheless the predictability was very low, as mercury cells have the tendency that their voltage drops very rapidly at the end of their service life. Therefore different methods have been developed to improve control of the pacemakers from the energy point of view. These methods are either X-ray analysis of the pacemaker batteries, transtelephone monitoring or patient owned test devices. The following papers will show, how all these methods work and how the social system reacts on them. Though these new methods have been developed with the Mallory mercury cell in mind, they are also very apt for their application with the new lithium powered (Greatbatch, SAFT) pacemaker generation.

Fortunately it can be stated, that up to now these new lithium cells have never failed within an implanted pacemaker. But there is still uncertainty, whether this good performance will last until the projected end of life of these pacemakers. This experience is still to come. And therefore, especially in regard to the pacemaker electronics, that must work for a much longer time than before, a thorough follow-up must go on.

Instead of 3 to 4 years, pacemaker electronics will have to perform for more than 10 years now. That means, that the chance of the electronic circuit to fail is much higher than in recent times. A very close look must be taken to the pacemaker performance to discover as soon as possible, whether a pacemaker is going to deviate from its designed parameters. And so Photoanalysis which was pushed to the background since the time pacemakers have a defined voltage-frequency relationship, is gaining more interest again.

When talking about pacemaker performance it can be seen, that the new pacemakers that are on the market now, are performing worse than they did many years before. This is especially true for the rate stability. A few years ago it was guaranteed that a pacemaker would pace with a long-term stability of 1 ms from beat to beat. Therefore, if such a pulse generator would speed up only for a few milliseconds this was a safe indication that a malfunctioning of the electronics was going to occur and the unit could be removed immediately.

Today pacemakers of many manufacturers have the tendency to drift or fluctuate as it is called. This means that valuable time is spoiled until the examining physician can decide whether a pacemaker behavior is normal or out of the limits. In this respect a critical statement about the AAMI (Association for the Advancement of Medical Instrumentation) should be made. The standards that have been established by this organisation should be more strict because for example a long-term stability of 2% is not good enough. Regarding preciseness of operation it must be considered that the test apparatuses for the pacemakers must at least be as precise as the pacemaker itself. So these gadgets at least should comply to the GMP (Good Manufacturing Practices) of the FDA (Federal Drug Administration). It is very doubtful whether this has been considered by all distributors.

Besides all the just mentioned deficiencies of pacemakers it must be agreed that the quality of these units has been much improved over the last years. But as a result of the prolonged service life, the time within which failures may occur is much longer as well. And also the timespan within which a system failure might be encountered will be very long and therefore a large number of pacemakers may be involved in such a problem. Though at least in the United States an agency like the FDA is checking the pacemaker companies regularly to assure that minimum standards of good manufacturing practice will be established, pacemaker failures never can be abolished completely. Just recently a company had to inform physicians about thousands of units that might be malfunctioning.

In Europe or in other parts of the world no such supervising agencies like the FDA are in existence. Therefore the medical and engineering community must establish their own warning system. Such a system could consist of a national pacemaker registry, to ascertain that all known pacemaker malfunctions will be reported to a central data bank.* Thus statistically reliable data could be accumulated within a short period of time. The next papers will give some results of these projects.

In this context it must be considered that such a central registry has a tremendous impact on the pacemaker industry. It would be very likely that a company that might be criticized by this agency might get into serious economic trouble. Therefore all data must be checked thoroughly prior to any comment on the quality of a certain product.

* In the meantime the Working Group Cardiac Pacing of the European Society of Cardiology (established April 1977) has initiated some of these programmes. (Th.)

In some cases however this criticism might be of no economic influence. This is the case, when companies are a dominant factor on the world market. Then no market reaction would be possible due to insufficient replacement units by the competitors. This fact should be considered when either talking about manufacturer control or when selecting a pacemaker brand.

Nevertheless a central data acquisition agency could collect so much data, that the pacemaker clinics could be informed and warned about impending failure modes in time.* One problem for these data centers would be the question about the qualification and selection of the participating hospitals. Of course it would be very important that as many hospitals as possible would participate. On the other hand only a few pacemaker clinics are able to really analyse technical problems and to distinguish between low input sensibility of a pacemaker and a low intracardial potential, for example. There is no doubt that many malfunctioning pacemakers have been replaced by new units without being regarded as malfunctioning. And in addition many statistics do not consider pulse generators in dead patients that have failed or at least would have failed if the patient would have lived long enough.

Therefore the collected data will always be better than the real pacemaker failure rate. This emphasizes that it is important to analyse the sampled material exactly. It should be mandatory, that all pacemakers that are explanted due to assumed malfunctioning will be sent to a testing station prior to sending them back to the manufacturer. And this independent agency should be supervised by a scientist that is not directly connected with pacemaker implantation to avoid a preference of any pacemaker make. In Germany such an investigating service is under construction.

How important it will be to collect data on a wide scale is well known. Not only that in recent times tremendous pacemaker failure series have been discovered by the FDA but also that many pacemaker series have been malfunctioning without any timely information to the pacemaker community. And how fast statistically significant data can be collected on such a national or international basis could be observed in Germany, when in 1973 at a national pacemaker meeting many physicians heard about pacemaker problems in many hospitals, which the distributor claimed not to know of. So within 1 hour sufficient data was collected to take preventive steps.

For the follow-up of pacemakers, pacemaker data sheets must be available. Today there are about 20 to 30 manufacturers on the market with about 150 different models. That means that within the next 5 to 10 years there will be at least 500 different pacemakers implanted, as the companies introduce new mo-

* In the meantime the Working Group Cardiac Pacing of the European Society of Cardiology (established April 1977) has initiated some of these programmes. (Th.)

dels every year. If information about these pulse generators shall be collected and this is necessary because it is unknown which pacemaker will be implanted in a patient that is moving in from a different community, a tremendous amount of catalogues and literature must be compiled.

But the worst is still to come. It is well known that some, if not to say many pacemakers, deviate from the performance that can be found in the original data sheets. And the manufacturers are very reluctant in updating their data. So for the national or international pacemaker registry there is still another important task. That means to control and update the data sheets to give a fair chance to follow up pacemakers in a correct way. This service has now been established in Germany by the German Working Group for Pacemakers.

As a summary of this preface it should be stated, that the methods of pacemaker follow-up have changed in the past and will change in the future. But there is no evidence, that pacemaker follow-up can be neglected in the near future.

SIGNIFICANCE OF PHOTOANALYSIS IN A PACEMAKER SURVEILLANCE SYSTEM

H. ECTOR, A. AUBERT AND H. DE GEEST

On the first pacemaker colloquium, organised by Vitatron in Arnhem, the Netherlands 1975, we had the occasion to discuss the reliability of our pacemaker surveillance system (1). This reliability clearly improved in 1975 and 1976. In these last two years 114 pacemaker replacements were carried out at St. Raphael University Hospital in Leuven.

Table 1 gives the reasons for pacemaker removal in these 114 cases. We had 86.8% elective replacements and of these 31.6% can be considered as prophylactic. In 55.2% a decision for replacement was based on changes noted in final clinic analysis. The incidence of late electrode malfunction was 8.8%. Sudden pacemaker failure occurred in 5 cases.

Table 1. Reasons for pacemaker removal in 114 cases

	Number of cases	%
Elective replacements:		86.8
Changes noted in final clinic analysis	63	55.2
Patient's or physician's choice	36	31.6
Sudden pacemaker failure	5	4.4
Late electrode malfunction	10	8.8
Extrusion	0	

Table 2 illustrates the value of different parameters in predicting imminent battery failure. In 63 out of 68 cases where no prophylactic replacement was performed a correct prediction of imminent battery exhaustion was made. When calculated in this way the reliability of the pacemaker surveillance system comes to 92.6%. In 62 cases we noted a change in pacing rate and/or photoanalytic data. Loss of R wave detection was the only change in one case.

Table 3 shows the changes noted in the final clinic analysis, when a decision for replacement was taken. In this figure we only consider these 63 cases, where an imminent pacer failure was predicted. In 90.5% of these cases there was a distinct alteration in pacing rate. Only in 5 cases we needed photoanalysis as the exclusive

Table 2. Value of parameters in predicting imminent battery exhaustion

Manufacturer	*General Electric* *Ventr. As.*	*Ventr. Inh.*	*Medtronic* *Ventr. As.*	*Ventr. Inh.*	*Vitatron* *Ventr. As.*	*Ventr. Inh.*	*Total*
Unexpected failures	3	1	0	0	1	0	5
Prophylactic replacements	10	4	2	9	3	8	36
Correct predictions based on pacing rate and photoanalysis	9	23	3	3		24	62
Loss of R wave detection as the only change		1					1
Reliability of a pacemaker clinic in predicting imminent battery failure:	9/12	24/25	3/3	3/3		24/24	63/68
	In 63 out of 68 cases, where no prophylactic replacement was performed a correct prediction of imminent battery exhaustion was made. The reliability of the follow-up system was 92.6%.						

Ventr. As. = ventricular asynchronous; Ventr. Inh. = ventricular inhibited.

Table 3. Value of parameters in predicting imminent battery exhaustion

Manufacturer	*General Electric* *Ventr. As.*	*Ventr. Inh.*	*Medtronic* *Ventr. As.*	*Ventr. Inh.*	*Vitatron* *Ventr. As.*	*Ventr. Inh.*	*Total number of cases*	%
Number of correct predictions	9	24	3	3		24	63	100
Alteration in pacing rate								
present	9	23	1	2		22	57	90.5
absent	0	1	2	1		2	6	9.5
Photoanalytic data								
exclusive diagnosis	0	0	2	1		2	5	7.9
additional information	3	13	1	1		14	32	50.8
unchanged	2	8				6	16	25.4
unknown	4	3		1		2	10	15.9
Loss of R wave detection								
only change		1					1	1.6
additional information		5				2	7	11.1

Ventr. As. = ventricular asynchronous; Ventr. Inh. = ventricular inhibited.

diagnostic tool. In another 32 cases (50.8%) a change in photoanalytic parameters offered some additional information.

Table 4 summarizes the total significance of photoanalysis for both follow-up periods 72-74 (1) and 75-76. In the period 75-76 an exclusive diagnosis by photoanalysis alone was made in 8 cases. Besides the 5 cases of battery depletion, there are 3 cases of lead malfunction, diagnosed by photoanalysis. When we compare the two follow-up periods, we can conclude that photoanalysis is still contributing in a very similar way to the quality of a pacemaker surveillance system. As a diagnostic tool photoanalysis is useful as well for some types of lead malfunction as for a number of battery failures. The reliability of a pacemaker clinic and the safety of the pacemaker patient completely depend on the quality of the pacing system. One of the major features for a pacing device are reliable and simple end-of-life indicators. Our feeling is, that in the future photoanalysis will continue to give an interesting contribution in the prediction and recognition of these surprises, which have always been a challenge for pacemaker manufacturers and clinicians.

Table 4. Significance of Photoanalysis in detecting pacing defects

Follow-up period	*72-74* *Number of cases*	*75-76* *Number of cases*
Battery exhaustion, predicted by photoanalysis alone	6	5
Lead malfunction		
high relative threshold*	2	1
broken insulation	4	1
incomplete wire fracture		1
Abnormal impulse shape	1	
Additional information about battery exhaustion	27	32
Conclusion		
Exclusive photoanalysis diagnoses	13	8
photoanalysis useful	40 (27 + 13)	40 (32 + 8)

* As measured by the Vitatron pacemaker analyzer MPA 1.

Reference

1. Ector, H., Emmerchts, C., De Schepper, S., De Geest, H., The reliability of the pacemaker surveillance system at St. Raphael University Hospital, Leuven, Belgium; In: Norman, J. and Rickards, A. (ed.), Proceedings of the pacemaker colloquium, *Arnhem, the Netherlands*. P. 149, (1975).

PACEMAKER FAILURE DETECTABLE BY RÖNTGEN ANALYSIS

W. DU MESNIL DE ROCHEMONT AND U. MÖDDER

Roentgenologic examination is an important means in follow-up of patients with an implanted pacemaker. In pacemaker malfunction it often provides confirmation of the underlying defect.

The correct intracardial position of the electrode has to be documented early after implantation by radiographs in two planes. The catheter should run through the right atrium in a gentle curve and the electrode tip should lie transversely at the apex of the right ventricle and be slightly wedged beneath the trabeculae. The lateral chest examination is as important as the frontal view. The catheter has to lie anteriorly and at some distance from the chest wall.

The radiographic documentation of the total pacemaker system soon after implantation is important as a control for radiologic studies in identifying pacemaker failure (1, 2). Some roentgenologic findings in pacemaker malfunction are listed in Table 1.

Table 1. Roentgenologic findings in pacemaker failure

A. Catheter

1. primary malposition: coronary sinus or loops in the heart cavity
2. dislocation with or against the direction of blood flow: outflow tract, truncus pulmonalis, pulmonary artery, right atrium, vena cava, hepatic vein
3. penetration into the myocardium
4. perforation of the myocardium
5. sharp angulation of the catheter
6. lead fracture
7. changes in the subcutaneous loops and/or intracardial course of the catheter with or without dislocation of the electrode tip, indicating traction on the lead (after replacement of the pulse generator)

B. Pulse generator

1. battery exhaustion
2. rotation of the generator with coiling of the lead wire and retraction of the electrode tip or fracture of the lead (pacemaker twiddler's syndrome)

A frontal projection alone cannot define good, poor or false catheter position. In Fig. 1 both catheters run almost parallel. It is a patient with severe mitral stenosis and calcifications in the wall of the enlarged left atrium. The upper

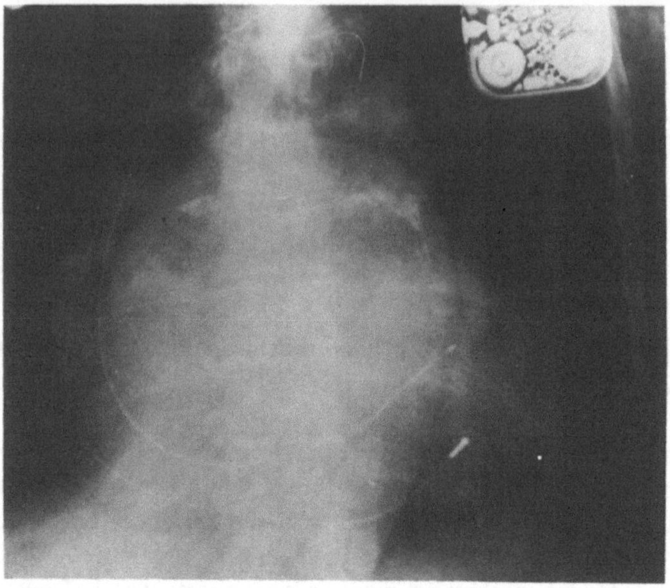

Figure 1. Two catheters running almost parallel in the frontal plane; the bipolar temporary electrode (upper one) lies anteriorly, the permanent unipolar (lower one) in the coronary sinus (see lateral projection Fig. 2).

bipolar temporary electrode by the lateral projection is proven to lie anteriorly. The unipolar permanent electrode was placed lower and the temporary electrode was removed after the frontal picture was taken. The lateral projection later shows a false position of the catheter in the coronary sinus (Fig. 2). This demonstrates that we cannot be sure about the correct position of the electrode by looking just at the frontal plane.

Dislocation of the catheter is the most common cause of pacemaker failure (3). A dislodgement is possible with the direction of blood flow into the outflow tract, the truncus pulmonalis and the pulmonary artery or against the direction of blood flow into the right atrium, the vena cava or hepatic veins.

There may be a slight angulation of the catheter loop as it crosses the tricuspid valve. Any sharp bending and close abutment of the tip against the ventricular wall with every systole can lead to penetration and perforation of the myocardium and finally entrance of the catheter tip into the pericardial space. Even without fluoroscopy we can anticipate an intracardial kinking of the catheter if the radiograph shows a motion unsharpness 5-7 cm proximal of the catheter tip especially in the lateral view. In combination with a wide curve of the catheter in the right atrium with the catheter running close to the myocardium along the right contour of the heart, we might expect penetration or perforation of the tip of the electrode.

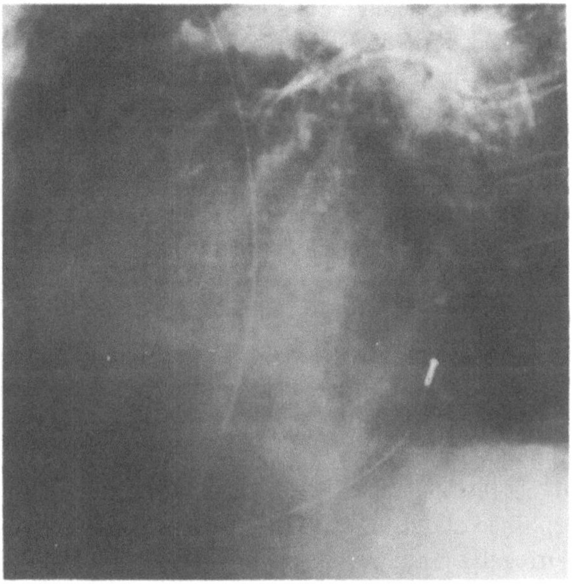

Figure 2.

Penetration of the electrode tip may be readily seen in the standard projections. But the catheter tip might appear to be in adequate position with no change of position as compared with previous films. In this case fluoroscopy and spotfilms taken in different projections may show the tip close to the cardiac surface suggesting a penetration into the myocardium anteriorly. An angulation of the tip indicates a complete perforation of the myocardium with the elecgrode tip lying in the pericardial space. In pacemaker malfunction fluoroscopy and spotfilms in several oblique projections are essential even though the standard projections do not show any abnormalities. Free flotation of the catheter inside the right ventricle may be detectable only by fluoroscopy.

If there is a sharp angulation of the catheter we always have to look for damage to the leads. Lead fractures actually are rarely seen in intracardial electrodes since these contain very fine, coiled electrodes, and fractures may be evident only on direct inspection or radiography after removal from the patient. The larger diameter of epicardial electrodes make them more adaptable to roentgenologic identifaction of fracture. Besides the flexion-tension of the epicardial electrode close to the costal margin is due to fixation greater than in intracardial electrodes. To determine if electrode wire breakage has occurred, slightly overpenetrated films of good quality are essential (4).

Changes in the subcutaneous loops and the intracardial course of the catheter with or without dislocation of the electrode tip indicate traction on the lead for instance after replacement of the pulse generator. Often we do not pay enough attention to these little changes. A slight variation in the intracardial course of the catheter and the electrode tip contacting the endocardium in a different angle may lead to a rise in threshold.

Roentgenographic information about the pulse generator is rather limited. The type of pulse generator can be identified from its shape, the position of the individual batteries and the picture of the electronic circuit using a pacemaker control table.*

In pulse generators with mercury cell batteries we are able to study signs of battery depletion. Mercury batteries contain two radiopaque ring electrodes, a central zinc anode with a hollow core and an outer ring made from mercuric oxide. Both rings are separated by a radiolucent electrolyte (5, 6).

In new batteries the rings are clearly defined. With battery discharge, metallic mercury is deposited about the inner electrode, which loses its smooth border and becomes irregular gradually opacifying the electrolyte. Finally liquid mercury enters the hollow core and obliterates it.

In order to visualize this change, the roentgen-ray beam must be directed perpendicularly to the long axis of the cell. Optimum position may be determined fluoroscopically and then high kv roentgenograms are made. Unfortunately this technique has a low degree of reliability in accurately predicting pulse generator depletion. In the new lithium power sources there is no possibility of radiographic study of pacemakers for signs of battery depletion.

Changes in the position of the pulse generator are not as infrequent as one may expect. A slight movement does not have any serious effect on the electrode. Six times we noticed in our patients a rotation of the pulse generator within its pocket with traction on the lead, sometimes retracting the electrode tip and with damage to the insulating sheath of the catheter. Rotation occurred either spontaneously or as a result of repeated twiddling on the part of the patient. We saw this pacemaker twiddler's syndrome with several different types of pulse generators (7, 8, 9). A round pulse generator may rotate clockwise several times, coiling the lead wire and retracting the electrode. In one patient the electrode tip was retracted into the neck adjacent to the phrenic nerve and the brachial plexus. The patient had epigastric jerking movements, occasional spasms of involuntary inspiration and movements of the right forearm. The rotation of the pulse generator in this patient was spontaneous.

* H.K. Schulten, O. Baldus, D.W. Behrenbeck, Univ. of Cologne, Dept. of Medicine and Cardiology (Prof. Dr. H.H. Hilger): Schrittmacher Kontrolltafel Ed.: Pharma Beiersdorf, 2000 Hamburg, FR Germany.

An 80-years-old patient with a pulse generator, which had a straight take-off of the lead, told us, that he was disturbed by the "foreign body" under the skin and that he had turned it several times. The lead wire was coiled around the straight take-off part of the wire and there was damage to the insulating sheath (Fig. 3).

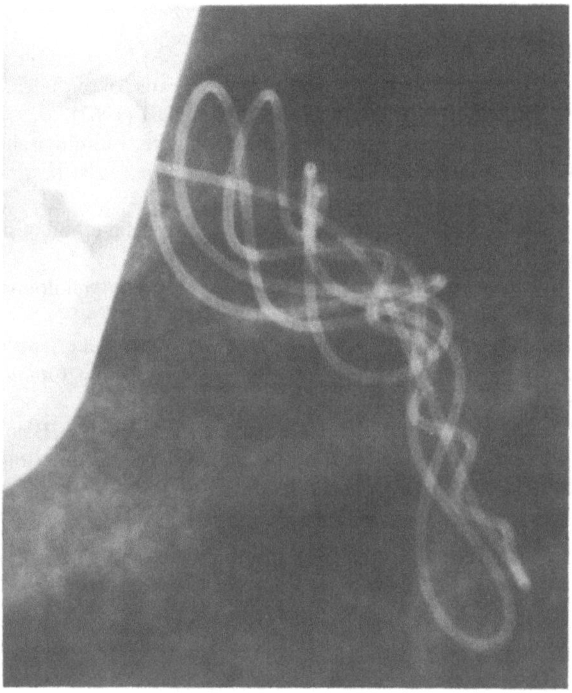

Figure 3. Pacemaker-twiddler's-syndrome.

There are a number of predisposing factors for this complication:

- Firstly inadequate fixation of the transvenous lead at the side of introduction,
- secondly the form of the pulse generator and
- thirdly factors of the pacemaker pocket. There appears to be a tendency for fluid accumulation and enlargement of the pocket in the initial stages of healing. Once we noticed a hematoma in a case where rotation of the battery occurred later.

The pocket should be tightly fitting initially. The use of a firm compression dressing for several days postoperatively is important.

Roentgenographic studies are one important part in the follow-up of patients with pacemaker treatment. In case of pacing failure radiology can substantially aid in identifying the underlying cause.

References

1. McHenry, M.M. and Grayson, C.E., Roentgenographic diagnosis of pacemaker failure. *Amer. J. Roentgenol.* 109, 94 (1970).
2. du Mesnil de Rochemont, W., Röntgenbefunde bei Schrittmacherpatienten. *Röntgen-Bl.* 29, 5 (1976).
3. Schaudig, A., Zimmermann, M., Thurmayr, R. and Beyer, J., Komplikationen der Schrittmachertherapie. *Internist* 18, 25 (1977).
4. Parsonnet, V., Gilbert, L., Zucker, I.R. and Asa, M.M., Complications of the implanted pacemaker, a scheme for determining the cause of the defect and methods for correction. *J. Thoracic and Cardiovasc. Surg.* 45, 801 (1963).
5. Gebhard, M. and Zwicker, H., Über eine einfache radiologische Methode, den Entladungszustand von Herzschrittmacherbatterien zu bestimmen. *Fortschr. Röntgenstr.* 113, 434 (1970).
6. Short, W.F., Schloss, J. and Morse, D.P., An improved method of pacemaker roentgenography. *Amer. J. Roentgenol.* 112, 571 (1971).
7. Grosser, K.D. and Friedmann, G., Klinische und röntgenologische Befunde bei intracardialem Schrittmacher. *Med. Welt* 19, 856 (1968).
8. Bayliss, C.E., Beanlands, D.S. and Baird, R.J., The pacemaker-twiddler's syndrome: A new complication of implantable transvenous pacemakers. *Canad. Med. Ass. J.* 99, 371 (1968).
9. Schulten, H.K., du Mesnil de Rochemont, W., Jochem, W., Baldus, O., Grosser, K.D. and Behrenbeck, D.W., Störung der Schrittmacherstimulation durch Rotation der Batterie (Pacemaker-Twiddler's-Syndrome). *Med. Welt* 26, 1406 (1975).

TRANSTELEPHONE PACEMAKER MONITORING *

SEYMOUR FURMAN

The function of pacemaker systems has always been variable and patients with implanted pacemakers have had intercurrent events which affect the interaction of the pacemaker system and the patient. Their welfare has required continued observation to reduce the incidence of sudden and unpredicted failure of the pacing system, to detect substandard performance of some units, and to produce maximum longevity of those units capable of prolonged operation.

Pacemaker failure

Until recently, the average longevity of implanted pulse generators was so short and the spread of failure so wide that adequate follow-up involving direct patient contact was not feasible for large numbers of patients (1, 2). One could accept a high incidence of undetected failure as well as short maximum longevity if units were removed electively at some specific period such as at the 50% failure time or follow the implanted pacemaker carefully with periodic telephone transmissions (3).

The present availability of newly designed pulse generators operating on lithium based cells rather than mercury zinc has caused a substantial change in the behavior of implanted pulse generators and, consequently, the failure patterns which must be detected (2) (Fig. 2).

For example, the pattern of mercury zinc cell pulse generators implanted since 1969 established an average longevity of 18-36 months with the initial failures appearing within the first three months after implant and enough failures appearing soon thereafter to require monitoring from early after implant. During 1976 the average pulse generator longevity for battery depletion for those generators removed during that year was 35.8 months, but enough electronic failures as well as battery depletions occurred so that the average longevity of failed generators (for all causes) was 33.4 months. The standard deviation of the mean was 10.7 months so that ± 2 SD extends from 12 months after implant until 45

* Supported in part by U.S. Public Health Service Grant No. He-04666-16.

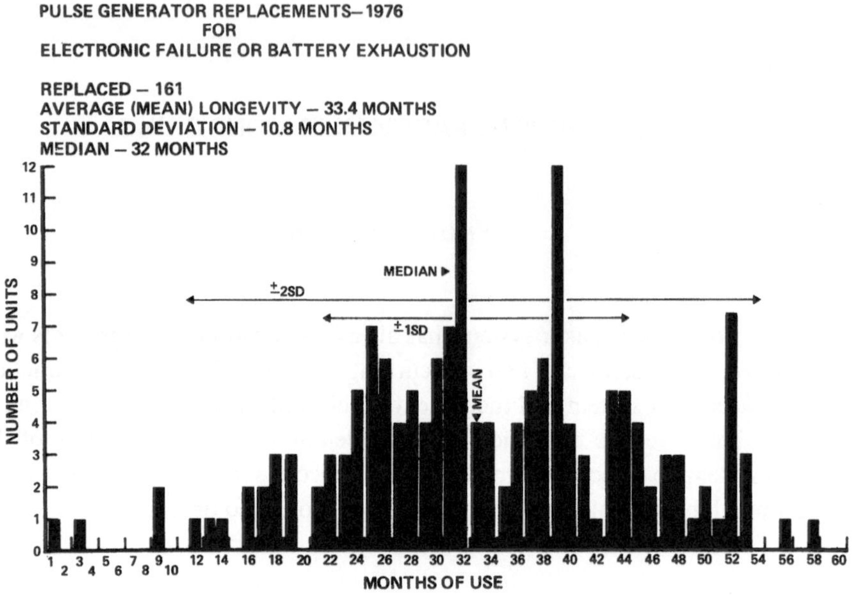

Figure 1. The superimposition of cumulative survival curves for all mercury-zinc powered pulse generators used since 1969 and of lithium-powered pulse generators since 1974 shows a distinct change in longevity anticipation. With such different failure patterns, different follow-up is required.

months after implant (Figure 2).

These were pulse generator failures only and do not relate to overall system failure which includes a substantial portion of electrode malfunction (4).

In a review of transtelephone monitoring in the general population, electrode problems occurred in 9.5% of all implants and 10% of all failures were reported during the initial telephone contact, *whenever* that occurred after implant, so that a substantial number of patients had no cardiac control at all for an unknown period after implant and before the initial telephone contact (5).

A more recent review (6) confirms that 340 pacer systems malfunctioned out of 1705 followed over a four-year period. 9.7% of all system failures occurred within one week of implant and 41% of failures were caused by battery exhaustion and 59% from other causes. Five percent of failures were deemed to be related to electronic component failure and four percent to arrhythmias which were not pacer related. Fifty percent of all failures were caused by lead distraction, high threshold, poor sensing, or fracture. None of these failures are affected by longevity of the power source.

During analysis of 1873 pulse generators implanted during an F. D.A. sponsored registry,* from Juli, 1974 to December, 1976, 88 (4.7%) failed, only 13 for

* Food and Drug Administration Contract # 223-74-5199.

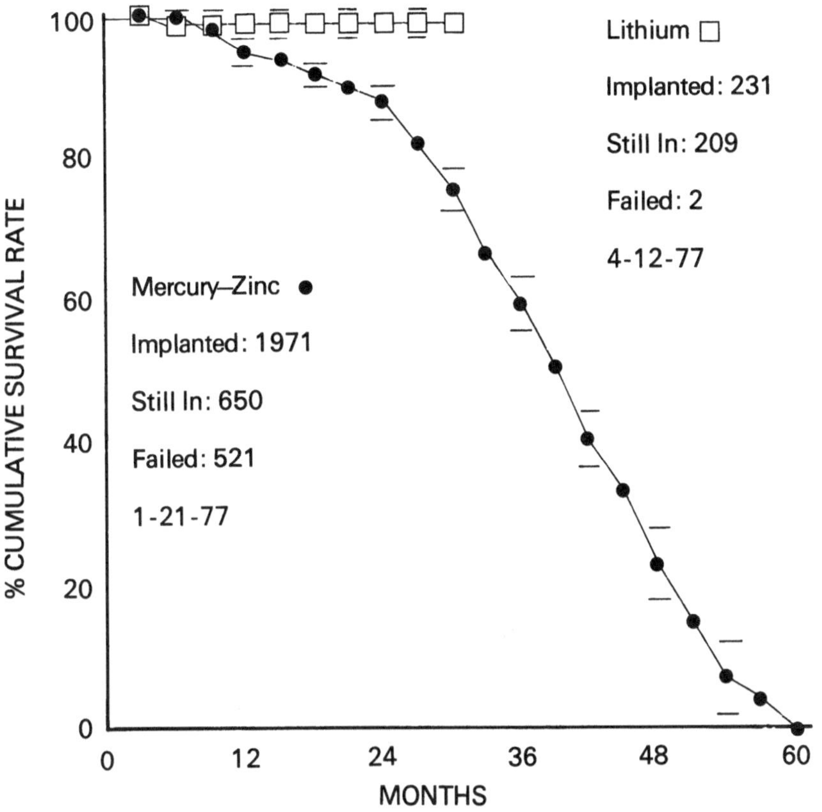

Figure 2. In 1976 pulse generators removed for electronic failure or battery depletion fell into an approximation of a normal distribution with a mean at 33.4 months of use and a standard deviation of 10.8 months.

battery exhaustion and 74 for component failure, with one having both component and battery failure. Lead failure occurred in 98 (11.6%) patients of 844 initial implants. Electrode malposition was concentrated during the first post-implant days, but fracture, erosion, infection and high threshold arose late after implant as well as early (7).

All three sets of data indicate that the problems related to implantation of a cardiac pacemaker have not been fully resolved. All data which does exist indicates that pulse generator longevity can be increased by careful follow-up and that electrode problems remain to be detected by follow-up.

Projection of decreased need for monitoring is based on far less data and on the implicit acceptance of manufacturers' projections in a highly competitive industry.

Purposes of transtelephone monitoring

1. Careful follow-up to provide maximum patient safety and longevity of the pacing system (8);
2. Careful observation of pulse generator series which are suspect, on a recall list, or are beginning to show early and as yet indistinct signs of malfunction;
3. Monitoring of the ECG where an intercurrent arrhythmia is suspected;
4. Follow-up as a laboratory resource for physicians who do not provide their own follow-up but do make decisions concerning the patient;
5. Extension of pacer follow-up to remote areas which are not well served by face to face clinics and for patients who are unable to travel.

Varieties of transtelephone monitoring

Rate Only

Initial monitoring was rate only; no indicator of ventricular capture existed. It depended for effectiveness on the presumption that a pacer impulse consistently provided ventricular capture once an electrode had become chronic and demonstrably stable. In only one instance did an error occur in which stimuli did not produce a ventricular response. This approach is now obsolete (9).

Rate and Non-ECG Indicator of Ventricular Capture

Two varieties of non-electrocardiographic indicator of ventricular capture exist.

1. Rate and digital plethysmography was adapted from the rate only technique because of the occasional need to determine whether ventricular capture had occurred. This technique is somewhat better than rate only but almost certainly has an incidence of false positive and negative which has never been reported (10).
2. Rate with detection of pacing and tracking pulses used in two different pulse generators (11). There is no indicator of ventricular capture by the pacing stimulus. A spontaneous beat has a shorter duration pulse placed into it which the telephone monitor can distinguish. It is assumed that the tracking pulse responds to spontaneous beats but this is not certain.

Rate and electrocardiogram

This technique, which is the most widely used, provides the pacemaker rate during the free running and magnet modes and a simultaneously transmitted electrocardiogram to confirm capture and sensing. This technique provides the universally understood indicator of cardiac activity and is sufficiently simple so that individual patients can have the device at home (12).

Rate, electrocardiogram and electronic analysis

This is the most sophisticated system of data transmission and provides the greatest amount of data. Since the technique is complex and the transmitter is costly, the patient must visit a peripheral facility from which data is transmitted to a central facility (6).

Electrocardiography in transtelephone monitoring

The ECG monitors provide data and artifacts similar to that of conventional electrocardiography which can indicate failure to sense, pace, or both, as well as clear-cut indication of normal function (Figure 3).

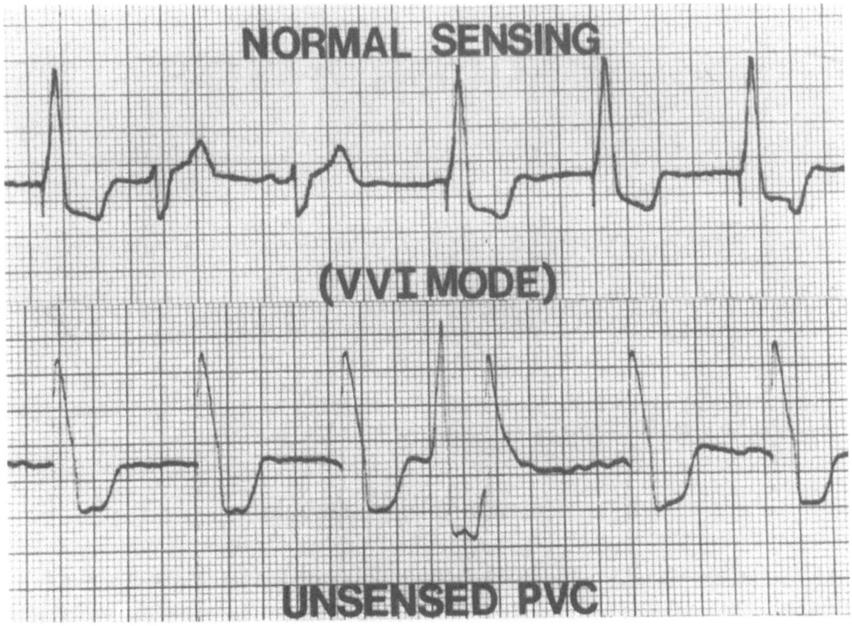

Figure 3. A ventricular inhibited pulse generator operating normally above, and at a later date with an unsensed premature ventricular contraction. Transtelephone monitoring.

Perhaps the most serious artifact is that caused by the single lead one in which electrodes are placed on both limbs. The pacemaker artifact or the QRS complex may be isoelectric or indistinct. Telephone line noise, muscle artifacts and electrical transients may occur as well as 60 Hz interference. If the pacemaker rate in the magnetic mode must be determined, the patient places the magnet over pulse generator. If a tremor is present it will be transmitted to the ECG and if the patient cannot accurately place the magnet, an incorrect rate may be found (Figure 4).

The induction of a competitive pacemaker rhythm is benign though findings may include premature ventricular contractions, runs of ventricular tachycardia, the presence of atrial fibrillation, etc.

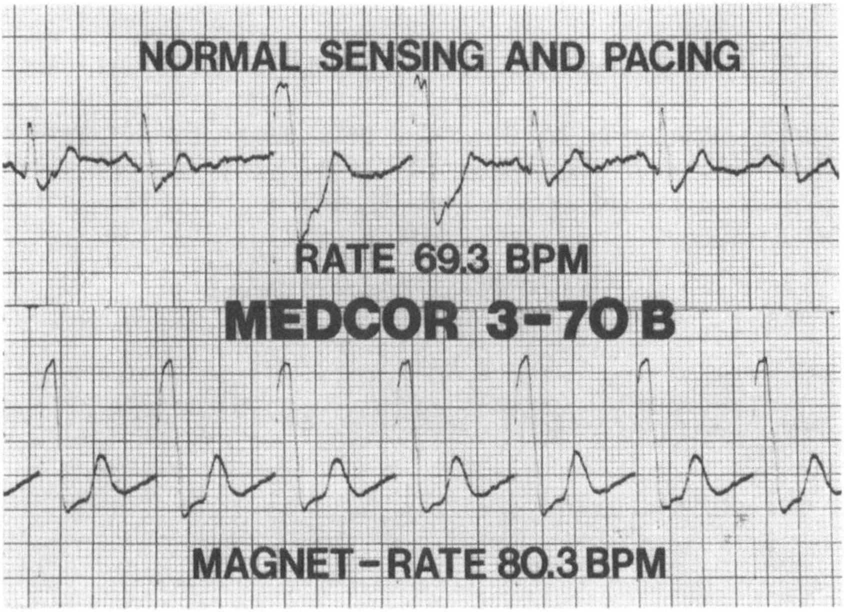

Figure 4. Normal operation of a pulse generator with one free-running rate demonstrating normal sensing and pacing and another with a more rapid rate in the magnet mode.

The monitoring schedule

The schedule should conform as much as possible to the anticipated failure pattern of the generator and the lead system. Where a pulse generator system is newly available and no clear-cut pattern is known, a decision can be made to monitor according to a previous projection. If the unit is known to be in danger of premature power source depletion or electronic failure more frequent monitoring can be undertaken.

There are today two dominant power sources, the mercury zinc battery which is still used and useful for short duration (13) application (3-4 years) and the variety of lithium based cells for smaller or longer lasting generators.

For both series the patient should be monitored weekly after implant for one month to detect electrode failure. If the electrode remains stable less frequent monitoring can begin. For the mercury-zinc cell pulse generator, weekly monitoring is begun at 30 months in anticipation of the steep rate decline accompanying battery depletion. For the lithium based power source which shows a progressive rather than a sudden decline, monitoring monthly begins at 30 months (Table 1).

Table 1. Telephone monitoring schedule

Months	*1972*	*Months*	*1975*
1- 6	Q 2 Mo.	1	Weekly
7-15	Q 1 Mo.	2-18	Q 2 Mo.
16-17	Q 2 Wk.	19-24	Q 1 Mo.
18-	Weekly	24-30	Q 2 Wk.
		30-	Weekly

Results

Only three errors have been made by our program, two with rate only monitoring with a normal rate but without consistent capture and one patient in whom rate was stable and ventricular capture consistent during each transmission. As battery voltage had declined intermittent pacing and asystole were demonstrated on subsequent direct examination. The error rate for transtelephone monitoring is thus 3 out of 524 patients followed to pulse generator replacement or 0.56%.

Of 1191 patients followed since October 1969 failure was detected in 524, sudden loss of pacing after a satisfactory transmission in 8 and lead fracture in 16. Death occurred in 163, though in none was there any evidence of relation to pacer malfunction. Despite careful follow-up, 151 patients terminated monitoring, the majority for vacation travel which they did not want to interrupt; a few others because they tired of consistent monitoring and others at the election of the pacer staff. The last group were pacers in a careful observation or "recall" status in which we had decided that sudden electronic failure might occur between calls.

The overall error and undetected cessation of pacing rate (for all causes) for transtelephone monitoring is 5% (27 of 524) for patients followed to generator replacement. If the calculation is of all patients monitored and one assumes no sudden deaths were pacer related, then it is 2.3% (27 of 1191) (Table 2). In either event it provides far greater safety than can be achieved without a follow-up system.

Because of the ability of transtelephone monitoring to provide careful, extensive follow-up, readily performed by technical staff supporting the cardiologist and surgeon, its utility remains great. Such follow-up allows development of an accurate base of data concerning pacemaker function. It should be extended to include additional patients, but the call schedule should be so modified to reflect the power source in the pacer being followed. It is inappropriate to test a lithium-powered pacer as if it were powered by a mercury-zinc battery. Once this is accomplished appropriate utilization can be achieved.

Table 2. Transtelephone monitoring 1191 Patients – 10/13/69 – 1/13/77

	Failures Detected	524
	Errors (TTM – Rate Only)	3
	Loss of Pacing (IAIT)	8
	Lead Fracture	16
	Dead (Pacer O.K.)	163
Elective End of TTM	151	
	Presently Active	326

References

1. Parsonnet, V., Myers, G.H., Gilbert, L. and Zucker, I.R., Prediction of impending pacemaker failure in a pacemaker clinic. *Amer. J. Cardiol.* 25, 311 (1970).
2. Escher, D.J.W. and Furman, S., Oscilloscopic and recent other methods of implantable pacemaker follow-up. *Ann. Cardiol. Angéiol.* 20, 503 (1971).
3. Morse, D.P., Tesler, U.F. and Lemole, G.F., The actual lifespan of pacemakers. *Chest* 64, 454 (1973).
4. Lillehei, R.C., Romero, L.H., Beckman, C.B. et al., A new, solid-state, long-life, lithium-powered pulse generator. *Ann. Thorac. Surg.* 18, 479 (1974).
5. Mugica, J., Dubos, M. and Duconge, R., Etude de la survie cumulée de 1697 stimulateurs cardiaques. *Arch. Mal. Coeur* 69, 1051 (1976).
6. Parsonnet, V., Gilbert, L. and Zucker, I.R., Natural history of pacemaker wires. *J. Thorac. Cardiovasc. Surg.* 65, 315 (1973).
7. Furman, S. and Escher, D.J.W., Transtelephone pacemaker monitoring: five years later. *Ann. Thorac. Surg.* 20, 326 (1975).
8. Mantini, E.L., Majors, R.K., Kennedy, J.R. and Lebo, G.R., A recommended protocol for pacemaker follow-up: an analysis of 1,705 implanted pacemakers. *Ann. Thorac. Surg.* (In press).
9. Bilitch, M., Furman, S. and Parsonnet, V., Twelve months experience with commercially available cardiac pacemakers: a multicenter study. *Amer. J. Cardiol.* 37, 121 (1976).
10. Furman, S., Escher, D.J.W. and Parker, B., The pacemaker follow-up clinic. *Progr. Cardiovasc. Dis.* 14, 515 (1972).
11. Furman, S., Parker, B. and Escher, D.J.W., Transtelephone pacemaker clinic. *J. Thorac. Cardiovasc. Surg.* 61, 827 (1971).
12. Pennock, R.S., Dreifus, L.S., Morse, D.P. and Watanabe, Y., Cardiac pacemaker function. *J.A.M.A.* 222, 1379 (1972).
13. Grunkemeier, G.L. Dobbs, J.L. and Starr, A., Statistical analysis of pacemaker follow-up data: rate stability and reliability. *Circulation* 53, 241 (1976).
14. Furman, S., Transtelephone observation of implanted cardiac pacemakers. *Med. Instrum.* 7, 196 (1973).
15. Ruben, S., Sealed zinc-mercuric oxide cells for implantable cardiac pacemakers. *Ann. N.Y. Acad. Sci.* 167, 627 (1969).

PACEMAKER FOLLOW-UP BY A SELF-CHECK SYSTEM

CH. HIMMLER, K.F. SEIDL, H. PRÄUER AND A. WIRTZFELD

It is generally accepted that an implanted cardiac pacemaker should be replaced as soon as one of the cells that a conventional pacemaker consists of is exhausted or – in the case of Lithium batteries – if a certain voltage drop has occurred. Generally about 90-95% of all pacemaker exchanges are necessary because of battery exhaustion (1, 5, 8). Various methods have been developed to detect early battery depletion; repeated checks in specialized pacemaker clinics using impulse and rate analysis (1, 3, 5) or transtelephone monitoring techniques (4) are the most common methods.

The efficiency of these methods, however, particularly towards the end of the expected time of pacemaker life seems to depend rather on the frequency (2, 4) of checks being performed than on the chosen individual method itself (3, 8).

With the rapidly growing number of pacemaker patients weekly checks by telephone or monthly clinic visits put much strain both on the clinic and the patient (10, 12). That's why we prefer to make the patient himself take part in his pacemaker surveillance. To ask the patient to count his pulse rate carefully every day turned out not to be very successful because on the one hand many patients are unable to count their pulse rates exactly enough and because on the other hand the method of pulse counting is not applicable to patients with pacemaker-independent cardiac activity.

Therefore, we use a patient-owned pocketable monitoring system (6, 11, 12) which enables the patient to check exactly his pacing rate at home. We wish to report on our experience with this method of patient self-check which has been in use at our institution since four years till now.

This monitoring system, called Pace-Guard, is based on a simple and practically interference-free electronic system which compares the pacing interval with a limiting rate individually adjusted to the patient and his pulse generator. We chose the pacing rate as the parameter for surveying the pulse generator's function because this parameter can easily be measured and is dependent on the battery capacity as well as on the undisturbed function of the generator's circuit (1, 5, 7).

The principle of our control system is as follows: by means of a clinic-owned Pace-master-unit the doctor at first determines the pacemaker's individual pacing interval with a precision of 1 msec. Then he sets two limiting intervals on the Pace-Guard unit, one indicating the upper and the other the lower limit which will be accepted as the normal range of this pacemaker. As long as the pacing period falls within this range, a green light on the Pace-Guard signals normal function; the light will turn to red however, as soon as the period exceeds or falls below the limiting range by more than 1 msec.

When using the Pace-Guard, the patient puts a magnetic electrode on the skin directly above the pulse generator thereby reverting a demand pacemaker to asynchronous pacing. At the same time a sensor electrode is touched, which switches on the Pace-Guard unit and closes the circuit so that the pacer's electric signals can be detected galvanically. The handling of the Pace-Guard is very simple indeed because no figures have to be read but only a light watched for. It is practically impossible for the unit to be used incorrectly. This monitoring system enables the patient to check his pacemaker everywhere and at any time.

We asked our patients to apply the monitoring system once a day for a few seconds and to come to the clinic within 2 days in case the red light flashes up, indicating a drop in voltage or a disturbed pacemaker function.

In addition we called in the patients for a routine clinical check every 4-6 months for wave form and ECG analysis and general check-up. Because of this optimal combination of patient self-control and clinical examination it is no longer necessary even at the expected end of the pacemaker lifetime to see the patients more frequently and the rate of 2-3 clinic visits per year can be maintained indefinitely.

The sensitivity of our monitoring system lies in the order of 200 mV and consequently it can only control unipolar pacemakers but these pacemakers are used almost exclusively in Germany as well as in other countries, at least in Europe. Because of this intentionally low sensitivity, the Pace Guard is able to detect not only changes in pacing rate but also a critical drop of voltage such as occurs with a broken electrode or an isolation defect. In this situation neither the green nor the red light will flash anymore and this will cause the patient to come to the clinic.

Until now we have provided this monitoring system to 533 patients who carried different pacemaker models of Biotronik, Cordis, Elema, Medtronic and Vitatron. 182 of these units had to be replaced so far. In 178 patients the indication for the replacement was battery depletion and in 176 of these patients the battery exhaustion had been signaled before any symptoms endangering the patient had developed so that elective replacement could be performed. Let's now consider the 2 other cases of exhausted batteries, which had not been signaled by the Pace Guard in time: In the first case the limiting rate had been set incorrectly and in the second case 2 battery-cells had run down by the time the patient was admitted to the hospital and loss of capture due to the drop in pacer output had developed.

Three patients had a broken lead yet only one of them developed a syncopal attack; the two other patients were symptom-free as they had sufficient pacemaker independent cardiac activity; they came to the clinic nevertheless because the Pace Guard had stopped flashing altogether. The results of Pace-Guard monitoring of these 533 patients shows the table 1.

Table 1. Results of Pace-Guard monitoring of 533 pacemakers

	Pat.	*elective replacement*	*failures*
Battery depletion	178	176	2
electronic failure	2	2	–
lead fracture	3	–	3
false alarm	–	–	–
patient died	41	–	–
PM still operative	312	–	–

If we consider only those pacemakers which were removed because of a battery depletion and compare them to a second group of pacemaker-patients, which we had followed prior to the advent of our self-check system by conventional methods including ECG-, rate- and photoanalysis, the efficiency of the combined use of clinic analysis and patient self-check is quite obvious (Table 2): as you see on the table the failure rate of over 10% which is comparable to the results reported by other centers using the same techniques (2, 3, 5, 7, 10) could be reduced to 1.1%.

The following table (Table 3) shows the lifetimes of our 176 electively replaced pulse generators at the time of the indicated battery exhaustion. It shows that the actual lifetime of the conventional pacemakers ranges from 11/2 to 5 years in about 95% of the cases. Prophylactic replacement after a certain lifetime for example after 18 to 24 months, as it was propagated some time ago, cannot be

Table 2. Results of Pacemaker follow-up (Battery-exhaustion only)

PM replacement	*Clinic analysis only*	*Patient self-check combined with clinic analysis*
Elective	212 (79,1%)	176 (98,87%)
prophylactic	31 (11,6%)	–
emergency	25 (9,3%)	2 (1,13%)
number of cases	268 (100%)	178 (100%)
failure rate without prophylactic replacement	10,5%	1,13%

Table 3. Life-span of electively replaced pacemakers (Battery depletion)

Time (months)	*number of PM*	*% per year*
0- 6	1	1,1
6-12	1	
12-18	5	10,2
18-24	13	10,2
24-30	29	49,4
30-36	58	49,4
36-42	31	31,2
42-48	24	31,2
48-54	8	7,9
54-60	6	
Sum	176	100%

accepted any more. Without patient self-check weekly transtelephone monitoring or monthly clinical checks would be necessary after a pacemaker lifetime of two years. This implies that these patients would require around fifty telephone calls or twelve clinic visits per year for the rest of their generator's life, which may take another 3 or even 4 years. This strain on the clinic as well as on the patients is reduced to a great extent by means of the patient self-check, as I have explained just now. At the same time the patient is protected against unexpected premature battery failure or unexpected electronic malfunction in a very efficient way.

The patients themselves welcomed very much indeed the new method of pacemaker control realizing its expanded safety and appreciating the fact that we could dispense with monthly clinic appointments which we had performed prior to the advent of the Pace-Guard system. The patients took their monitors on longer travels and we have some patients who were caught by the red signal while abroad, broke their journey and returned to Munich the next day for pulse generator replacement.

In summary therefore our experience with the patient self-check Pace Guard system to date indicates that a patient-oriented method of pacemaker surveillance combined with conventional clinic follow-up possesses great reliability and efficiency, superior to or at least comparable to other follow-up methods which are far more elaborate. For the first time full use of the battery's capacity has been possible without risking the patient's health. Although patient self-check cannot and should not replace careful patient follow-up, it adds a significant measure of safety to existing techniques.

References

1. Escher, D.J.W., Follow-up of the patient with an implanted cardiac pacemaker. *Med. Conc. Cardiovasc. Dis.* 43, 77 (1974).
2. Frick, M.H., Efficiency of a pacemaker clinic to prevent sudden pacing failures. *Brit. Heart J.* 35, 1280 (1973).
3. Furman, S., Escher, D.J.W. and Parker, B., The pacemaker follow-up clinic. *Progr. Cardiovasc. Dis.* 14, 515 (1972).
4. Furman, S. and Escher, D.J.W., Transtelephone monitoring of implanted cardiac pacemakers. In: *Cardiac Pacing*, p. 429. Editor: H.J.Th. Thalen, Van Gorcum, Assen (1973).
5. Hager, W. and Seling, S., *Praxis der Schrittmachertherapie*. F.K. Schattauer, Stuttgart (1974).
6. Himmler, Ch., Wirtzfeld, A. and Lampadius, M., Kontrolle implantierter Herzschrittmacher durch Patienten-eigene Testgeräte. *Verh. Deutsch. Ges. Inn. Med.* 81, 155 (1975).
7. Irnich, W., Probleme der Schrittmacherüberwachung. *Intens. Med.* 10, 95 (1973).
8. Parsonnet, V., Pacemaker surveillance. *Chest* 61, 203 (1972).
9. Parsonnet, V., Magnet Pacemaker Reversion. *Jama* 224, 1428 (1973).
10. Parsonnet, V., Furman, S. and Smyth, N.P.D., Implantable cardiac pacemakers: status report and resource guideline. *Am. J. Cardiol.* 34, 487 (1974).
11. Wirtzfeld, A., Lampadius, M., Pace Guard, ein neues Gerät zur Selbstkontrolle implantierter Herzschrittmacher. *Dtsch. med. Wschr.* 98, 2402 (1973).
12. Wirtzfeld, A., Lampadius, M. and Himmler, Ch., Patientenorientierte Herzschrittmacherüberwachung mit dem Pace-Guard-System. *Dtsch. med. Wschr.* 99, 2606 (1974).

DISCUSSION IX. FOLLOW-UP METHODS

CHAIRMAN: S. FURMAN *(New York, U.S.A.)*

J. MEIBOM *(Copenhagen, Denmark):* I would ask Dr. Himmler: How much does your Pace Guard cost?

CH. HIMMLER *(Munich, F.R. Germany):* The cost of the Pace Guide is approximately $ 300.

J. MEIBOM *(Copenhagen, Denmark):* I have also a question for Dr. Ector. On two of your slides, you have a column called "Additional Information on Exhausted Batteries"; what do you mean by that?

H. ECTOR *(Louvain, Belgium):* I consider as additional information the fact that the patient was referred to the hospital because of an alteration in pacing rate. The photo-analysis did confirm exhaustion of batteries. I have to add to my presentation that we instruct our patients to take their pulse twice daily. This is a way of auto-control that seems to me reliable. Not so reliable maybe as the Pace Guard system, but it works.

CHAIRMAN: Thank you. I think the next question will be from Dr. Green.

G.D. GREEN *(Glasgow, Scotland):* I would like to challenge the first speaker, Mr. Lampadius, most strongly. He made a blanket condemnation of mercury pacemakers, on the basis that the mode of rundown of the mercury cell was bad, that is, it is a plateau and then it drops suddenly. The point is that, of course, one has not one cell in a mercury generator, but several cells, and the probability of all four or five cells going simultaneously is in fact very small. So, theoretically I challenge him. I challenge him in practice from experience with hundreds of mercury cell generators in Glasgow, where in fact the first step – that is, one cell has failed but the output is still being sufficient to allow pacing to continue – has, of course, been detected at pacemaker clinics. The mode of rundown of a battery has not been mentioned so far but this is one of the most important things to bear in mind in connection with pacemaker clinics: if the mode of natural rundown of the battery is bad, then you are wasting your time having pacemaker clinics.

CHAIRMAN: Since you have challenged, are you going to choose your weapons also? I think that is your option.

G.D. GREEN *(Glasgow, Scotland):* No.

CHAIRMAN: Dr. Lampadius, will you respond to that?

S. LAMPADIUS *(Munich, F.R. Germany):* There is not much response necessary. Just a question. Did you ever see a patient come back to your hospital with a syncope that was not paced anymore because of two batteries failing at the same time?

G.D. GREEN *(Glasgow, Scotland):* My point is that the number which come back for those reasons is in fact very small indeed. A high percentage of those do come back in that condition because the threshold has gone up at the same time. So the battery voltage has come down and it has been rather unfortunate that the threshold has also gone up. But, in general, emergency admission from battery depletion – at least with the type of generators we have used in Glasgow, i.e. mercury-cell generators – is rare. The mode of battery rundown is most important for the choice of the type of lithium pacemaker you are going to implant.

CHAIRMAN: Dr. Goldman?

B.S. GOLDMAN *(Toronto, Canada):* I am interested in the cost of telephone monitoring in the European centers that have reported the use of some form of telephone check. Although I am a proponent of telephone monitoring in North America, it has been suggested that the cost of these calls, over the patient's lifetime, can often exceed the benefit in terms of cost saving from a replacement. Who picks up the charges for this?

A. WIRTZFELD *(Munich, F.R. Germany):* I never made such a calculation, but this is actually not the problem. The problem, at least in our country, is: who pays for the telephone and for the calls. The patients are usually insured, and the insurance companies will not pay for this.

B.S. GOLDMAN *(Toronto, Canada):* Are you saying that, as far as the insurance companies are concerned in Germany, whether they are governmental or private, they do not recognize telephone monitoring as a legitimate medical expense.

A. WIRTZFELD *(Munich, F.R. Germany):* That is correct. They do not. At least not to the extent that they will pay for it.

CHAIRMAN: That seems to be a good extent. Dr. Ector, did you have a comment to make?

H. ECTOR *(Louvain, Belgium):* As you could see on your way to Brussels, Belgium is a small country. I can assure you that with many general practitioners, there is some ECG control available. Even when telephone monitoring is a very good surveillance system, I think that, in Belgium, the need for telephone monitoring is less because of the availability of ECG control by general practitioners and by cardiologists. I think that for a good cooperation with the referring physicians, it is better that the patient is controlled by the general practitioner or by the referring cardiologist than by telephone.

R. DODINOT *(Nancy, France):* Our goal is to try to give patients safety without making them slaves of a pacemaker clinic, either by telephone or by coming for a photo-analysis. To have a self-check for a patient is very useful. What we also have is a telephone free of charge where the patients call once a month or once every three months, in the case of lithium batteries. So we can have a patient self-checking system combined with a telephone system, which allows the patient freedom without obliging him to go to the clinic too often. This seems to be reliable and very economical.

M. LEVANDER-LINDGREN *(Stockholm, Sweden):* Someone asked for economic calculations with regard to telephone checkup. I can give you such a calculation. We have now made about 4.000 telephone checkups. After the first thousand, we began calculations. Then we found, that we had saved about S. Kr.70 for every pacemaker generator with regard to prolonged life. We saved about S.Kr.80.000 with regard to travel expenses, but Sweden of course is a country with long distances.

CHAIRMAN: It is possible then that this would be especially suitable in a country with long distances.

M. LEVANDER-LINDGREN *(Stockholm, Sweden):* Yes, it might be. It is very uncommon that you can tell the administration of a hospital that you have bought equipment that really saves money. You can do this with telephone checkup.

H.J.TH. THALEN *(Groningen, The Netherlands):* I would like to ask a question to Dr. Wirtzfeld and to all Europeans. I think that the difference between patient follow-up is that, in the European setting, we had photo-analysis, or at least pacer clinics, a bit earlier than the United States had. In the United States, they did not start with photo-analysis, but with the telephone system. In Europe the insurance companies are paying for the visits to the pacemaker clinics. We can use the telephone system to decrease the patient load of the follow-up clinics. Now as we are going to pacers that function for four, five, six and seven years, and that are electronically most probably more reliable and as we are going to a further increase in the number of pacemaker patients, I think the telephone system could be a nice addition to the clinic, through which the patients' visits to the clinics could be diminished. It makes a big difference if a patient has to come by cab for the visit – all paid by the insurance company – or has the telephone system. When you talk to the insurance companies, you can point out to them that it will cost them less with most probably the same safety with less burden for the patient. I would suggest – I do not know if you have already done this, Dr. Wirtzfeld – that, in Europe, we talk to insurance companies to get telephone analysis paid for by them. Telephone analysis is also coming to Europe.

S. LAMPADIUS *(Munich, F.R. Germany):* I am rather doubtful as to whether telephone monitoring will be the best solution for the future. We should talk about pacemakers lasting ten years. We do not know, for instance, when an electronic failure will occur. That should mean, at least every week for ten years, a telephone call, if you really want to be sure, because you never know when electronic failure is going to occur. I am talking from the viewpoint of the patient with a pacemaker and I really would like to be sure. It would be a tremendous work load for the hospital, a tremendous cost. So, I think patient's own test devices might take care of follow-up needs and of battery and electronic malfunctions. This is much cheaper and should be considered.

H.J.TH. THALEN *(Groningen, The Netherlands):* I would like to make a comment on that. You stated that the patient has to phone every week, because there might be an electronic defect. If that is the case, then we are doing a bad job at the moment, because patients are now visiting the clinics only – let us say – every fifth month the first and the second year. But so far the clinics have detected about 90-95% of the defects via the system they have now. So I do not think you have to start this business of a telephone per week for ten years. It would be too expensive. I think we should be reasonable and look at the cost benefits as outlined also by Dr. Levander-Lindgren. But I also agree that there is some place for patient self-check devices, perhaps in addition to the clinic systems for checks in between, depending upon the type of pacemaker and patient.

CHAIRMAN: To step out of the role of moderator, I would say that, in our experience, we do not believe that weekly telephone calls would be especially necessary. We believe, to this time, since we are on a very extensive telephone monitoring system, that there seems to be no replacement for a human analysis of the maximum amount of data. We believe that the analysis by the trained specialist in cardiac pacing is far more valuable than the machine analysis by a patient who may or may not interpret the data correctly, no matter how simply it is provided. However, that remains a topic for future discussion. I thank all of the panellists for their contributions and close this session.

Section X

COMPUTER APPLICATION IN PACEMAKER REGISTRATION AND FOLLOW-UP

COMPUTER APPLICATIONS FOR THE CONTROL OF PACEMAKER PATIENTS: REMARKS AND PERSONAL EXPERIENCE

G.A. FERUGLIO

For an effective follow-up of large groups of pacemaker-patients (PMP) and for evaluation of the results of permanent pacing on a reliable statistical basis, many pacemaker centers in the world are now using some computer system. Actually, many problems and questions in pacemaker treatment can be solved by electronic data processing, such as: 1) storage in limited space and immediate retrieval of all pertinent data; 2) lists, tables and graphs for routine clinical and administrative work; 3) expedite and safe dealing with recurring alarms from industry; 4) statistical models for pacemaker longevity, to be utilized for determining optimal check-up intervals and elective replacement time; 5) control of pacemaker performance data given by the manufacturer; 6) statistical analysis of survival time, mortality rates, pacer and electrode function time, complications, patient risk, etc.

There is no standard type of computer system for processing pacemaker follow-up information. Apparently, each clinic has developed its own system and program, according to local computer facilities and specific needs for service and/or research (1-8).

However what to store and how to store data in a computer aided pacemaker clinic, still represent a problem which deserves much attention and study.

It appears obvious that all and only essential clinical and technical data are to be stored and that such data must be immediately retrievable 24 hours a day. Moreover this information must be kept in storage for a long period of time (usually for 5-10 years or more). Therefore suitable types of memory are needed and, in order to save costly memory space, special care is required in selecting the information and programming. Furthermore, it is generally believed that a patient data system with structured display records, designed to give comprehensive and surveyable information, immediately retrievable on video display or printed sets, seems to offer the most convenient solution.

In our institution the pacemaker clinic, covering over 600 patients in need of a regular follow-up, is linked to a live patient data system. Such a system, called G/3-Informatica Friuli-V. Giulia, is mainly devoted to in-patient management; it operates on a regional scale since 1974 and is based on a IBM 370/125-duplex computer. The system consists of a general data base (fig. 1), for all patient

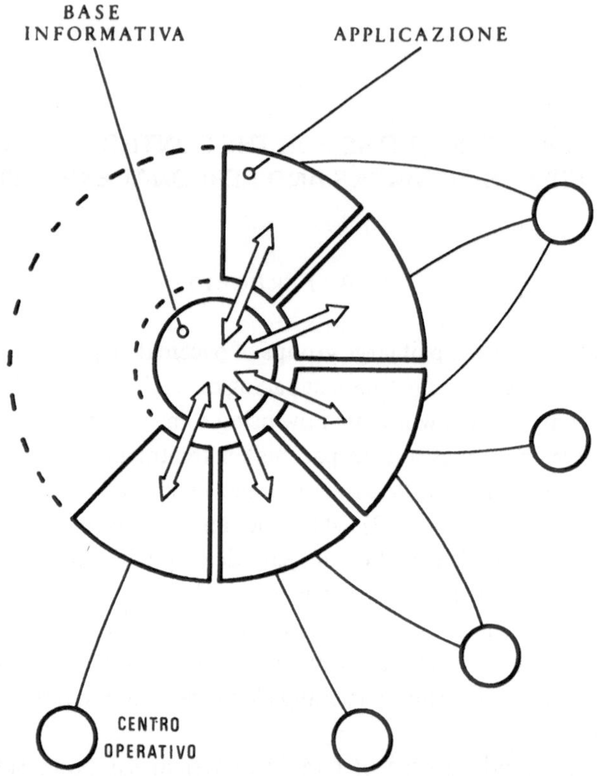

Figure 1. Diagram of the patient data system G/3-Informatica Friuli-V. Giulia. The system consists of a general data base, for all patient hospital admissions in the Region, and of a series of particular applications including a pacemaker follow-up system.

admissions in the hospitals of the Region, and of a series of specific applications including our pacemaker follow-up system.

This type of solution, compared to a dedicated system, has a great advantage in that it allows an easy interchange of information concerning pacemaker patients with other departments and hospitals.

The pacemaker follow-up application is based on two main on-line programs and a series of batch programs. One of the two on-line programs (PMRG program) is used for registration of new implants; the other (PMCT program) for regular check-ups and replacements. By means of simple on-line transactions the programs allow storage and retrieval of all pertinent data concerning each pacemaker's life while the batch programs are used for searches on stored information and data of interest.

Input and retrieval of information are made on-line through a conventional video-keyboard (fig. 2). Data to be stored are collected on a series of four stan-

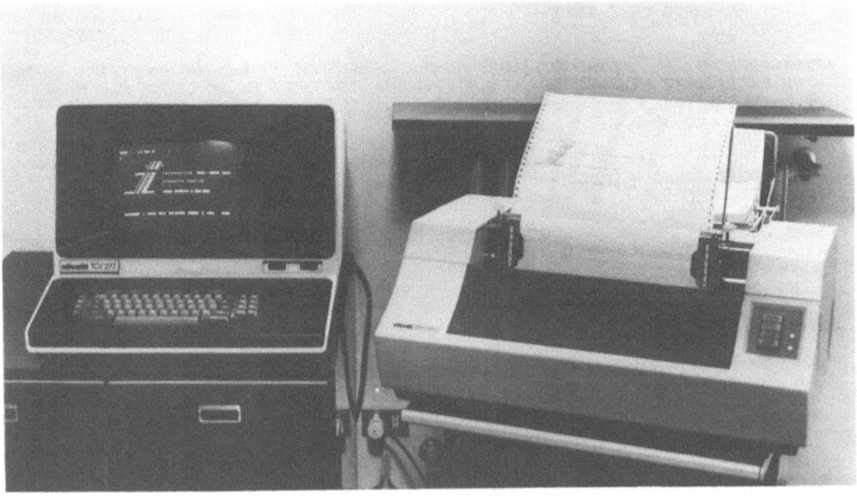

Figure 2. Input and retrieval of information are made on-line through a conventional video-keybord. Reports generated by the computer can be printed out when necessary.

dardized formats. These have fixed headings with coded alternatives and limited space for comments in free text. In figures 3, 4 two samples of such formats (for new implants and for routine controls) are presented. When storing the information some items must be filled in compulsorily. The program does not proceed without such data. For retrieval, reports generated by the computer will appear on CRT display and will be readily printed when necessary.

```
NUMERO SANITARIO CBME 907347 VHA                          NUMERO DI REGISTRO 01. 00500
CABAS/VIRGILIO                                                       M  13/12/1907

START 09/05/77       DIAGNOSI: BAV COMPL. DEGENERAT    DURATA MALATTIA: 00/00/10
 1 PM E  1 CONTR REGISTRATI.  PM ATTIVO DAL 19/05/77 AL 10/06/77 PER MESI  0. 21
----------------------- P R I M O   I M P I A N T O -------------------------

DATA IMPIANTO: 19/05/77 OPERATORE GM
INTERVENTI NN                          ANESTESIA LOCALE     DEGENZA  25 GIORNI

ELETTRODO: MARCA ELEMA             MODELLO 7/62             -TIPO UNIPOLARE
          SEDE ATRIALE  VENTRICOLARE  EPICARDICA              VIA CEFALICA DX

GENERATORE:MARCA ELEMA             MODELLO EM177            ALIM. MERCURIO
           TIPO FISSO  INIBIZ. VENTRIC.   SINCR. VENTRIC.

AMPIEZZA STIM. CA   DURATA   TEMPO DIMEZZ.  FREQ.   PERIODO   T. M. I.  SOGLIA ST.
    5. 1 VOLT       0. 6 MS     0. 4 MS      68 M'   869 MS      0 MV   1. 1 VOLT

SOLO IN CASO DI REIMPIANTO: CATETERE :
IN SITO     RIPOSIZIONATO     RIPARATO      SOSTITUITO     NUOVO CATET.

                                   ********** DATA PRIMO CONTROLLO 30/05/77
```

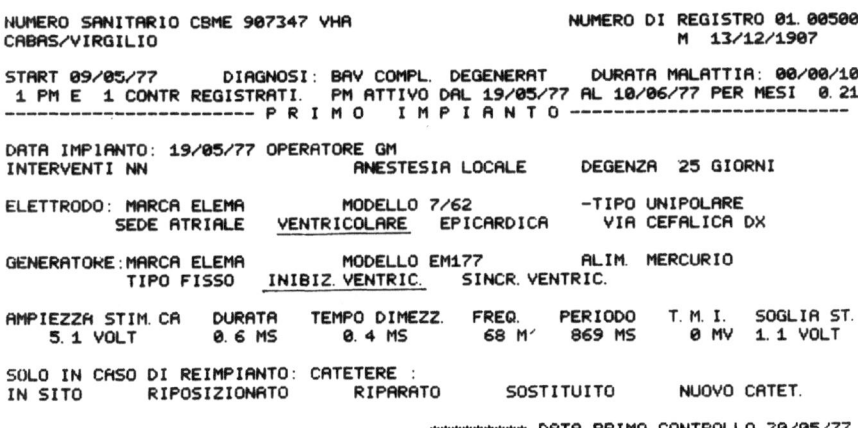

Figure 3. Printed set for a pacemaker implant.

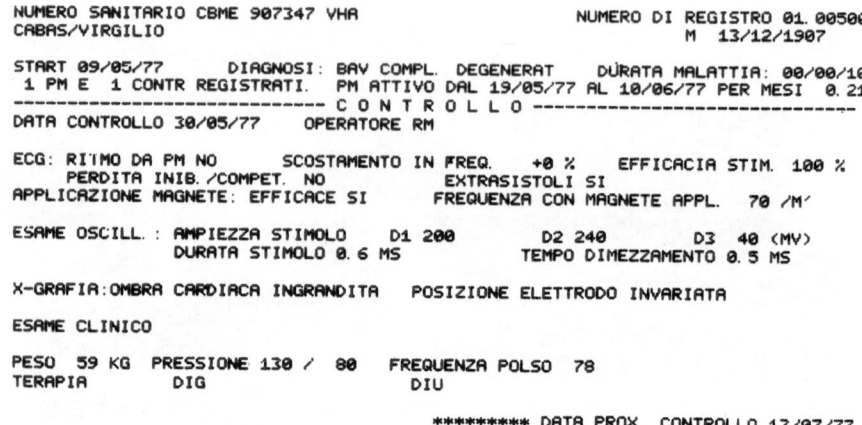

```
NUMERO SANITARIO CBME 907347 VHA                          NUMERO DI REGISTRO 01.00500
CABAS/VIRGILIO                                                       M  13/12/1907

START 09/05/77       DIAGNOSI: BAV COMPL. DEGENERAT     DURATA MALATTIA: 00/00/10
 1 PM E  1 CONTR REGISTRATI.  PM ATTIVO DAL 19/05/77 AL 10/06/77 PER MESI  0.21
---------------------------- C O N T R O L L O -----------------------------
DATA CONTROLLO 30/05/77    OPERATORE RM

ECG: RITMO DA PM NO      SCOSTAMENTO IN FREQ.   +0 %    EFFICACIA STIM.  100 %
    PERDITA INIB./COMPET. NO             EXTRASISTOLI SI
APPLICAZIONE MAGNETE: EFFICACE SI      FREQUENZA CON MAGNETE APPL.  70 /M'

ESAME OSCILL. : AMPIEZZA STIMOLO    D1 200         D2 240         D3  40 (MV)
                DURATA STIMOLO 0.6 MS            TEMPO DIMEZZAMENTO 0.5 MS

X-GRAFIA:OMBRA CARDIACA INGRANDITA   POSIZIONE ELETTRODO INVARIATA

ESAME CLINICO

PESO  59 KG  PRESSIONE 130 /  80   FREQUENZA POLSO  78
TERAPIA        DIG                  DIU

                                   ********** DATA PROX.  CONTROLLO 13/07/77
```

Figure 4. Printed set for a routine control.

The batch programs are about a dozen, divided into five groups: a) to produce lists, tables and graphs for routine clinical and administrative work; b) to obtain special lists for handling the recalls from industry; c) to control pacemaker performance data; d) to analyze various parameters such as survival time, mortality rates, complications, pacer and electrode function time; e) miscellany.

The programs have been established according to peculiar needs of the pacemaker clinic. Registration of a new pacemaker requires only 97 bytes of memory to store pre-implant clinical and ECG data, and 103 bytes for implant data. Another 103 bytes are required for each control so that when a pacemaker is replaced after an average of 20 clinical regular check-ups it takes a little more than two Kbytes of memory altogether. And this is a rather little memory space if we consider that the average capacity of a disc memory is usually 100 Mbytes. In our system, therefore, one single disc can provide storage for over 40,000 pacemakers.

The computer edits coded information to surveyable reviews. Stored data, when needed, can be transferred on tapes, punched cards, etc. and analysis of data can be carried out by using also minicomputers.

Our experience is not too large at the present time; nevertheless our results can be summarized as follows:

- no more uncontrolled drop-outs in our patient follow-up;
- no missing charts and vital information in our files;
- no uncoordinated program resulting in too numerous emergency replacements;
- two recalls from industry, handled within a matter of days;

- no tedious and unreliable statistics made by paper and pencil;
- time saved and cost reduction.

Our system acts as the initial data base for a regional and, further on, for a possible national pacemaker registration plan. The system and programs may be applicable to other centers wishing to avail themselves of the technique.

References

1. Feruglio, G.A., Lestuzzi, F., Carminati, D., La gestione automatizzata dell'ambulatorio dei portatori di pacemaker all'Ospedale Civile di Udine. *Friuli Medico*, 32: 99, 1977.
2. Goldman, B.S., Noble, E.J., MacGregor, D.C., Morrow, J.D., Covvey, D., Heller, J.C., Taylor, K.W., Conceptual development of a university pacemaker centre. In: H.J. Th. Thalen (Ed.), *Cardiac Pacing*, Assen 1973.
3. Levander-Lindgren, M., Paperless records: data display records for patients with cardiac pacing. In: *Vth Internat. Symposium on Cardiac Pacing*, Abstracts, pag. 71, Tokyo 1976.
4. Parsonnet, V., How to detect pacemaker failure: techniques used in office practice and in a pacemaker clinic. In: L.E. Meltzer and J.R. Kitchel, Current Concepts of Cardiac Pacing and Cardioversion, Philadelphia 1971.
5. Schaudig, A., Zimmermann, Thurmayr, R., Kreuzer, E., Reichert, B., Computer applications for monitoring of pacemaker patients. In: M. Schaldach and S. Furman, *Pacemaker technology*, Berlin, Heidelberg, New York, 1975.
6. Starr, A., Dobbs, J.L., A computer-assisted pacemaker follow-up system. In: *Vth Internat. Symposium on Cardiac Pacing*, Abstracts, pag. 71, Tokyo 1976.
7. Svorcik, C., Netusil, M., Naprstek, Z., Pacemaker clinic in Prague.In: H.J.Th. Thalen (Ed.), *Cardiac Pacing*, Assen 1973.
8. Welti, J.J., Fontaine, G., Bonnet, M., Kevorkian, M. Piogger, G., Computer application for the control of an important group of pacemaker patients. In: H.J.Th. Thalen (Ed.), *Cardiac Pacing*, Assen 1973.

COMPUTER STORAGE OF PACEMAKER DATA

ANTHONY RICKARDS

A computer based pacemaker record system has been designed at the National Heart Hospital to process the large amount of technical information derived from the local pacemaker service.

In the design of such a system consideration must be given to the function of a pacemaker data base. Possible uses are:

1. Calculation of reliability and survival of generators and electrodes.
2. Logging of modes of pacemaker failure.
3. Storage of clinical information relating to the patient population.
4. Use of the data base to organise follow-up in the pacing clinic.
5. On-line analysis of electro-stimulograms in the pacing clinic.

In the system to be described uses 1, 2 and 3 were incorporated into the system from the initial design. Use 4 implies much greater use of pacing clinic based terminals and although not technically difficult requires computer hardware expansion. Use 5 has not yet been considered.

System description

The pacing program is run on a Hewlett-Packard computer system. The central processor is a 32K 2100A series computer with 4 × 2.5 M bytes discs as mass storage peripherals. The prime function of this particular machine is to provide on-line analysis of cath lab information (5600 system) and the computer is also linked to the public telephone service and a number of interactive video terminals to allow access to and interrogation of a catheter data base consisting of approximately 4 800 cases on line.

The computer operates in a Real-Time environment and this is capable of performing a number of tasks in addition to the prime function described. One 2.5 M byte exchangeable disc is designated as the "spare" disc not used by the catheter system and it is this disc which contains the pacemaker data.

The minimum requirements therefore are a 2.5 M byte rapid access mass-storage device, a 10 K Fortran IV programming area and an interactive display terminal.

The mass storage area is designated as a single file containing 9696 ×128 word data blocks. A 500 block header contains 11 words per patient in sequence thus allowing more than 5000 patient indices. The first word of each header contains the packed first two letters of the patient name and the subsequent 10 words point to the data blocks containing the information for that patient. A minimum of 128 and a maximum of 1280 words may be therefore used by each patient with the current configuration.

Each patient record is organised so that the first 30 words contain basic and non-recurring information (Table 1). The symptom, pre-pacing ECG and aetiology items are coded data which point to a 32 character string stored in the pacemaker codes section of the disc stored in blocks 9500 onwards.

The details of the recurring intervention data are shown in table 2. Each of these records occupy 70 computer words and are used for all types of intervention from electrode reposition to new system implantation. Not all the questions are required to be answered and the interactive program forms the questions according to which option is selected on entry into the program (Table 3). Thus in the maximum of 1250 words available to each patient 17 interventions can be described.

Table 1. Patient data

Name: Mythical patient
ID: 123456
Hospital:National Heart Hospital
Year of birth: 1901
Sex: m
Date of first implant: 21, 4, 77
Symptoms: Syncope
Free-pacing ECG: Left anterior hemi block
Aetiology: Ischaemic – anterior infarct

Additionally each patient record may contain a number of 10 word follow-up records shown in table 4. The information in the record can be used to produce lists for the pacing clinic and to check for patients overdue for follow-up.

Conclusions

The system described has been designed within a number of constraints dictated by finance and the local uses of the computer system. The information stored is compact and access to the system and entering of patient data are rapid and do not require form-filling. An example of a survival survey run of Vitatron 42 and 43 RT pacemakers is shown in table 5. Computation and output of the information took approximately 30 seconds.

Table 2. Intervention data

Date of intervention: 21, 4, 77
Type of system: A-V sequential
Generator manufacturer: VI
Generator type: 55RT
Generator serial: 1234
Generator site: abdominal – sub muscular
Electrode approach : Thoracotomy to LV
: bipolar
Electrode manufacturer: CO
Electrode type: epicardial
Electrode serial: 1234
Extension-adaptor used: N

	Voltage	current	Pulse Width
Threshold 1:	.50	1.20	.50
Threshold 2:	1.00	.50	.50
Threshold 3:	5.40	2.15	.15
Output data 1:	5.40	.60	.50
Output data 2:	4.00	.80	.50

Endocardial R + S voltage: 8.0
Endocardial ST elevation: 12.0
Atrial electrode approach: epicardiol to la
Atrial electrode manufacturer: CO
Atrial electrode type: EPI
Atrial electrode serial: 1234
Atrial voltage threshold: 1.20
Atrial electrogram: 4.00
Pacing stimulus interval: 858
Pacing pulse width: .50
Pacing stimulus escape interval: 906
Pacing stimulus interference interval: 912
General anesthesia: Y
Temporary electrode: ?

on 22, 4, 77 Generator removed. Infection-ulceration
Electrode removed. Elective with generator change

Table 3. Pacemaker program options

1. View or edit this file
2. Add clinic follow-up data
3. Run survey programs
4. Pacemaker change
5. Pacemaker and electrode change
6. Reposition pacemaker
7. Reposition electrode
8. Electrode change
9. Close this file
10. Stop

Table 4. Follow-up data

Date of follow-up:	Day, Month,
ECG:	Code
Pacing stimulus interval:	MS
Pacing pulse width:	MS
Relative output:	%
Relative threshold:	%
Time to next visit:	Months

Table 5. Pacemaker survival survey

Run on day 292 year 1977
Generator MFG: VI
Generator type: 42RT
Generator type: 43RT
Total 615 generators exposed for 8308.1 months – average 13.5 months

		Cumulative Survival Calculations								
Age		*	Codes A to D		*	Tot	Expos	Fail	Surv	Surv
	N	A	B	C	D	T	X	F	S	S1
0- 3	615	11	6	4	5	22	606.5	.008	.992	.992
3- 6	589	63	2	1	0	65	556.5	.000	1.000	.992
6- 9	523	60	2	2	0	62	492.0	.000	1.000	.992
9-12	459	113	0	1	0	113	402.5	.000	1.000	.992
12-15	345	72	0	1	0	72	309.0	.000	1.000	.992
15-18	272	98	1	0	0	99	222.5	.000	1.000	.992
18-21	173	93	0	0	0	93	126.5	.000	1.000	.992
21-24	80	58	0	0	0	58	51.0	.000	1.000	.992
24-27	22	22	0	0	0	22	11.0	.000	1.000	.992

STORAGE, EVALUATION AND APPLICATION OF DATA IN A PACEMAKER CLINIC

A. SCHAUDIG, R. THURMAYR, M. ZIMMERMANN AND J. BEYER

In our pacemaker clinic, we are using EDP since 1969. It is our experience that large numbers of pacemaker patients can be managed and evaluated effectively only with computer application.

First question: How do we store data? We (1) designed 3 different marker sheets – one for initial hospital admission, one for operative pacemaker procedures and one for re-admittance (table 1).

Each marker sheet has a capacity of 80 different bytes. The data are transferred off-line to punch cards by an electronic reader, the punch cards then being used to put all the information into EDP storage. The first step is extensive checking for formal errors; cases of re-entry are compared with previously stored data. The second step consists of filing the checked data. Patients are identified by consecutive numbers, so that new information on a patient who is already represented in the bank will be stored under his number, and this sequentially; this implies that the logical structure of the file is patient-related. In addition to entries for first implantation or replacement, the file is also updated with implantation or replacement; the file is also updated with follow-up information from the clinic or the physician in charge. All data on patients who are dead, cared for in another institution, or have dropped out of the study, remain in the file. The time interval between patient treatment and input of information into the data bank amounts to two weeks.

Second question: What do we store?
All identification data of the patient, his or her consecutive file number, the diagnosis and additional diseases, risk factors, etiology, type and degree of heart block, indication for implantation, case history and important data of the physical examination are set down in the marker-sheet for "first admittance." Also, the referring physician and the mode of follow-up are recorded. The second marker-sheet is used for all kinds of surgery in connection with implantation and replacement, incision, vein used for catheter insertion, threshold in V and mA, R wave potential, rate and length of stimulus, type of testing device, manufacturer, type and number of impulse generator and of electrode, site of pacemaker implantation and many other items.

The third marker-sheet serves for data collection from different sources.

Table 1. Flow diagram of the EDP system (data collection, data input and error checking, patient-related data storage, evaluation and application) for our pacemaker clinic.

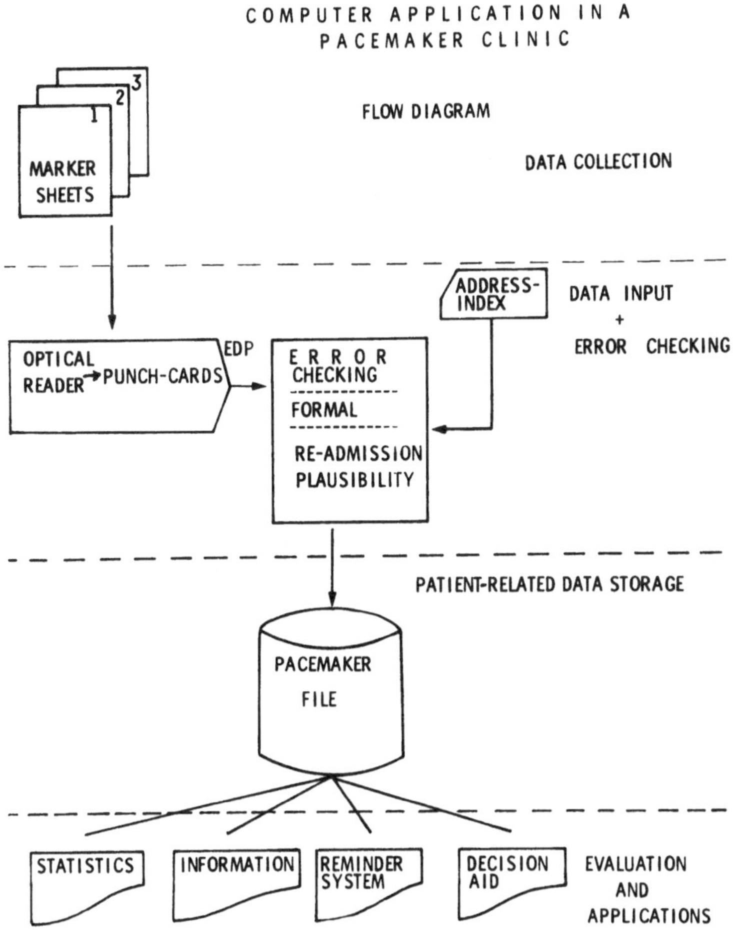

Mostly, it is used for re-admittance: In addition to important findings, the indication for in- or out-patient treatment, general and local physical status, indication for replacement, technical data of pacemaker and/or electrode are filled in. There are also markers for reports on patients controlled by a third party and for dropped-out patients. There is a whole section in this sheet concerning circumstances and cause of death, whether pacemaker-related or not, whether the pacemaker system was functioning or not, the postmortem report and so on.

In the course of time, we have changed many marker symbols, adapted others for better handling and omitted some because of inconvenience or errors. Up to now, with this 3-sheet system, we have been able to cover completely the case histories of all of our 2180 patients, the patients having an average of 4 admittances (table 2). The drawbacks of the system will be discussed later on.

Third question: How do we evaluate the data?
In order to retrieve and interpret the variables stored (table 3), we developed 7 EDP programs, i.e., patient survival, pacemaker lifetime, electrode lifetime, pacemaker complications, electrode complications, threshold increase and mortality. Of course printouts of contingency tables for each pair of variables wanted and single-variable scanning are additionally available.

Table 2. Application of marker sheets. For the initial treatment the "first admission" – and the "Surgery" – sheet are used. On all other occasions (in- and out-patients) the sheet "Re-admission" is needed, frequently in combination with the "Surgery" – sheet.

	MARKER SHEET	INITIAL TREATMENT	FURTHER TREATMENT + SURGERY	FURTHER TREATMENT NO SURGERY	COMPLICATIONS END OF FOLLOW-UP DEATH
1	FIRST ADMISSION	X			
2	SURGERY	X	X		
3	RE-ADMISSION ---------- FOLLOW UP		X	X	X

It is not possible to explain all the programs in this paper. But, as an example of the versatility of our system, some aspects of the patient survival and the pacemaker lifetime programs will be discussed. There is no general agreement on how to calculate survival time of pacemaker patients or the lifetime of pulse generators. There are different statistical approaches in use, but still many pacemaker centers compute mortality by taking the number of all patients treated and the number of patients deceased, and calculating the percentages. But pacemaker patients are people with different observation times and in different stages of

Table 3. For reasons of statistical evaluation 7 EDP-programs have been developed.

EDP - PROGRAMS FOR

1. PATIENT SURVIVAL
2. PACEMAKER LONGEVITY
3. ELECTRODE LONGEVITY
4. PACEMAKER COMPLICATIONS
5. ELECTRODE COMPLICATIONS
6. THRESHOLD RISE
7. MORTALITY

Table 4. Calculation of pacemaker longevity, adapting the BMD 0 1 S-program (DIXON). Labelling columns 4, 5, 6 and 7 (counting from left) with 3 indicates that routine exchange, number of patients dead, loss of follow-up and observation period not ended within one interval – are dealt with as a sum in equation $l_x = \boxed{1} - 1/2\ \boxed{3}$.

MEDTRONIC DEMAND

	[1]	[2]	[3]	[3]	[3]	[3]	[4]	[5]	[6]	[7]
Time interval	Functioning at begin of interval	Loss of function during interval	Routine exchange	Pat. died	Loss of follow up	Observ. not ended	Effect.nr. of units observed	Proportion of unit failure	Proport. functioning	Cumulative proportion functioning
days							$l_x = \boxed{1} - 1/2\ \boxed{3}$	$q = 2/l_x$	$p = 1-q$	$P = p_1 \cdot p_2 \ldots$
90	41	2		3	1	8	35	0,057	0,943	0,943
180	27			1		13	20	0	1	0,943
270	13					1	12	0	1	0,943
360	12	1		1		1	11	0,090	0,910	0,858
450	9					2	9	0	1	0,858
540	7			1	1	3	5	0	1	0,858
630	2					2	1	0	1	0,858

treatment, e.g., patients with first implants for different periods of time, others with a second pacemaker, and so on. The same considerations must be applied to deceased patients. Also, dropped-out patients have to be taken into account.

For these reasons, we chose a statistical program from the University of California to evaluate the cumulative survival time of patients with varying observation periods.

Table 4 shows the Cutler-Ederer method of calculating the so-called cumulative survival curve, according to the BMD program 0 1 S of the University of California (2, 3). The accumulated length of observation of each patient is divided into 90-day intervals, and the number of patients in each interval is arrived at by due consideration of mortality, drop-out and terminations of observation periods. In accordance with the laws of probability, the survival rates from all observation periods are multiplied with one another, resulting in the so-called cumulative survival curve. This program also determines the standard error involved.

Table 5 shows the program for pulse generators. We tested the validity of this program for pacemakers, comparing the results with performance data released by one manufacturer. In figure 1, our results are plotted against the results obtained for a certain demand pacemaker model.

Table 5. Calculation of pacemaker longevity, adapting the BMD 0 1 S-program (DIXON). Labelling columns 4, 5, 6 and 7 (counting from left) with 3 indicates that routine exchange, number of patients dead, loss of follow-up and observation period not ended within one interval – are dealt with as a sum in equation 1_x = [1] – 1/2 [3]. (This is a calculation done 6 years ago).

MEDTRONIC DEMAND

	[1]	[2]	[3]	[3]	[3]	[3]	[4]	[5]	[6]	[7]
Time interval	Functioning at begin of interval	Loss of function during interval	Routine exchange	Pat. died	Loss of follow up	Observ. not ended	Effect.nr. of units observed	Proportion of unit failure	Proport. functioning	Cumulative proportion functioning
days							l_x = [1] -1/2 [3]	$q=2/l_x$	$p=1-q$	$P=p_1 \cdot p_2 \cdots$
90	41	2		3	1	8	35	0,057	0,943	0,943
180	27			1		13	20	0	1	0,943
270	13					1	12	0	1	0,943
360	12	1		1		1	11	0,090	0,910	0,858
450	9					2	9	0	1	0,858
540	7			1	1	3	5	0	1	0,858
630	2					2	1	0	1	0,858

The cumulative survival curve for 2058 consecutive patients is shown in figure 2. The mean general 5 year survival rate is 62%, the 10 year survival rate 43%. The latter result is obtained from a rather small number of patients. Over the years, our experience with computing survival rates has shown that an increasing num-

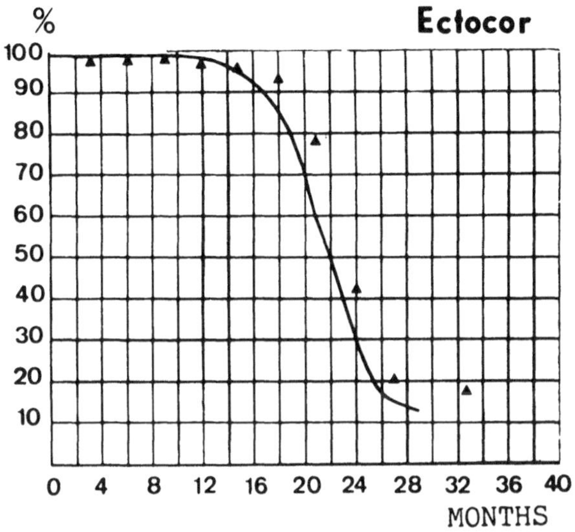

Figure 1. On the diagram Cordis-Ectocor performance values (---), as obtained from the manufacturer, are plotted against our data (▲).

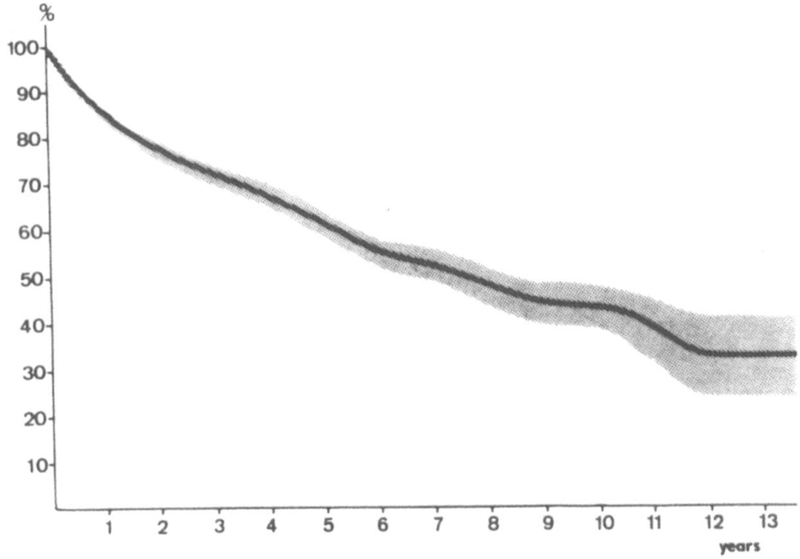

Figure 2. Cumulative survival curve of 2058 consecutive patients (Dept. of Cardiac surgery, University hospital Munich). (July 1962- October 1976).
The shaded area represents double standard error.

ber of patients tends to improve the results. Hence, we believe the 10 year-results to be better than estimated. The versatile layout of our system allows for stratification of the results. The cumulative survival curve may be evaluated separately for male and female patients (figure 3), for patients with and without Adams-Stokes attacks (ASA) (figure 4), and for different age groups (figure 5). Of course, one could obtain survival curves for different age groups stratified for sex, ASA, type and degree of block, brands of pacemakers used, mode of electrode application and so on, simultaneously but for such extensive stratification, the number of our patients – now 2180 – is still too small to yield significant results.

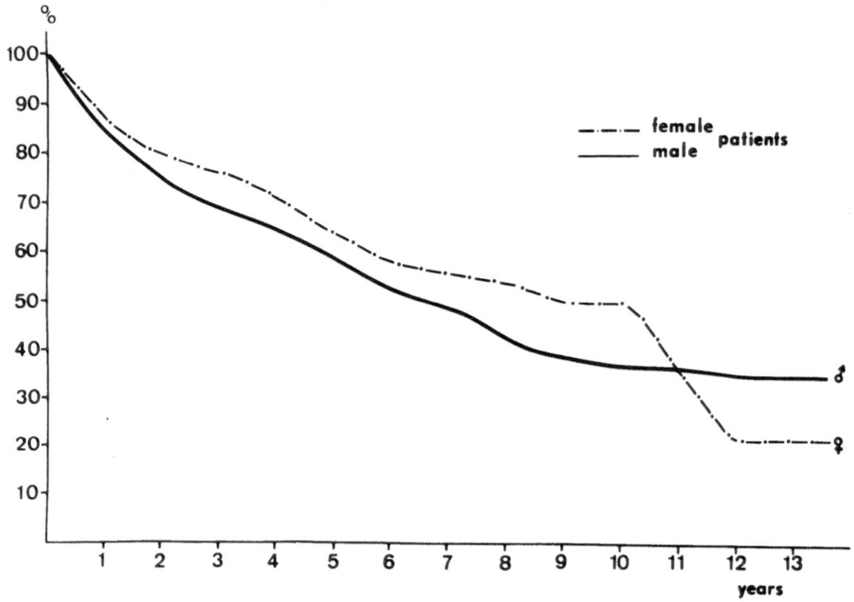

Figure 3. The cumulative survival curve of Figure 2, stratified for male and female patients. (July 1962-October 1976). The deviation of the curves is not of statistical significance.

Aside from statistics, our system supplies us with decoded information on all patients. As soon as new data are fed into the file, we receive printouts of the abridged version of all patients' updated case history (figure 6). We do not yet have terminals for dialogue EDP in our pacemaker clinic. However, the constant availability of pertinent data greatly facilitates daily handling of patients and the office work involved.

To streamline the latter, a reminder system was built up to supervise out-

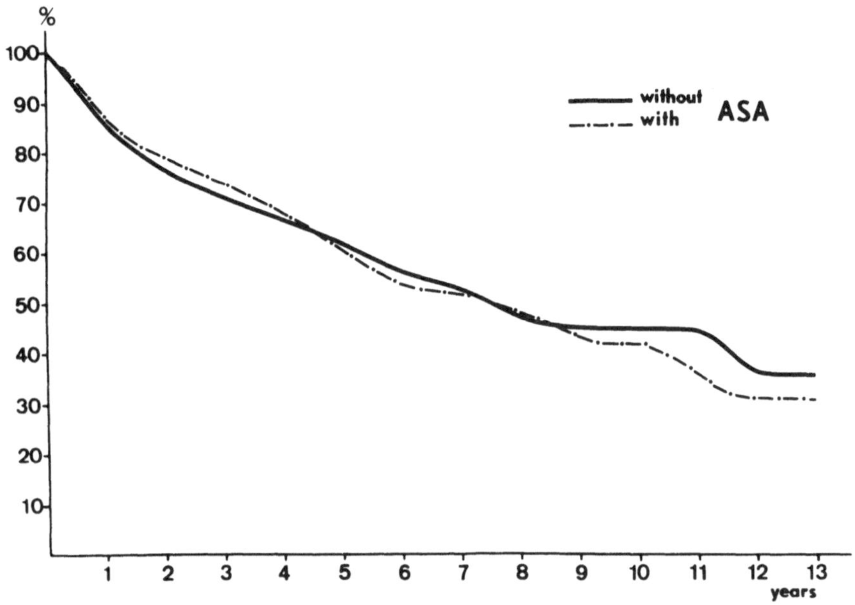

Figure 4. The cumulative survival curve of 2058 consecutive patients of Figure 2, stratified for patients with and without ASA. There is no significant difference between the two curves.

patient checks 3, 12, 18, 21 months etc. after pacemaker implantation or replacement.

The reminder system (figure 7) is started every mid-month and identifies all patients to be called in for checks during the following months. The reminder program requires the current date from the computer, so that it needs no control from the users. The addresses of the respective patients are printed on sticker labels and supplied to us for mailing.

Last but not least, our computer aided documentation system can be used for research projects. Some aspects of statistics are utilized in this respect, as mentioned before. Recently, we have created a decision aid which computes 5 year survival probabilities for individual patients with the aid of discriminant analysis (figure 8). Up to now, we can predict the probability of death within 5 years with only 69% accuracy.

However, we hope to improve the program to yearly survival probabilities of individual patients by refining the discrimination analysis used for classification, and by developing better statistical approaches. Other research projects concern simplification of data collection, specific programs, and a nation-wide data file.

Finally, we want to add some remarks on the economic aspect of EDP in

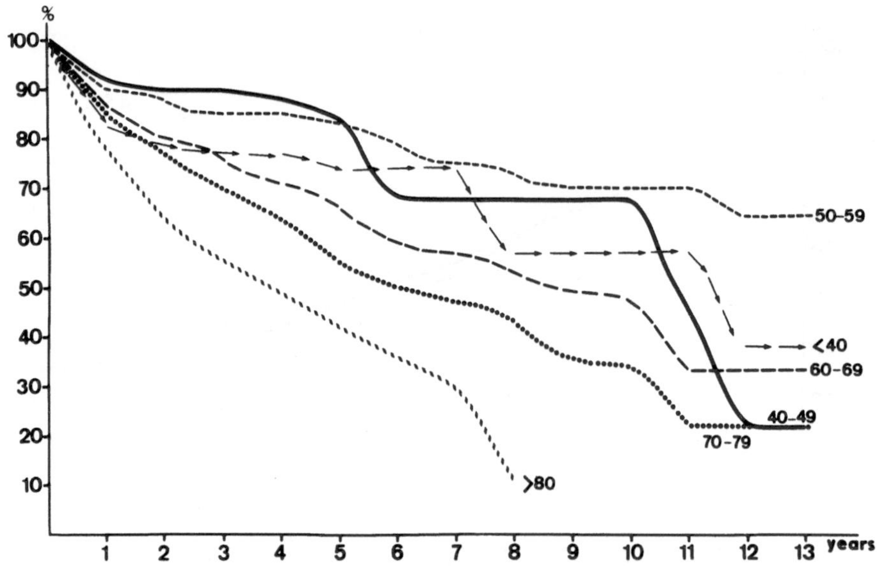

Figure 5. The cumulative survival curve of Figure 2, stratified for 10 year age-groups. (July 1962-April 1977). Because of the small numbers, patients up to 40 years of age are collected in one group. The best results are obtained in the 50-59 years age-group.
The curves are not age-adjusted.

```
GESCHLECHT                            2 MAENNLICH
OPERATION --------------        1888 PATIENTEN-NR ---------
AUFNAHME-NR.                          1 NR.
OPERATIONS DATUM                   2710 TAG UND MONAT
OPERATIONSJAHR                       75 JAHR
OPERATIONS NR.                        1 NR.
ANAESTHESIE                           3 LOKAL
ENDOCARDIALE SONDE                    2 RECHTS
VENE                                  3 CEPHALICA
ELEKTRODENTYP                         1 UNIPOLAR
ELEKTRODE                             3 ELEMA
IMPULSGEBERFABRIKAT                   5 VITATRON
REIZART                               1 R-WELLE BLOCKIERT
FREQUENZ                             72 SCHLAEGE PRO MINUTE
KRANKENBLATT-NR.                   9999 ZAHL
KRANKENBLATT-NR.                     75 JAHR
IMPLANTATIONSSEITE                    2 RECHTS
IMPLANTATIONSTIEFE                    1 SUBCUTAN
IMPLANTATIONSORT                      1 PECTORALIS
ENTLASSUNGSART                        2 VERLEGT IN AND. KLINIK


WIEDERHOLUNG ***********        1888 PATIENTEN-NR **********
AUFNAHME-NR.                          2 NR.
```

Figure 6. Section of a decoded printout of an abridged patient's case history.

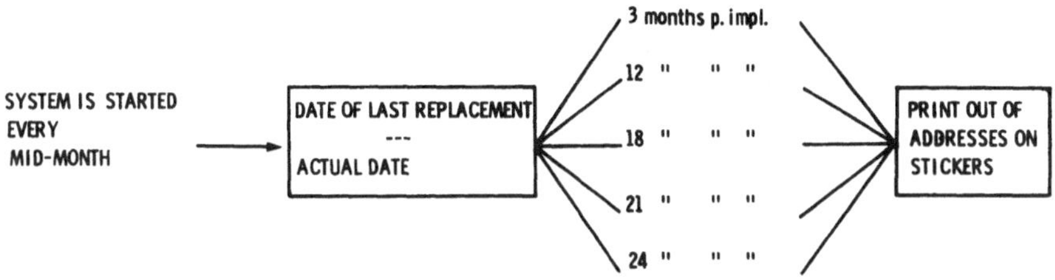

Figure 7. Reminder-system for routine follow-up in a pacemaker clinic.

Prediction of 5-year-survival probability

69 % accuracy for all patients

84 % accuracy for 15 % of patients

Figure 8. Prediction of 5-years-survival probability as a decision aid is still too insignificant.

pacemaker data collection and evaluation. Our system was initiated in 1969, and we have experienced some problems: our marker sheets had contained many unnecessary items, whereas many important ones were missing. Handling of the sheets is still rather troublesome. After some attempts to introduce improvements such as data collection using computerized surgical reports and physicians' letters, we reverted to our old system. We still think it must be improved, but we have learned that EDP makes data collection easier and more economical only when used very carefully indeed. Then, computerized storage, retrieval and evaluation of data distinctly facilitates pacemaker treatment, as against conventional record keeping and calculation.

References

1. Zimmermann, M., Die Verwendung der EDV zu Ergebnis-beurteilung chirurgischer Schrittmachertherapie. *Med. Inaug. Diss.*, München 1971.
2. Cutler, S.J., Ederer, F., Maximum Utilization of the Life Table Method in Analyzing Survival. *J. Chronic Dis.*, p. 699-712, (1958).

3. Dixon, W.J., "BMD Biomedical computer programs." Health sciences computing facility, Department of Preventive Medicine and Public Health, School of Medicine, University of California, 1964.

DIGITAL COMPUTERS IN PACEMAKER ANALYSIS

GEORGE MYERS AND VICTOR PARSONNET

I. Introduction

At present computers are used in two areas of pacemaker analysis: clinic operation and data surveys. In a pacemaker clinic, typically it is used to measure and record data from patients in a specific area for the purpose of diagnosis and treatment. An example is the clinics at the Newark Beth Israel Medical Center and its affiliates that maintain surveillance on more than 2,000 patients in New Jersey. A data survey, by contrast, samples data from a wide geographic area, and is not used specifically for treatment or diagnosis. Examples are the Computer Pacemaker Registry of the Food and Drug Administration and the World Surveys of Pacing made for the recent Tokyo meeting.

While studies of this type can be done with "pencil and paper", a computer becomes absolutely necessary when large patient populations are involved, or information is required rapidly.

This paper will review the current status of both areas, and will discuss future prospects and needs.

II. Current status of surveillance systems

Most clinics acquire data non-invasively and use the computer for data storage, retrieval, and display. Usually, data is inserted into the computer manually, but in some centers automatic or semiautomatic procedures are used.

There are three current approaches to using a computer in a surveillance system: (1) Batch processing; (2) Real-time with manual insertion of data ("semi-automatic"); (3) Real time with data inserted by means of analog-digital converters ("automatic").

In the batch-processing procedure, data collected in the normal way are periodically (daily, weekly) processed by the computer. This technique is useful for maintaining historical files, but because of time lag, is not useful for patient diagnosis.

In the "semi-automatic" mode, digital information is inserted into the computer immediately *after* it is collected, and the processed data is then available shortly afterwards for use in both patient diagnosis and historical records. In the "automatic" procedures, the data are transmitted directly into the computer. This method requires less time for data insertion, and is less prone to human error. However, in many cases the time required to insert the data manually is much *less* than the time required to prepare the patient and make the measurements, so the time saved by going to automatic methods is small, while the added expense in equipment may be large. Each situation has to be judged by its own costs and benefits.

Semi-automatic procedures at our Center are typical of many such clinics (1). Electrocardiographic leads are attached to the patient by a technician. Measurements taken of the amplified wave shape include impulse interval, amplitude, and duration. These data are automatically recorded on a printer and the artifact is photographed. An ECG rhythm strip is analyzed for sensing, competition, and capture. If there are no natural heartbeats and a demand pacemaker has been implanted, external overdrive (EOD) is used to test the sensing circuit. The data are then inserted into the computer and a report is produced immediately. The comparison of present data with all previous data immediately highlights trends, and failing pulse generators are easily detected. An average examination takes four minutes.

The computer also provides other services; it automatically writes letters to referring physicians in which the findings of the clinic are concisely summarized. There are also numerous retrieval and statistical programs, some of these are listed in Table 1.

In addition to these capabilities, new features are now under development: In the telephone monitoring program, linear regression is used to predict the next pulse interval to be measured, based on the previous 20 readings. The "out of limits" values are based on the variability of past measurements and known characteristics of the pulse generator. A typical series of measurements is shown in Fig. 1. If the measured interval falls outside of these intervals, the pulse generator is identified as "potentially failing," and the patient is asked to come to the hospital for a more detailed examination. Soon we will also have automatic insertion of digital information into the computer.

Because of the necessity for operator intervention, neither the waveform analysis with A/D conversion or the ECG analysis can be called fully automatic. However, these partially automated techniques do point the way to the future.

Using the computer in this way also does not appear to be capable of saving much examination time on the average, although, of course, a considerable amount of time may be saved with a particular patient. Most of the time spent during an examination is spent taking the electrocardiogram, performing EOD, adjusting scale factors, photographing the waveform, and assembling the ECG

Table 1. A list of some of the retrieval, inventory, and statistical programs used in the Pacemaker Clinic at the Newark Beth Israel Medical Center.

PRESENT REPORT PROGRAM

4/6/77

A. CLINIC REPORT - (INDIVIDUAL PATIENT) REPORT USED IN CLINIC-ON LINE

B. DELINQUENCY REPORT - SHOWS PATIENTS WHO HAVE NOT VISITED CLINIC IN 4 MONTHS... USED TO ENSURE FOLLOW-UP PATIENTS-WEEKLY.

C. WEEKLY LISTING OF PATIENTS WHO RECEIVED CLINIC TESTS-ON REQUEST (INCLUDES SCHEDULED WEEKLY CLINIC AND PRIVATE CLINICS.)

D. CLINIC RETRIEVAL REPORT - USED TO PRINT CLINIC DATA ON ANY PATIENTS-ON REQUEST.

E. ACTIVE FILE REPORT - ALPHA LISTING BY PATIENT OF NAME, BIRTH DATE, PACEMAKER TYPE, LEAD TYPE, IMPLANT DATE, PRIMARY DIAGNOSIS AND REFERRING M.D.-MONTHLY.

F. ACTIVE PATIENT LISTING BY PACEMAKER TYPE INCLUDING SUMMARY OF DISTRIBUTION-QUARTERLY, AS REQUESTED.

G. PACEMAKER CODE LIST - LIST OF THE CODES USED TO IDENTIFY THE VARIOUS PACEMAKER TYPES-ON REQUEST.

H. LETTER TO REFERRING M.D.

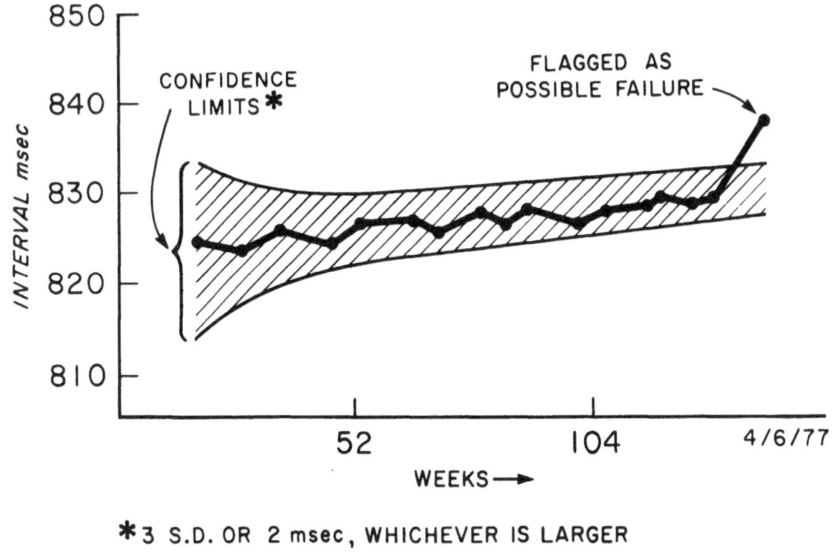

Figure 1. The computer determines when a pulse generator monitored over the telephone is about to fail by determining when a measured interval does not lie on a straight-line projection of the previous 20 intervals. Because the intervals do not lie exactly on a straight line, an interval has to be outside of the confidence limits to be a possible failure.

strip and photographing onto the final report. It does not appear likely that the additional automation materially speeds procedures in view of the large amount of operator interaction and manual processing required.

It should be noted that there are really two parts to a pacemaker evaluation, waveform analysis and electrocardiogram interpretation. Some centers have made progress in automating one or both of these aspects.

Methods are described by Black and Collins (2), and Grant and Hanson (3) for A/D conversion, but both systems require operator intervention to adjust scale factors or to indicate artifact polarity. Black and Collins photograph the display of the waveform and the computer report from the cathode ray tube. Although Grant and Hanson do not use the computer for graphic depiction of the waveform, they analyze the waveform for decay of the flat top. They have also automated the electrocardiographic interpretation. Computer interpretation of pacemaker function from an electrocardiogram is considerably simpler than the general case of computer electrocardiogram interpretation, because in the case of pacemakers it is only necessary to determine the occurrence of the R wave, the artifact, and the time relation between them. Thus, an R wave without a succeeding artifact indicates that the pacemaker is sensing, while an artifact *with* a succeeding R wave indicates that the pacemaker is capturing. An R wave with no preceding artifact indicates competition. It is relatively easy to detect, by means of a computer, an R wave or an artifact. However, it is sometimes quite difficult to distinguish the R wave immediately following a paced beat from the "tail-off" of the artifact. Similarly, fusion beats can sometimes appear to be unsensed R waves. Grant and Hanson do not discuss these problems explicitly, but their computer report only indicates the ratio of artifacts to captures and the percentage of R waves which are not followed by artifacts. It thus appears that it is up to the diagnostician to determine if the pacer is actually not pacing or not sensing. However, it is certainly true that these ratios provide a warning flag which is not easy to overlook. Furthermore, these are "fail-safe" indications – they will signal possible failure when the pacer may be functioning properly, but not the other way. Thus, there is little doubt that the computer ECG analysis is a valuable aid.

III. Current status of data surveys

Three different types of data bases for surveys are commonly used:

1. A random sample of all practitioners, as exemplified by the recent survey for the Tokyo meeting. (4)

2. A full sample of a small number of representative institutions, such as in the Pacemaker Registry of the Food and Drug Administration (FDA), which uses

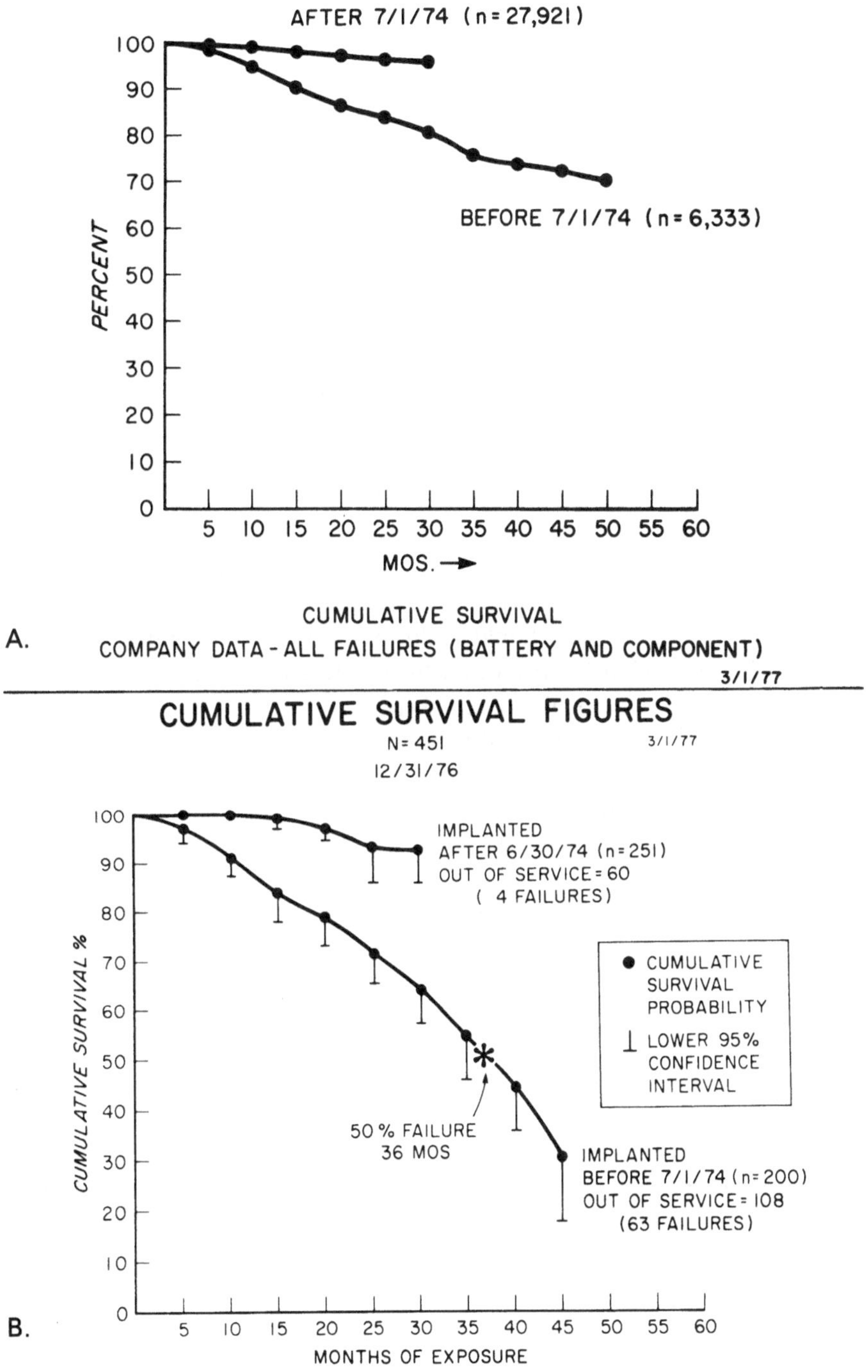

Figure 2. Comparison of actuarial survival curves, for one model pacemaker, showing difference between manufacturer's data (A) and data from registry (B).

all patient data from three large implanting institutions. (5)

3. An analysis of all devices in a certain class, such as manufacturers' registries.

The limitations and advantages inherent in each of the three techniques relate almost entirely to the methods of data acquisition.

The sampling technique, which uses a questionnaire, covers a wide geographical area and a broad range of physicians, but contains hidden biases and cannot be relied on for quantitative answers. Most respondees do not have ready access to detailed statistics concerning their own practices, but must rely on memory and impressions. There is also a problem in setting up the sample, such as the desire to canvass all practitioners in a particular class, "all physicians implanting bipolar pacemakers," or "all physicians implanting at least five pacemakers a year." In practice, it is usually impossible to learn who these physicians are. Instead, alternate methods are used, such as polling all cardiac surgeons, or obtaining lists from societies or manufacturers. Such lists invariably omit some who should be polled, while including many who should *not* be polled. The use of selected lists, such as those from a professional society, omits those who are not members of the society, who often are less sophisticated in their techniques and therefore whose practices should really be included. Questionnaire surveys, therefore, give much better results for treatments and procedures, and are weak on data concerning particular pacemakers.

Notwithstanding all of these difficulties, broad sampling surveys do give valuable information on how specific problems are attacked by different practitioners and on the effects of differences in patient populations.

Manufacturers try to maintain records on all their pacemakers, usually in a computer. In general, such lists do provide an excellent source for information concerning early failures, but are quite *in*accurate for failures after this time, and do not contain data on other pacer problems. Adequate information is obtainable in only about 25% of the pacemakers sold, and is of high quality in only about 10% of cases. (6) Figure 2 shows how much manufacturer's data can differ from registry data.

Surveys based on detailed data from a few institutions give highly quantitative data on a 100% sample of all patients and procedures falling within the group under examination. This all-inclusiveness leads to a major problem: the large mass of collected data limits the number of centers, practitioners, and patients. The limiting factor is usually the time and money available for reducing the data. Despite problems, however, a computerized statistical analysis of clinical results gives the most accurate and unbiased data on pacemakers available.

With such rapid reporting the FDA registry has already detected early pulse generator problems before the general recognition of the problem, even though the study was limited to only three centers. An example is shown in Figure 3 in which two almost identical pulse generators revealed important differences in actuarial survival. It is apparent that one of them was much less reliable, and the problem was in the unit with a unipolar lead. With this knowledge, the trouble was traced to the connector, and then corrected.

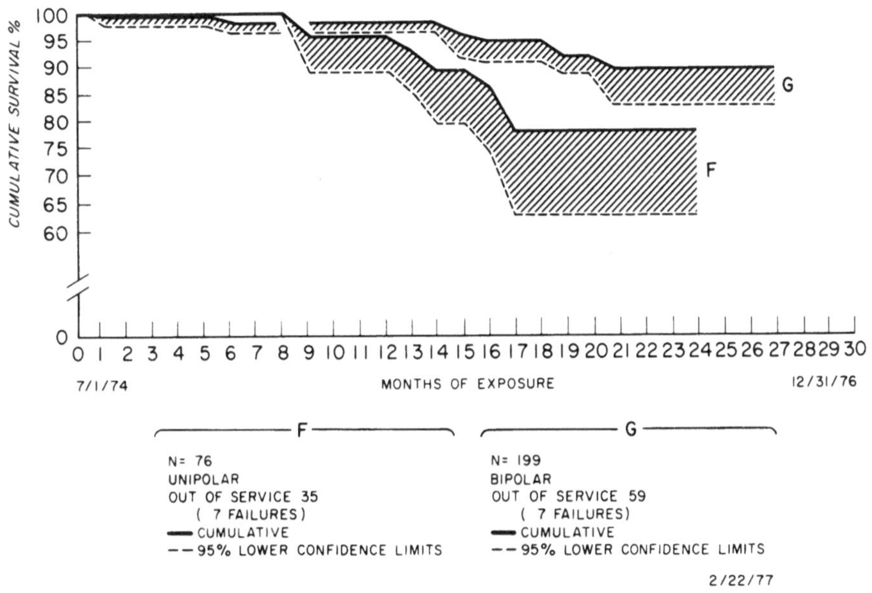

Figure 3. Cumulative survival curves for two pulse generators differing only in the type of lead used. The problem with the unipolar system was traced to the connector.

IV. The future

The principal change to be foreseen in surveys is "standardization" of a data base. Unfortunately, efforts to accomplish this have so far been unsuccessful. Until now, most effort has been devoted to automating measurement procedures, and diagnosis is still done principally by the physician; but clinics are likely to see more automatic diagnosis in the future. The dividends can be expected to be high here, because most test results are "normal," so a procedure which can distinguish normal from abnormal with a high degree of reliability can save large amounts of physician time. A reasonable next step would be automatic data acquisition devices which would permit a computer direct access to pacer parameters. If this could be done by a telephone monitor, the advantages would be even greater.

References

1. Parsonnet, V., Myers, G.H., Gilbert, L., Zucker, I.R. and Shilling, E., Follow-up of Implanted Pacemakers. *Amer. Heart J.*, 87, 642 (1974).
2. Black, J.L. and Collins, D.W.K., Computerized Assessment of Cardiac Pacemaker Performance. *Int. J. Bio-Medical Computing*, 7, 163 (1976).
3. Grout, Michael, and Hanson, S., A Totally Computerized Cardiac Pacemaker Surveillance System. *Computers and Biomedical Research*, 8, 580, (1975).
4. Hori, M. and Furman, S., World Survey on Long Term Follow-up of Cardiac Pacing. *Cardiac Pacing Proc. Vth International Symposium*. Y. Watanabe, Ed. Excerpta Medica, 555, (1977).
5. Bilitch, M., Escher, D., Furman, S., Parsonnet, V., "Twelve Months Experiences with Commercially Available Cardiac Pacemakers – A Multi-Center Study"(Abstract) *Am. J. Cardiol.* 37, 121 (1976).
6. Greatbatch, W., Personal Communication.

THE NATIONAL PACEMAKER DATABANK

G.D. Green and G. Thompson

1. Introduction

Glasgow's Pacemaker Databank has been operating for over a year (1). It arose, first, because of the need to have an ever increasing amount of data on pacemakers regularly updated and readily available for use at Pacemaker Clinics and on other occasions; secondly, because of the need for computer analyses of the basic data. Within a short time the concept and advantages of a National Pacemaker Data bank emerged and some progress has been made in this direction in that a number of hospitals in the U.K. (plus several in Australia) are now having their data processed in Glasgow.

The computer print-outs which are currently being issued to hospitals consist of two parts. The first part is an alphabetical list of patients, with dates of birth and serial numbers for easy location of patients in Part 2. Part 2 is more comprehensive and includes details about the pacemakers and their performance in terms of implant lifetimes.

The next stage in our development programme is to provide a computer print-out which will include some clinical data and it is our proposals for this more comprehensive and better databank which are outlined below.

2. Collection of data

Three forms have been designed to collect data about pacemaker patients and their implants. Clinical data have been selected recently following consultations with medical colleagues in Glasgow and elsewhere, whereas pacemaker data have been chosen from experience with the existing databank.

Forms 1 and 2 are completed at the time of the primary pacemaker operation. Form 3 is completed at any "Subsequent Event," as explained in section 3.

If after submitting a form to the Databank Controller an error is discovered, or data becomes available which was not available hitherto, then the error or omission can be rectified by submitting another form which clearly indicates which are corrected or additional data.

Many of the items on the forms need no explanation, but comments are necessary on some of them.

3. Patient data – form no. 1 (Figure 1)

Card 1

Each patient is given a National Pacemaker Databank Number (Spaces 2-8). This seven digit number is issued by the hospital where the patient receives his first pacemaker, from a block of numbers allocated to that hospital by the Databank Controller. This unique number which has a "check-digit" incorporated in it together with other stringent programming safeguards ensures that a particular patient's data are not corrupted by data from another patient.

An Event (Spaces 9 and 10) is defined as any of the following:

(1) a pacemaker related operation

(2) the death of a patient

(3) a decision that a patient has become lost to follow-up.

Clearly, the primary pacemaker operation is Event No. 1. The Hospital Code Number (Spaces 11 to 16) is also a unique number given to a hospital and this may be issued by a Government Department, as in the U.K., or if necessary such a number can be allocated by the Databank Controller.

The Hospital Case Sheet Number (Spaces 17-22) is the number issued by a hospital to a particular patient for internal administrative purposes.

Card 2

This card enables the clinician to identify the reasons for implanting a pacemaker, the electrocardiographic diagnosis and the etiology of the cardiac disturbance.

4. First event data – form no. 2 (Figure 2)

Card 3

Card 3 (Spaces 25 to 55) refers mainly to the generator and the site of implantation of the generator. The three letter code (2) is used to identify the kind of generator which has been implanted.

Space 24 enables a clinician to indicate whether a patient is apparently pacemaker dependent. Any patient who has been having Stokes-Adams attacks

PACEMAKER DATABANK FORM - No 1 (PATIENT DATA)

NATIONAL PACEMAKER DATABANK No. | EVENT No. | HOSP. CODE No.	Card 1 ⎵ ⎵⎵⎵⎵⎵⎵⎵ 0 1 ⎵⎵⎵⎵⎵⎵	1-16
HOSPITAL CASE SHEET No.		17-22
SURNAME		23-38
FIRST NAME		39-50
INITIALS OF FORENAMES		51-54
DATE OF BIRTH		55-62
SEX : (1) Female (2) Male		63

Card 2 : 1-16 as for Card 1

REASONS FOR PACING — 17-22

(1) Poor exercise tolerance (2) Easy fatigability
(3) Dizziness (4) Syncope
(5) Congestive cardiac failure
(6) Palpitation
(7) None - prophylactic implantation
(8) Other

TYPE OF CARDIAC DISTURBANCE

Atrio-ventricular Block — 30-35

(o) Stable (1) Intermittent
(2) Third degree (complete)
Second degree (incomplete, partial)
(3) - Mobitz (Type II)
(4) - Mobitz (Type I) (Wenckebach)
(5) First degree

Bundle Branch Block — 40-46

(o) Stable (1) Intermittent
(2) Right bundle branch block (RBBB)
(3) Left posterior hemiblock (LPH)
(4) Left anterior hemiblock (LAH)
(5) Left bundle branch block (LBBB)
(6) Intra-ventricular conduction defect. (7) Other

Supraventricular Bradycardias — 50-55

(o) Stable (1) Intermittent
(2) Sinus bradycardia (3) Sinus bradycardia/tachycardia syndrome
(4) Sino-atrial block
(5) Sinus arrest (6) Other

Supraventricular Tachycardias — 60-67

(o) Stable (1) Intermittent
(2) Atrial flutter
(3) Atrial fibrillation
(4) Atrial tachycardia
(5) Junctional tachycardia
(6) AV nodal re-entry tachycardia
(7) Extra nodal re-entry tachycardia
(8) Other

Idioventricular Rhythms — 68-69

(1) Ectopics (2) Tachycardias

ETIOLOGY OF CARDIAC DISTURBANCE — 70

(1) Idiopathic
(2) Congenital
(3) Surgical
Ischaemic post myocardial infarct
(4) - inferior posterior
(5) - anterior
(6) - not specified
(7) Other

Date — Signature

Figure 1. Patient Data – Form No. 1.

PACEMAKER DATABANK FORM No 2 (FIRST EVENT DATA)

Hosp. Case Sheet No. ________________ Patient's Name ________________

Card	Item	Columns
Card 3 (1–16) as for Card 1	Date of implantation	17–22
	Anaesthetic : (1) general (2) local	23
	Apparently pacemaker dependent : (1) yes (2) no	24
	Generator manufacturer	25–26
	Type of generator (Three letter code)	27–29
	Model designation	30–38
	Serial number	39–47
	Basic generator rate at body temp.	48–50
	Pulse duration	51–53
	Location : (1) left pectoral (2) right pectoral (3) abdominal (4) other	54
	Depth : (1) subcutaneous (2) submuscular (3) within rectus sheath (4) other	55
Card 4 (1–16) as for Card 1	Lead manufacturer	17–18
	Type of lead	19–21
	Model designation	22–30
	Serial number	31–39
	Serial number	40–48
	Atrial lead (or indifferent lead) manufacturer	49–50
	Model designation of atrial (or indiff. lead)	51–59
	Serial number of atrial (or indiff.) lead	60–68
	Placement of endocardial ventricular lead :	
	Side : (1) left (2) right	69
	Vein : (1) ext. jug. (2) int. jug. (3) cephalic (4) subclavian (5) other	70
	Depth : (1) anterior clavicle (2) posterior clavicle	71
	Placement of myocardial/epicardial ventricular lead	
	Access : (1) left thoracotomy (2) median sternotomy (3) subxyphoid (4) other	72
	Ventricle : (1) left (2) right	73
	Placement of Atrial Lead	
	Side : (1) left (2) right	74
	Access : (1) ext. jug. (2) int. jug. (3) cephalic (4) subclavian (5) other vein (6) thoracotomy	75
	Atrium : (1) left (2) right	76
	Form of pacing : (1) bipolar (2) unipolar	77
Card 5 (1–16) as for Card 1	Pacing threshold values	
	(1) Ventricle (2) atrium (3) both	17
	Measuring instrument used	18–24
	Current (mA)	25–28
	Voltage (V)	29–32
	Pulse duration (mS)	33–35
	Current (mA)	36–39
	Voltage (V)	40–43
	Pulse duration (mS)	44–46
	Sensing Signals	
	(1) ventricle (2) atrium	50
	Measuring instrument used	51–57
	Voltage (mV)	58–60

Date Signature

Figure 2. First Event Data – Form No. 2.

PACEMAKER DATABANK FORM – No. 3 (SUBSEQUENT EVENT DATA)

Hosp. Case Sheet No. ____________ Patient's Name ____________

NATIONAL PACEMAKER DATABANK NO.	EVENT No.	HOSP. CODE No.	Card 6		1–16

HOSP. CODE NO./HOSP. CASE NO. 17–30

(If operation is taking place in diff. hosp. from previous one).

Patient presentation : (1) Re-operation before leaving hosp. after previous event. 31

(2) via pacemaker clinic (routine appt.)
(3) " " " " (special appt.)
(4) elective re-operation (5) emergency admission

Date of event* 32–37

Anaesthetic : (1) general (2) local 38

Apparently pacemaker dependent : (1) yes (2) no 39

Allocation of Implant Lifetime codes and other codes

Generator 40–49

Date for determining generator implant lifetime – if different from above* 50–55

Lead 56–65

Date for determining lead implant lifetime – if different from above* 66–71

Card 7 (1–16) as for Card 6

Generator manufacturer 17–18
Type of generator (Three letter code) 19–21
Model designation 22–30
Serial number 31–39
Basic generator rate at body temp. 40–42
Pulse duration 43–45
Location : (1) left pectoral (2) right pectoral (3) abdominal (4) other 46
Depth : (1) subcutaneous (2) submuscular (3) within rectus sheath (4) other 47

Card 8 (1–16) as for Card 6

Lead manufacturer 17–18
Type of lead 19–21
Model designation 22–30
Serial number 31–39
Serial number 40–48
Atrial lead (or indifferent lead) manufacturer 49–50
Model designation of atrial (or indiff.) lead 51–59
Serial number of atrial of atrial indifferent lead 60–68
Placement of endocardial ventricular lead :
Side : (1) left (2) right 69
Vein : (1) ext.jug. (2) int.jug. (3) cephalic (4) subclavian (5) other 70
Depth : (1) anterior clavicle (2) posterior clavicle 71
Placement of Myocardial/epicardial ventricular lead:
Access : (1) left thoracotomy (2) median sternotomy (3) subphyxoid (4) other 72
Ventricle: (1) left (2) right 73
Placement of atrial lead
Side : (1) left (2) right 74
Access : (1) ext.jug. (2) int.jug. (3) cephalic (4) subclavian (5) other vein (6) thoracotomy 75
Atrium : (1) left (2) right 76
Form of pacing : (1) bipolar (2) unipolar 77

Card 9 (1–16) as for Card 6

Pacing threshold values (1) ventricle (2) atrium (3) both 17
Measuring instrument used 18–24
Current (mA) 25–28
Voltage (V) 29–32
Pulse duration (mS) 33–35
Current (mA) 36–39
Voltage (V) 40–43
Pulse duration (mS) 44–46
Sensing signals (1) ventricle (2) atrium 50
Measuring instrument used 51–57
Voltage (mV) 58–60

Date Signature

Figure 3. Subsequent Event Data – Form No. 3.

ought to be classified as such. Some others, who may not have had such symptoms become apparently pacemaker dependent after only a short period of temporary pacing.

Card 4

This card (Spaces 17 to 77) refers to the pacing lead, or leads, and the means of access to the heart. It may be helpful in certain circumstances to specify the form of pacing (Space 77). For instance, two myocardial leads might be implanted, one to give unipolar pacing, the other being held in reserve for future use.

Card 5

Pacing and sensing values are specified on this card. Ventricular pacing threshold are always stated first (Spaces 25 to 35), followed by any atrial threshold values (Spaces 36 to 46). The minimum value of the sensing signal (ventricular or atrial) is specified in spaces 58 to 60). In all cases the instrument used should be specified. (Spaces 18 to 24 and 51 to 57).

5. Subsequent event data – form no. 3 (Figure 3)

Card 6

When a patient has another Event associated with the same hospital there are no difficulties in completing the first line (Spaces 2-16) and the second line (Spaces 17-30) is irrelevant.

When a patient is operated on following formal transfer to the hospital the patient's National Pacemaker Databank Number (Spaces 2 to 8), the last Event Number (Spaces 9 and 10) and the former Hospital Code Number (Spaces 11 to 16) will be readily available in the latest print-out issued to that hospital. Spaces 17-30 refer to the hospital where the latest operation is taking place.

When re-operation takes place in a hospital without formal transfer having been arranged Form 3 should be completed, as far as is possible, and then sent to the former hospital, assuming that the patient will be returning to that hospital for further follow-up.

Patient presentation (Space 31) has been divided into five categories.

Spaces 40 and 56 on this card are amongst the most important on Form 3. These are reserved for the major implant lifetime codes, namely F, I, C and E. When a patient dies the code D is entered in Spaces 41 and 57. A whole range of minor codes have been introduced which can be entered in Spaces 42 to 49 and 58 to 65. Most of these are easy to remember such as BVR which means Battery Voltage Reduction.

The dates associated with the codes I, C and E are the same as the Event date (Spaces 32 to 37), but the code F should sometimes be linked with an earlier date. For instance, the first indications of battery voltage reduction might be detected some time before re-operation takes place. In the case of an insulation failure on a pacemaker lead reoperation might be delayed for many months until an indication of sufficient battery voltage reduction makes re-operation imperative. Thus, Spaces 50 to 55 and 66 to 71 have been reserved for the relevant dates associated with the major code F.

Spaces 50 to 55 are also used to record the date of death of a patient. (There is no need to repeat the date in Spaces 66 to 71).

Cards 7, 8 and 9

Card 7 is similar to Card 3 except that the first three lines of Card 3 have been omitted. Cards 8 and 9 are identical to Cards 4 and 5 respectively.

6. Major implant lifetime codes

Four major implant lifetime codes are used in the databank. These are:

Failed Implant Lifetime (Code F)
Incomplete Implant Lifetime (Code I)
Curtailed ,, ,, (Code C)
and Elective ,, ,, (Code E)

These have been carefully explained elsewhere (3).

7. Transfer of data – form no. 4 (Figure 4)

The only point to emphasise in connection with the simple Transfer Form is that it should be sent without delay to the Databank Controller once a decision has been made to transfer the future care of a patient to another hospital.

8. Retrieval of data

Figure 5 shows how input data will be presented in the computer print-out. It includes no Pacemaker Clinic data. However, in due course another form – Form

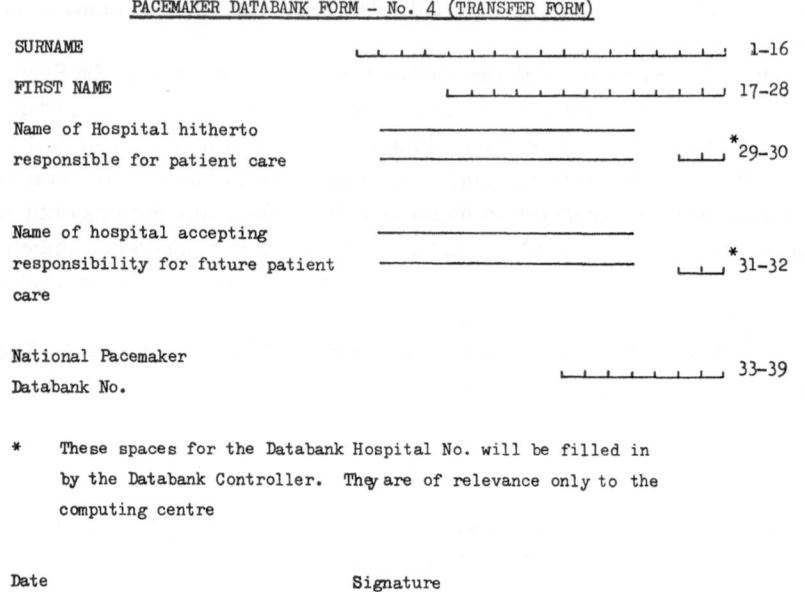

PACEMAKER DATABANK FORM - No. 4 (TRANSFER FORM)

SURNAME		1–16
FIRST NAME		17–28
Name of Hospital hitherto responsible for patient care		*29–30
Name of hospital accepting responsibility for future patient care		*31–32
National Pacemaker Databank No.		33–39

* These spaces for the Databank Hospital No. will be filled in by the Databank Controller. They are of relevance only to the computing centre

Date Signature

Figure 4. Transfer of Data – Form No. 4.

No. 5 for "Subevent Data" will be introduced for use at successive Pacemaker Clinics. Only a few additional items will be added from the Pacemaker Clinics.

Print-outs of collated data on all aspects of pacing become easy once appropriate retrieval programs have been written. A whole library of analysis programs will also be available so that any hospital will be able to have its own data analysed with minimum effort and cost. The print-outs and analyses provided for any hospital will, of course, remain confidential to that hospital.

It is, however, proposed to retrieve some data from the databank on a national basis. The larger number of implants when aggregated nationally will provide better statistical data than when considered on a hospital basis. National Pacemaker Statistics could be presented in an Annual Report.

9. Computing time

Experience with the existing databank suggests that about 12 hours of computing time will be required each month to process all the data on all the patients in the United Kingdom at the present time.

```
<-------------PATIENT'S NAME-------------> DATABANK    DATE  OF
SURNAME              FORENAME        INITS  NUMBER       BIRTH

WALKER               JOHN            J       59918 B   29 07 1892
WATSON               MARGARET        MR      52745 M   16 11 1899
WATT                 WILLIAM         W       71789 H   14 08 1914
WEDDERBURN           ANGUS           AO     123456 A   01 12 1907
WEIR                 BRIAN           B       72504 V   31 04 1902
WHITEHOUSE           MARY            M       67415 L   04 12 1911
WHITTERS             JEAN            J       67747 A   17 03 1910
WILLIAMSON           FRED            F       70914 E   22 11 1905
WOOD                 BETTY           B       73265 W   11 12 1912
WRIGT                LESLIE          LF      12345 A   23 04 1900
------------------------------------------------------------------------------------------------------------

DATABANK                               + APPARENTLY PACEMAKER DEPENDENT +
NUMBER - - 123456A  MALE

                       - REASONS FOR PACING -     - TYPE OF CARDIAC DISTURBANCE -     - ETIOLOGY OF DISTURBANCE -
NAME - - - WEDDERBURN
           ANGUS  AO     SYNCOPE                    STABLE THIRD DEGREE A-V BLOCK       IDIOPATHIC

D.O.B. - - 01.12.1907
                                             L E A D                                    G E N E R A T O R
HOSP     CASE                                                     IMPLANT                                                   IMPLANT
CODE     REF.NO  EVENT   DATE      MANU TYPE   MODEL    SERIAL NO SITE  LIFE(MONTHS)  MANU TYPE   MODEL    SERIAL NO SITE  LIFE(MONTHS)
G207H    285362  1 6    12.04.72     M   ENB  581858    1226061   LEJA  39   I          M   VOO   5862C    1E1650N   LPSM  39  F BVR
                                  TV(M5300)   1.0 MA   0.6 V   0.8 MS                 GEN.RATE  70PPM  DURATION 0.76MS
G207H    285362  2 6 RA 11.07.75                                         60   I          M   VOO   5912     000R7N    LPSM  21  I
                                  TV(M5300)   2.2 MA   1.2 V   0.8 MS                 GEN.RATE  70PPM  DURATION 0.76MS
------------------------------------------------------------------------------------------------------------
```

Figure 5. Example of two parts of computer print-out.

References

1. Green, G.D., Reekie, D., Computer Storage of Pacemaker Data. *Biomed. Eng.*, 10, 219 (1975).
2. Report of Inter-Society Commission for Heart Disease Resources. *Circulation*, L, (October 1974).
3. Green, G.D., Thomson, G., Proposals for an Improved National Databank: Clinical and Pacemaker Data. *J. Cardiovasc. Technol.*, 19, (1977).

IMPULSE ANALYSER-COMPUTER INTERFACE: A NEW WAY TO STORE PACEMAKER DATA

BERNARD J.L. CANDELON, ANDRÉ L. GRAULLE AND PIERRE F. PUEL

One important factor in the choice of a particular pacemaker is its performance following implantation. This parameter can only be assessed by a statistical analysis of data relating this performance and its evolution. This statistical analysis becomes very difficult because of the number of manufacturers and of different models. Only a computerized technique is able to help the doctor in this choice. A lot of pacemaker follow-up centers have a computerized technique for a long time. Different kinds of analysis can be performed: National, regional or clinical. It is the latter we choose in our department and we will present our system in this paper.

Material and method

In the case of statistical analysis of pacemaker data, one can separate data which has to be entered into the computer into two different groups:

– the *permanent data* include informations about the patient (name, birth date, etc...), presenting complaint (symptoms etc...), the pacemaker implantation (anaesthesia, pacemaker and lead positions, threshold, etc...) and the pacemaker and the lead themselves (manufacturer, model, type etc...).

– The *evaluation data* which include all electrical and timing parameters of the pacemaker spike which are the following:

- the pulse amplitude
- the pulse duration
- the pulse interval
- the pulse content which represents the area of the spike.

All these data have to be input into the computer in order to make a patient file. Input of these parameters is really the more arduous task in a computerized analysis. In our system, we simplified this task by performing it in part by the computer itself. Indeed, it is important to note that all the evaluation data are represented by mathematical numbers which can be directly coded in a computer form. Furthermore, these data are given at the output of a spike analyser. It is then easy to convert them into digital code and to input them directly into the computer. This is done automatically by means of an electronic interface between the spike analyser and the computer.

Permanent data have to be entered manually into the computer. This is done by means of a CRT keyboard through a conversational program. The complete system is represented on the diagram of figure I. The computer is a PDP8 of Digital Equipment Corporation which is connected to four units:

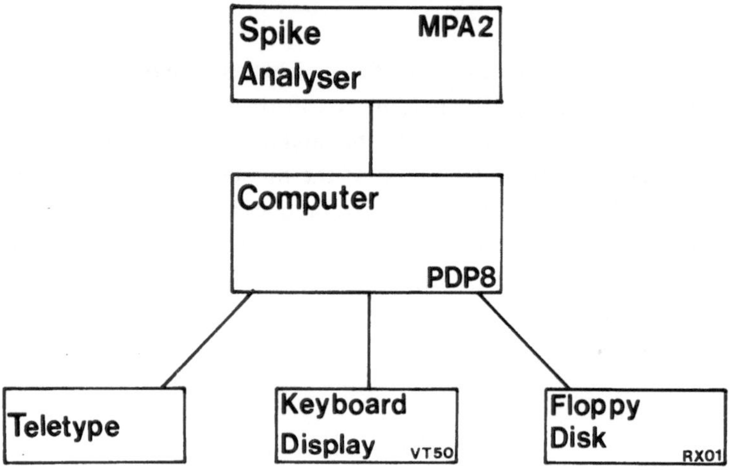

Figure 1. Pacemaker follow-up system and data analyser unit.

– the spike analyser (VITATRON MPA2) which is used for automatic input of evaluation data.

– A teletype (ASR 33) which serves as the output device to print the results of statistical analysis or of follow-up.

– A CRT Keyboard (VT50) utilised as a conversational terminal to input permanent data and also to control follow-up.

– A floppy disk unit (R X 01., 516 kilobytes) which allows the storage of patients data file.

The electronic interface between the MPA2 and the computer is described on figure 2. The MPA2 spike analyser provides a direct digital output which allows an interfacing with any kind of computer. Informations are coded in a 12 bits bus

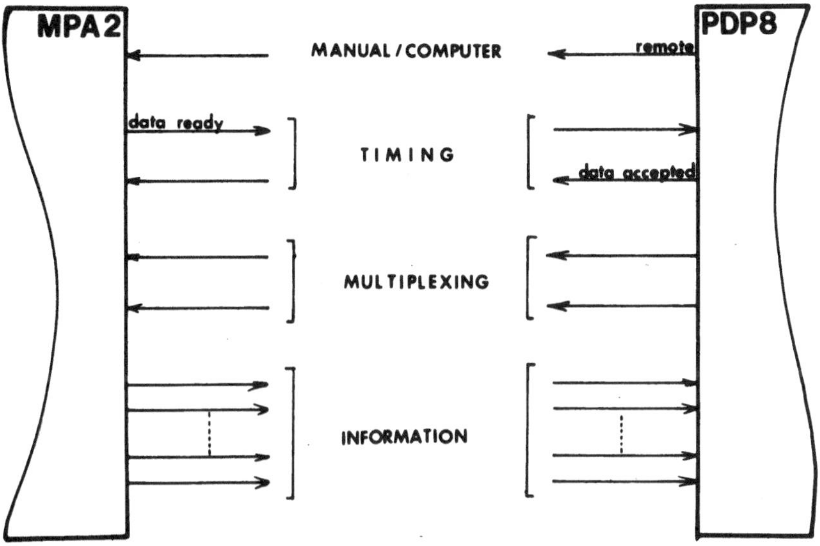

Figure 2. Analyser computer interface: diagram of logical signals.

(11 bits for data and one bit for the sign). In order to select the parameter to be sent to the digital output, two multiplexing signals must be input into the analyser. The transfer of information from the analyser into the computer is controlled by means of two timing signals. A REMOTE signal from the computer allows the automatic switching between manual and computer mode. In "manual mode," transmission of data is controlled manually and the value of every datum can be checked by means of a visual control. In "automatic mode" the computer controls the follow-up itself and data are transmitted automatically.

This system does not have only one purpose, I mean statistical analysis of pacemaker data. The other one, which is also very important, is the help to pacemaker follow-up and the automatic updating of the patient file.

Pacemaker follow-up

For computer analysis of pacemaker data, one can distinguish three important parts:

– the first pacemaker implantation: at this time, one has to create the patient file.

– the pacemaker follow-up: the file must be updated with the new values of electrical and timing parameters of the pacemaker spike.

– the pacemaker change: some permanent data have to be changed and some others cancelled.

A patient file is created by means of a conversational program at the CRT keyboard. An error checking is automatically performed at the input of permanent data. When a file is created, all the permanent data concerning the patient, the pacemaker implantation, the pacemaker and the lead are input into the computer which converts them into proper form for further storage on the disk unit.

The pacemaker follow-up is described in figure 3. The follow-up is done by a

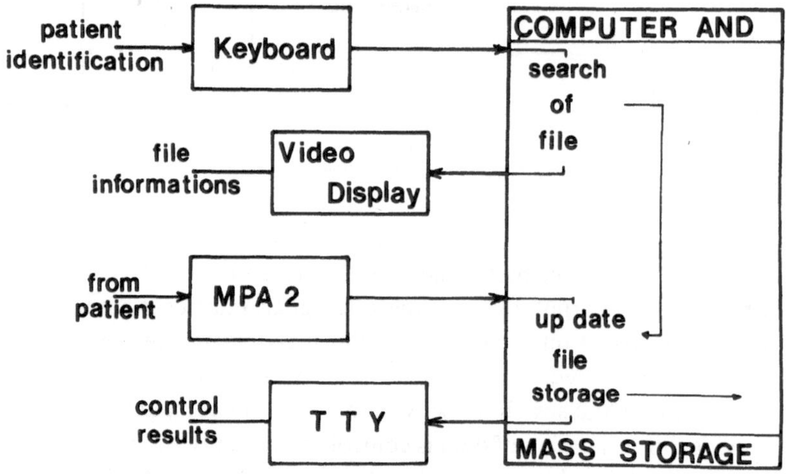

Figure 3. Real time pacemaker follow-up diagram and automatic updating of patient file.

real time program which controls the spike analyser. The patient file is specified to the computer by means of the name of the patient or an identification number at the keyboard. Then the computer searches the specified file in the storage unit. When it finds it, principal permanent informations are displayed at the CRT and also evaluation data of the first and the last controls. The system is then ready to accept the new values of the spike parameters. The computer loads these values automatically from the spike analyser. An average is made on the values of some cardiac cycles in order to minimize the error. When the parameters are measured, the file is automatically updated and the results of analysis are printed out at the teletype.

When the pacemaker or (and) the lead is changed some permanent data are changed through a conversational program at the CRT keyboard.

Advantages of this system concern two points: the first one is the real time follow-up with the automatic research of the patient file and the display of important data for the follow-up. The second one concerns the automatic transmission of evaluation data between the spike analyser and computer. This automatic transfer reduces the manual manipulation of data and so diminishes the error risk.

Application of such a system in a department of pacemaker follow-up is now possible because of the existence of low-cost fourth generation computers, like microprocessors and also of cheap mass storage units. It is evident that the capacity of storage is limited and also the capacity of statistical computation. But one must never forget the purpose of pacemaker data analysis. It is to help in the choice of a particular pacemaker for a given patient and the cost of such a study must not be out of proportion with the results obtained.

THE SIGNIFICANCE IN QUALITY CONTROL OF A COMPUTER FOR PRODUCTION- AND FIELD-DATA. COMPLETE TRACEABILITY, POSSIBLE OR NOT?

L.P. LOLKEMA AND P.A. VAN DER HEIJDEN

The use of a computer in Quality Assurance has become of great value, especially for traceability reasons. Traceability is the ability to recall under what conditions, standards, process-settings, the pacemaker and its components or materials have been made. One of the purposes of traceability, for instance in the case of pacemaker field problems, is to determine which other pacemakers are potentially involved to develop the problem. As you know, if such a problem can be localized, this is a great advantage for patients, doctors and also the pacemaker manufacturer. One can imagine, that a lot of system evaluation, process study, and organization work has to be done in order to arrive at a good working system. To store and process all the data a computer is almost a necessity. How far do we have to extend the traceability system? The more we can obtain now, the more profit we may get from it later. Complete traceability, however, is such a thing as zero defects: it is possible in theory, and one must make it as a goal to come close to it. We at Vitatron have a traceability system, for most parts and materials extended to the processes, raw materials, procedures and standards of our suppliers. This system is constantly updated and improved.

In this presentation, time is too short to give a complete view of all our activities in Quality Assurance. Therefore I will confine myself to remarking that all our procedures are based on the MIL-Standards for electronics, microelectronics and materials, together with the Good Manufacturing Practices and our own device procedures. To see to it that all procedures are followed and implemented properly, in our QA organization we have a Compliance Department.

To give you an idea how traceability works, as an example we will discuss a few components which are used in our pacemakers. First we want to discuss the feed-throughs. Feed-throughs have the function of feeding electrical signals from the pacemaker, which is in the hermetically sealed titanium housing, to the outside environment. The properties of the feed-throughs are very important because they must protect the pacemaker from moisture entering the can, even in very small quantities.

Before we approve a supplier for a component we go through a lengthy process of screening, agreeing on procedures, testing, evaluating, etc. When we get one lot of such components in our Incoming Inspection, we will give these feed-throughs a tag-number. Then we take a sample and subject it to destructive and non-destructive tests. This is based on an Acceptance Quality Level, the result giving a probability of what percentage of the lot will be rejected during further tests. The tag-number contains the code and lot number or the serial number of the supplier, and the amount received. Via this supplier information we will be able to recall under what processes the parts have been made, what materials have been used, from which lot numbers, etc. If after the sample inspection, it turns out that the lot is going to fail the agreed Acceptance Quality Level, we use a decision flow chart, which gives a safe way to select or accept the lot if only unimportant specification deviations are present. After passing the sample test the lot will be subjected to a 100% inspection which consists in this case mainly of a visual examination under a microscope, temperature shock, helium leak test, and some other tests, after which again a visual examination follows. The results must confirm the results of the sample tests.

Another important component we use in our pacemakers is the hybrid circuit. On these hybrid circuits are mounted flat-packs, containing the micro-circuits. In our Incoming Inspection we only open a sample of these packs. For these components we do quality audits at our supplier's plant.

From the tag-number we go to the block-number for efficiency reasons. This block-number is given also to other components on the pacemaker charts. Every pacemaker has such a chart on which all important data from assembly, processing, routing, welding, etc. are filled out. Many of these data also will be put in a computer for quick back reference when necessary. When the total electronics of the pacemaker have been assembled, a lot of data have already been filled out, but much further information has to be stored. For instance, when the pacemaker is welded into the can, the process conditions for that day are registered, the signature of the man who did the welding and inspecting is put down etc.

The computer we use for storing the information is the WANG 2200 computer. In this computer all data from returned pacemakers and process data are stored. The computer is programmed to obtain the following:

a The connection between significant data from returned pacemakers and waterbath results.

b The fast back-coupling to production or R & D if data indicate that improvements can be made.

c A faster statistical processing, where different end of life characteristics can be treated separately.

d A constant updating of the reliability and quality figures on the pacemakers.

Vitatron also uses another computer, the HP-9830. This computer processes data from pacemakers we keep in waterbaths. We have waterbaths operating at

37°C, 50°C, and 70°C from which we obtain important data regarding possible failure mechanisms in pacemakers. Many times, but not always, such phenomena can be accelerated so that design changes can be made, or evidence for certain design criteria can be obtained. The effectiveness of important changes can also be comparatively checked in this way. A certain percentage of the regular production of pacemakers is put into the waterbaths for traceability reasons.

With this I hope to have given you a little insight into the process of constant data gathering from which this is only a small but important part.

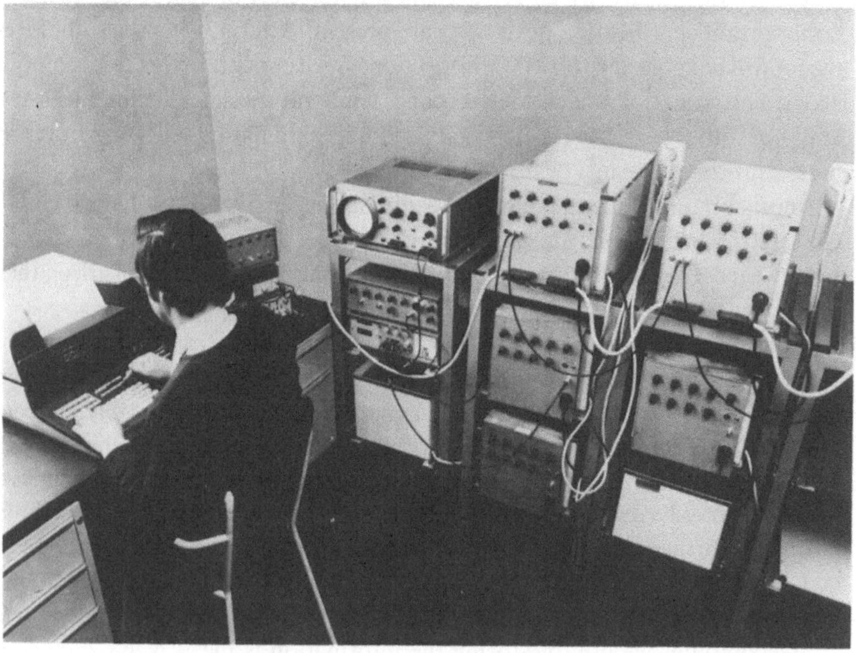

Figure 1. Computer control of pacemaker pilot series in watertanks.

References

1. Quality Control Handbook, section 9. J.M. Furman Ed. *Mc. Graw Hill*, New York (USA) 1972.
2. Reliability Engineering for Electronics Systems. R.H. Meijers, K.L. Wong and H.M. Gordy Ed. *John Wiley and Sons*, New York (USA) 1964.

DISCUSSION X. COMPUTER APPLICATION IN PACEMAKER REGISTRATION AND FOLLOW-UP

CHAIRMAN: G.A. FERUGLIO *(Udine, Italy)*

M. LEVANDER-LINDGREN *(Stockholm, Sweden):* Mr. Chairman, may I make some comments regarding the data display record. We have worked for the data display record since five years. We presented it for the first time at the IVth world meeting in Groningen and we think that our experiences have been very rewarding. I was very happy to find, Dr. Feruglio, that you have adopted about the same principles for your data system. Now our data display records have replaced the common record at the out-patient department. The structured and comprehensive record has made it much easier to make rapid and safe decisions regarding the patient. The nurse and the secretary are very happy with this system, because a lot of time is saved; they need no longer to look for and to handle the common manual records.

Last but not least, research work has been much facilitated. The computer makes searches, you can ask it for all patients who have had electrode dislodgement, and so on. It can search for important values. You get a list of the patients involved. You have all the records available when you want to work with that information. This is a very rewarding system.

CHAIRMAN: Thank you, Dr. Levander-Lindgren for your remarks.

G. FREUD *(Amsterdam, The Netherlands):* I should like to ask the various speakers about the clinical use of the computer system, one very practical question: How many man years were involved in developing the system? This is very important for the decision regarding copying one of their systems versus going on with your own system.

A.F. RICKARDS *(London, England):* Clinical use: the system is used by technicians and by nurses. It is used actively clinically in the sense that it replaces the notes of the patients who have got pacemakers. Development man years: about one-tenth of a doctor year, in terms of program writing. Commercial cost: about $ 20,000's worth of hardware.

CHAIRMAN: May I add to Dr. Rickards' figures that the costs in time and money are more or less the same in our experience. Nevertheless it must be pointed out that a system developed only for storing the data needed for routine work in the everyday practice, is useful but is not all. If one wants to go further and to use these data for statistical analysis, he needs additional work, batch programs and so on. Then, of course, the costs in time, manpower and money may increase.

Dr. Thalen has a question.

H.J.TH. THALEN *(Groningen, The Netherlands):* We, of the Dutch Working Group on Cardiac Stimulation, are starting computerization of the data of 68 clinics in The Netherlands. The problem is that we had a very nice system, like Dr. Green has, but that less than 40% of the clinics fill in these files.

It is not so much the implantation of pacemakers, but the administration, that takes up time. What I would like to know: Is it useful to have such complicated systems when you want an overall survey. You have all shown very nice computer programs, but there is not one of you – probably – who could bring us a computer program that could be used world wide, so that one way or the other we would have some possibility to provide worldwide data. We have many reports at international meetings, but it would be very nice to have the possibility of computing these data altogether. I would like to hear from the group. What do you think? Is it really worthwhile to have such a complicated system, as Dr. Green has, or should we go for a less complicated system in which we can cover almost all clinics?

V. PARSONNET *(Newark, U.S.A.):* I was going to ask the question myself: not only the financial costs but the physical and mental costs of getting programs like Green's working. I will give you an example. On the survey, with Bilitch and Furman, we have about ten pages of data. It looks very much like Dr. Green's, only it is longer. Just hundreds of data points. Our survey includes one center in California, one center in New Jersey and one center in The Bronx. It is not national in any sense of the word, it is just that the three centers have managed to put in clean information into the computer at great expense. It is very expensive to do it and what is more: to get the information clean. For example, we fill out all these forms ourselves – and I speak for the five of us – or we have a resident or a technician do it, but then it requires our personal review of every item before it gets processed and stored. I think it is a tremendous job.

We are, for example, concerned that we are only putting in X number of pacemakers or X number of pacemaker models and there are many other models about which we have no information at all. In order to get information like that, we are going to have to open this registry to other centers, four, five, six, ten other centers. The cost for doing that, training technicians, training other doctors, getting them to accept our format I think is exorbitant. So, I do not know what the end is. It is magnificent that so much of it has already been done. But, when you look at what has to be done in future, plus the changes in technology that are coming down the road. I see exhaustive work coming to us and perhaps we have to sit down another time to try to decide what reports are meaningful on a national level.

G.D. GREEN *(Glasgow, Scotland):* Mr. Chairman, I do not think it is difficult. The three forms which we have devised in Glasgow are fantastically simple. They look rather forbidding but in fact in each case, the number of spaces which have to be filled in is quite small. The forms have been designed to try to cover every contingency. Once one knows what one is doing, it takes less than five minutes – (three minutes I would guess – to fill in the second event form) at an operation. So, I do not know where the difficulty is.

What we have been doing – as I said – is to encourage clinicians to fill in the forms, by giving them a print-out on their own data. You see, people do not like filling in forms unless they are going to get something back in return. I do not know whether Dr. Sloman is in the audience, but he has been receiving print-outs on his own data for many months. Perhaps those interested would like to ask him afterwards for his views on the value of such print-outs. The second point about "going international" rather than "national" is that what we have done and are doing in Glasgow can be done by anyone who has a medium-size computer. Many of the programs are in fact available from the manufacturers, they are standard programs which need very little modification. There is only one bit of the program which has to be written. So, it is *not* expensive and there is no reason at all why anyone here from outside the U.K., who would like to adopt our system, should not do so, at very little cost. We will be glad to cooperate to the full with any of you.

H.J.TH. THALEN *(Groningen, The Netherlands):* I think there is one big difference, Dr. Green. You are promoting a system and you get clinics to adopt your system. However, what we try is to get an overall view from all clinics in The Netherlands and ask all clinics – also clinics not too much in favour of the administration load – to cooperate.

We have these files, like you have, and we worked on them for two years and sent them to all clinics. The experience is that you get back only 40% and of these 40% not all of them are filled in correctly. I really think it does not cost too much time, but, when you do 10 pacemakers a week, it is about five hours work, this can be too much for some. In theory, it is a nice system, in practice, it does not work.

G.D. GREEN *(Glasgow, Scotland):* If I may answer that, Mr. Chairman, I think the trouble is that you are probably trying to do too much too quickly. We are building ours up slowly. We are not pressuring people to join our databank. Before very long they will be knocking on our door and saying "Please can I join."

H.J.TH. THALEN *(Groningen, The Netherlands):* Practice has shown that now that we have a less sophisticated system, we get a 98% response.

CHAIRMAN: I would like to make a point before going on with the discussion. Of course there are several aspects of the problem of using computers in the pacemaker team. Please do not forget the most practical one which is that it helps us to handle a lot of information that we have and to alleviate the work. To answer partially the first question of Dr. Thalen, I will tell him that some material is here, at the disposal of the audience. Our program, as well as other programs are completely available for use in other laboratories, with just slight changes. We made our own program on the basis of the knowledge we gathered in the last couple of years and we are almost 100% happy with it. A summary is in the user's manual that I would like to put at everybody's disposal.

One question I would ask the members of the panel to answer: from which level of patient load do you think a pacemaker clinic is advised to go into computer management of its patient data?

G.D. GREEN *(Glasgow, Scotland):* We have clinicians on our system who are implanting a relatively small number of pacemakers each year, but they are delighted to be using the databank. Certainly, clinicians with larger numbers are equally delighted. Each end of the spectrum is pleased to have their own data analyzed and they will be glad to have it fed into a national databank.

A.F. RICKARDS *(London, England):* I think this pacemaker data business has two aspects to it. I am very sympathetic to Thalen's comments about forms. I dislike forms. I think if we were to try to run our system based on forms, inside the hospital, it would not work. The fact that we have an inter-active system, which structures the questions according to your answers, makes it relatively easy to use. I think there are two considerations. What does the hospital need? The pacing clinic, in general, needs the computer to replace the patients' notes so that it can look at the patients' information when they come up to the clinic. This is quite different from what a national data bank needs, which is very simple, minimum information about the generator and the patient, that, ideally, should be put in inter-actively with a telephone link system, and not require five forms to be filled out. I am quite sure, as Dr. Thalen has already told us from the experience in Holland, that the information you are going to get back will be of low quality and is going to require an awful lot of people, time and money to check out and of administration to make it worth having.

So, I think you have to divide up: what the hospital needs, what the nations need. Those are two quite different questions.

G.D. GREEN *(Glasgow, Scotland):* Mr. Chairman, may I answer that? We are including clinical data at the request of many clinicians. The pressure to have clinical data in the data bank is coming from the clinicians, not from the people such as myself. As regards the on-line databank I agree with you that the ideal national databank will be one with an on-line computer with terminals, including a visual display unit I am sure that will come, but we must walk before we can run.

A.F. RICKARDS *(London, England):* I distrust clinicians, as a clinician myself. I think if you go to a non-computing clinician and say: here is a super system that says your patient has got syncope, he is going to say he likes it. The proof will come in five years' time when he actually asks the question: how many of my patients who presented with syncope are in this situation? We have had some experience with a catheter reporting system. What happens is virtually nothing. They do not come back to you and ask the question. They are very enthusiastic in the beginning about storing a lot of clinical information, but when it comes to the crunch at the end they really are not very interested. You have been wasting your time.

CHAIRMAN: Are there any questions from the audience?

B. GOLDMAN *(Toronto, Canada):* It is a delight to see on the pacemaker data form a question which embarrassed me some four years ago in New York City, when I spoke clearly about the concept of pacemaker dependency. My definition, at that time, was that, if on an ECG sampling strip 50% of the complexes were pacemaker-induced, that patient was pacemaker dependent. I believe it was Dr. Bilitch who disagreed heartily with this and said that you must turn the pacemaker off and, if the patient starts to twitch and roll his eyes back, he is pacer dependent. I would like to ask the panel what you would do about that phrase: pacemaker dependent. We have decided to throw it out of our data base.

V. PARSONNET *(Newark, U.S.A.):* We believe in that terminology, largely because it affects our behaviour when we have a recall situation, our behaviour towards the urgency of the replacement of the pacemaker. If you have a minor rate interval change, you will have to make a decision as to whether this is important or not and it is much more important if the patient is going to keel over than if the patient is not likely to keel over. So, we make a value judgement in several ways. One is that if the patient had complete heart block, he may be pacemaker dependent. If at any time during pacemaker change, we find that we cannot wean the patient from the pacemaker and allow him to run at his own rate – whether it is idio-ventricular or a slow sinus rate – he is pacemaker dependent. In between that, we have a sort of pacemaker dependent score. In each of those clinics, we have a few seconds of rhythm strip. If the patient never has any idioventricular contractions at all, we put down: ten visits, zero episodes of competition. So he has been on a pacemaker 100% of the time, when seen in the clinic.

We try to make a value judgement in that way. We do not know of any absolute way you can do it, because whether or not the patient will faint depends upon how quickly that pacemaker fails, how quickly the rate drops and everything else. But I do think it is an important distinction to make and one must make it, in doing this kind of work.

CHAIRMAN: Is there any other member of the panel who wants to add something to this interesting topic?

J.G. SLOMAN *(Melbourne, Australia):* Well, if no one does, Mr. Chairman, may I say that I agree wholeheartedly with Dr. Parsonnet and for those very reasons. We are very careful to say "apparently pacemaker dependent." I guess you all know that, after reoperations when you switch off the pacemaker for a few seconds and you record a straight line or just P-waves, then you cannot go on but you must switch on again. You cannot really carry it to the ultimate test. So one says cautiously "apparently pacemaker dependent."

V. PARSONNET *(Newark, U.S.A.):* I am still back to Dr. Green on his argument on how easy things are. I do not really believe that a form like this is easy. For example, you look at your card number two. Somebody has to fill out the form which says: type of cardiac disturbance/atrial or ventricular block/stable or intermittent/third degree, second degree, Mobitz II, Mobitz I, first degree, on and on. Someone with enough brains and enough experience to recognize the classifications of various types of block will have to sit down with this form. We also have this kind of form and I can tell you that this is one of the weakest points of our system. I, as a busy surgeon, find it very difficult to get down and answer some of these questions and some I find very difficult to answer because I do not know enough. My internists, although they do profess interest, do not really care enough to sit down and make it out. Our cardiology residents hate the forms. So what finally comes out on the form, with check marks filled out in blanks is probably wrong. When we get back to doing our data retrieval and data analysis, we are going to have some very peculiar results. I do not believe this is easy and what one has to do is to make a value judgement as to what is really important for patient care, on the one hand, and clinical analysis and do just these things that are important.

For national surveys, what are the things we are really looking at? What our pacemaker generator survival rates are like? What our patients' survival rates are like? What the wire survival rates are like? What the dislodgment figures are like? Make your specific programs on the things that are of most value to the community. The rest of the stuff, we hope, which is in the computer is O.K. Someday we will get around to the details.

That is the way we have approached it. Do not think going at them all like this is going to be easy or cheap.

CHAIRMAN: I think Dr. Green wants to defend his form.

G.D. GREEN *(Glasgow, Scotland):* First of all I agree that this is the most controversial part of the form and I might add, this is the seventeenth issue of this form, – the seventeenth attempt to get it right after many consultations with clinical colleagues. I think we are just about there now, I certainly do not envisage any major change. But again, these forms were prepared at the request of clinicians and you cannot have it both ways, Dr. Parsonnet. This session was National Databanks with the Pacemaker Clinic in the background. Now if you want a national databank for analysis of generators, longevity statistics and so on, that is what we already have running in Glasgow. The reason why we have modified our program is so that the printouts and eventually the visual display units can be used at pacemaker clinics. The clinician, if he is a good one, should know or want to know quickly when the patient comes along, why, some months ago – some years ago in many cases – a particular patient had a pacemaker put in. If clinicians are unable or unwilling to fill in the Patient Data part of the form, that is all right – it is not an all-or-none situation. You fill in what you want to fill in and if you do not have the data or do not understand what has happened to the patient previously, leave a gap. The result is that there will be an omission of data in the printout. A National Databank for use at pacemaker clinics must include clinical information.

CHAIRMAN: Thank you Dr. Green. Following these remarks and before closing this session, one final comment. To the best of my knowledge this is the first time that people from different places and countries, physicians and engineers, meet officially to discuss the many aspects of computer application in pacemaker follow-up. The role of computers in pacemaker clinics appears to be well established by now. Various systems and programs are available today, for routine work and for statistical analysis. However the problem of what to store and how to collect data for a computer system is not yet settled and further experience and evaluation are needed. It appears clear that the needs of a single clinic, for its routine work, are different from those of a multicenter or national registration system. The latter for a single pacemaker requires much less information and only basic data. Therefore different types of programs are needed at different levels of application. New developments are expected in this field for the next few years. May we suggest for now to implement multicenter trials before starting any nationwide system of registration.

With this suggestion I close this session.

Thanks to the speakers and to all who have taken part in the discussion.

ROUND TABLE DISCUSSION

ROUND TABLE DISCUSSION

ROUND TABLE DISCUSSION. THE PACEMAKER CLINIC: ORGANIZATION AND PATIENT LOAD

Chairman: V. PARSONNET *(Newark, U.S.A.)*
Panel members: H. ECTOR *(Leuven, Belgium)*
B.S. GOLDMAN *(Toronto, Canada)*
J. MEIBOM *(Copenhagen, Denmark)*
J.R. MUIR *(Cardiff, England)*
I.J. PINTO *(Calcutta, India)*
F.A. RODRIGO *(Leyden, The Netherlands)*
A. SCHAUDIG *(Munich, F.R. Germany)*
R.J. ZOCHOWSKI *(Warsaw, Poland)*
P.M. ZOLL *(Boston, U.S.A.)*

CHAIRMAN: Let us start this panel with some experiences in the Toronto Pacemaker Clinic. Dr. Goldman will you start this discussion.

B.S. GOLDMAN *(Toronto, Canada):* I just wanted to show our experience in handling a volume of patients through a clinic, as is the theme of this panel, with a particular problem that has been alluded to only slightly during this symposium and that is the problem of the pacemaker alert or recall. Figure 1 shows the clinic volume at Toronto General Hospital over the past 13 years. Interestingly, after telephone monitoring our replacement rate, that is the solid bar dropped, but, over the subsequent three years: our pulse generator replacement rate tripled rather rapidly. The reason is the type of mail we received and which many people received: alerts, advisories, physician notification, performance up-date, recalls, whatever you wish to label them. Our experience was with eight separate recalls over a period of four years, that involved 469 units in our patient population. In fact, that was 1.3% of what I believe was the world recall number at that point in time. So, we had a very large number of patients to handle in our clinic framework. The 469 were subjected to increased surveillance but 18.5% of the patients with these alert pacemakers underwent an unpredicted failure. We were able to predict premature rate drop in 50% of them. In 11 we removed them rather abruptly when the manufacturer told us that there was a fear of catastrophic failure. Overall we replaced 184 pacemakers.

Our total experience with pulse generators over the past four years was 780 units. The unpredicted group – that is those that show loss of sensing or loss of pacing or both – is very high, about 25 or 26% because of the unpredicted group in the 184 recall pacemakers.

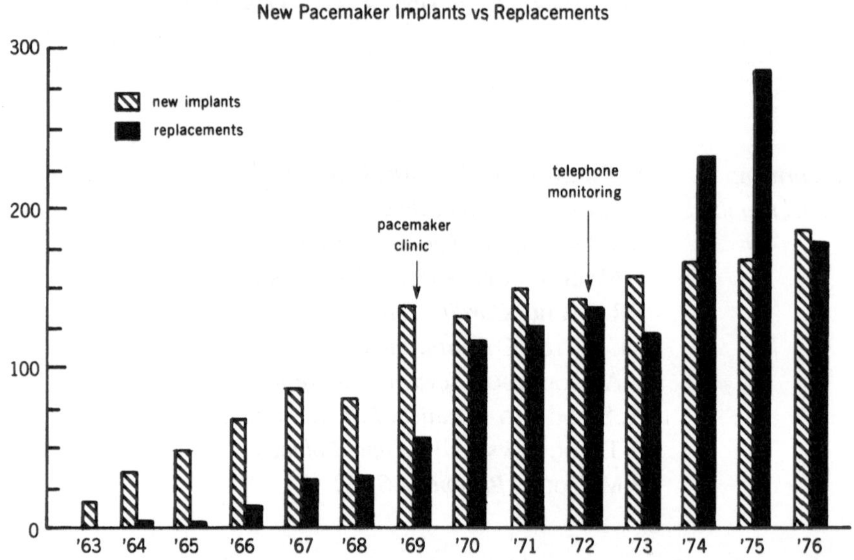

Figure 1.

The surveillance mechanism protected about 76% of the pacemaker patients. Although the remainder had some symptoms, only 11 required a temporary electrode. We do not know of any mortality that existed, in our attempts to survey these patients by telephone monitoring or by clinic visits.

We attempted to put together some guidelines for management that, I trust, are universal. As soon as a product problem is identified in North America, the manufacturer's responsibility is to notify the Food and Drug Administration. He may elect, at that time, to issue a press release to coincide with this notification. The next step is for the manufacturer to specify how the physician will be contacted, what action will be requested and how the manufacturer will verify that the physician has been notified. When the implanting physician becomes notified about the recall, it becomes his responsibility to verify the manufacturer's list of affected units and to make every effort to contact all the patients involved. Although the manufacturer himself may initiate the alert or recall, and make recommendations as to whether or not an individual pulse generator is going to be replaced prophylactically or subjected to increased surveillance, the decision really rests primarily with the clinic or with the implanting physician. Most pacemaker recalls, as you are aware, have not required surgical removal of the unit, but have required careful monitoring. We have shown that, despite the fact that unpredicted failures can occur with a frequency as high as 25%, morbidity is low, provided it is identified by early and frequent monitoring. Patients who demonstrate total pacer dependency should in all likelihood be handled more cautiously than those who have demonstrated a more consistently satisfying underlying rhythm. I think you also have to examine the mode of pulse generator failure, before you reach a decision regarding management.

If the incidence is not high, then a gradual rate change or a failure of sensing or pacing can be managed by increased surveillance. But, if there is an active failure mode, such as explosion or runaway or double pulsing, then the patient's well-being is obviously threatened and prophylactic replacement should immediately be considered. The physician should notify the patient and relatives of the problem and should obviously notify the outside physician.

We believe that good communication should be kept up with all government agencies involved; good communications with the news media, malpractice insurance carriers (if that happens to be a local problem) and, of course, the local hospital board. Our hospital board was extremely interested in our relationship with pacemaker companies at the time of the recalls. Provision of adequate follow-up facilities is an important statement. I think that the recalls should be modified according to one's experience and this relates to the observations that I made in the clinic as to how these pacemakers are performing. We have revised most of our recalls to our own satisfaction and have tried to avoid as many replacements as possible.

Lastly, as has been said before, some form of corroboration is necessary. The pacemaker should be returned to the manufacturer or followed by tank tests in the hospital itself and there must be some corroboration of the failure mode. It is only in this way that the manufacturer and the physician will acquire satisfactory information on failure modes in alerted pacemakers.

CHAIRMAN: Are there any questions or comments regarding the recall? From the panel? From the floor?

A.J. BLANKESTIJN *(Dieren, The Netherlands):* I think this is an interesting subject, not only for the clinicians, but also for the companies who sometimes have to handle these unfortunate situations. For us, as a company, it is always very difficult to turn the question back: What kind of responsibility can we reckon with from the clinicians's side? By analyzing certain problems and turning up the recommendations for the clinicians, we have to try to find out what the clinician is normally doing and what we can expect from him. In my opinion there should be certain standards of pacemaker follow-up, etc. on the clinicians' side, but sometimes there exists no follow-up at all.

CHAIRMAN: What percentage of recall pacemakers is the manufacturer likely to lose track of? If a pacemaker manufacturer sends out a recall notice, do you hear from half of the pacemakers, or three-quarters of them?

A.J. BLANKESTIJN *(Dieren, The Netherlands):* Our best results are 30%. The rest never respond. We have certain obligations, not only from an ethical standpoint, but towards the authorities who want to know where those failures are. But this is for us impossible because we just do not get the answers.

I think it is a problem, not just for the company, but also for the clinicians, because it can have very unfortunate effects for the patient. Then you get the unfortunate situation of recalls going into the press, radio, patients are alarmed and doctors get loads of worrying patients. A lot still has to be done. Corporations, companies, clinicians should get this type of negative information in the right way, to the right places. Then, if we ask for information, we should get the information back.

CHAIRMAN: Thank you. I would now like to go on to another speaker, who we are fortunate to have with us today, Dr. Pinto, from Calcutta, India, who has a few remarks to make about organization of the pacemaker clinics in India.

I.J. PINTO *(Calcutta, India):* We have certain difficulties in India, regarding implantation of pacemakers. First of all, the number of people who require pacemakers is less than in western countries, most probably because of the low age of survival. The socio-economic status is such that even the patients that require pacemakers cannot afford pacemakers. There is no National Health system that can give the patients pacemakers.

The distribution of the disease is peculiar. In Bengal, which is one of the east side countries of India, pacemaker insertion totals about 600 to 700 new cases a year, while in the rest of India it is probably less than 150. This and many epidemiological problems regarding the insertion of pacemakers need to be studied. Secondly, there are very few centers in India that implant pacemakers. I think that, altogether, there must be about seven or eight cities in the whole of India where pacemakers are being implanted. India is a large country and patients have to travel miles to come to the appropriate centers. Many of the centers like ours, where we do considerable amounts of cardiac surgery – do not have sophisticated equipment to assess pacemaker malfunction.

We have a certain follow-up system for our clinic. We ask the patients to come and see us once a month, if they are in the city. If they are out of the city, we ask them to send us electrocardiograms once a month. We study the electrocardiogram and send a report back to the patients' physician.

If a patient is in the city of Bombay and comes to us for an examination, we do a thorough clinical examination. We ask for some history of syncope and we take an electrocardiogram and study it for capture failure, sensing failure or combined failure. We study the artifact axis and we study the axis of the paced ventricular complexes. Then, we make an electrocardiogram with and without the magnet and we perform carotid sinus pressure in all cases, to find out possible malfunction of the pacemaker during the bradycardia. Finally we do a thorough stimulation test to find out the intrinsic rhythm. In those cases that are pacer dependent, we replace the pacemaker at the end of the warranty period. Those that are not pacer dependent are called regularly toward the end of the warranty period i.e. every two weeks, to do the test. With this test we try to prolong pacemaker lives, because the patients are poor and cannot afford a replacement.

In October we will have a meeting at which all cardiologists interested in pacing in India are going to meet. We have asked some foreign cardiologists to come, so we can get our data together and assess indications of pacing and improve our methods of pacing. The new Government is sympathetic to imported pacemakers. The previous Government was more keen on family planning. So we hope that, next year, we will be able to have better organized clinics and more possibilities to purchase foreign pacemakers.

CHAIRMAN: Clearly, pacemaker evaluation systems will not apply to every country. You have quite individual problems in India. I would now like to call upon Dr. Zochowski from the Department of Cardiology, University of Warsaw, who has some remarks to make about the organization of the national service in Poland.

R.J. ZOCHOWSKI *(Warsaw, Poland):* The cardiac pacing in Poland has been started in 1964, but on the larger scale it was initiated in 1965, when the Department of Cardiology (previous name: Institute of Cardiology) of the Medical Academy in Warsaw organized the first pacemaker clinic as well as the bank of pacemakers. Later on, implantation and/or follow-up centers were created in different regions within the country. Up to date, about 6200 pacemakers have been implanted in Poland including both first implantations and replacements. The total amount of pacemakers either fixed rate or on demand that have been implanted is shown in Figure 1. Our system of pacemakers distribution for the whole country assumes full centralisation. The only bank of pacemakers is located at the Department of Cardiology of the Medical Academy in Warsaw. It delivers all types of pacing equipment to all implanting centers in Poland.

Each first implantation is performed after a routine schedule. Urgent implantations occur very seldom. In case of life threatening situations temporary pacing via a bipolar electrode and an external pacemaker is advised. The network of 25 pacemaker implantation centers and 10 pacemaker clinics is spread almost uniformly over the country and endowed with necessary equipment for ECG, X-ray, and/or oscilloscopic measurements.

Indications for permanent cardiac pacing are similar to those which are set in different countries and are the same everywhere in Poland:

1. A-V block of the IIIrd degree with MAS attacks
2. Sick Sinus Syndrome/including brady-tachy/with MAS attacks
3. A-V block of IInd degree
4. necessity of digitalization in patients with total A-V block and Sick Sinus Syndrome even at the absence of MAS attacks.

This uniformity in indications for cardiac pacing is possible because of the system of meetings every second year. At these meetings cardiologists and other specialists like surgeons, engineers or technicians from different pacemaker clinics have the unique opportunity to exchange their experiences and attitudes and to discuss their problems and eventual difficulties.

It's worthwhile to note that qualifications for permanent cardiac pacing were usually preceded by causal treatment according to etiology of the illness. Yet, in an asymptomatic patient these qualifications have to be confirmed by different functional tests including atrial pacing, exercise test and His bundle recordings if necessary.

Examination and follow-up of the pacemaker patients include:

1. routine physical examination
2. standard ECG/for presence of capture and pacemaker synchronization
3. impulse analysis/rate duration, amplitude, time constant.

All patients are encompassed by a two level pacemaker checking system. The first one is performed by the General Health Service doctors, and contains routine physical examination and ECG only. The next level covers more precise examination with the measurements of all characteristic parameters of the pacemakers as pulse rate, pulse width and amplitude. They are done in a highly specialized center which acts as a superior unit within a nation-wide system of pacemakers' control.

In principle, we do not pay attention any more to conventional radioauscultation. However, specially manufactured beepers are an extremely important application in the telephone control system. So far transtelephone check-up is used in the terminal stage of battery life to avoid too frequent examinations but is still not everyday routine procedure.

Nevertheless, we plan to originate the production of beepers and to make the method of examination more popular very soon.

Although the pacemaker clinic of the Department of cardiology of the Medical Academy in Warsaw has played an exceptional role as pacing headquarters and superior consulting center for the country it has to perform also normal services and checks about 25-30 patients every day for the full control range. The check-up schedule contains the successive controls performed with the following time intervals:

1. immediately after implantation
2. months later
3. 18 months since the date of the manufacture of the pacer
4. every half year up to 80% of battery exhaustion
5. successive examinations individually/in accordance to the actually obtained measurements.

Nuclear pacemakers are controlled in an individual manner because of the small number and totally different life expectancy.

Complete lack of unexpected fatal cases due to battery exhaustion, has proved our system to be extremely efficacious. However sudden generator failures due to components damages that are practically unpredictable, occur but they are extremely rare, thanks to the technical improvement.

Also a majority of other complications within the pacing system electrodes dislocations, damages, and/or disconnections, have been diagnosed properly and in time, which enabled us to avoid unexpected serious consequences.

CHAIRMAN: Thank you very much, Dr. Zochowski, for your interesting presentation of the situation in Poland, that has been made also on behalf of Prof. Kraska and the Doctors Bukowiecki, Opolski, Pieniak and Radecki. Any questions or comments? Dr. Muir, I think you have a related topic to discuss. Would you like to present the way of handling pacemaker patients in Wales.

J.R. MUIR *(Cardiff, England):* Up to 1970 the incidence of pacing in Wales was very low. This was in line with the situation throughout the rest of the United Kingdom. The implantation rate was running at approximately ten new patients per million, per annum. In 1971 a new University Hospital was opened, with a new university cardiac department. As a result, there has been an explosion of permanent pacing within Wales.

This University Hospital serves a population of approximately 2,000,000, which is just over three-quarters of the total population of Wales. Figure 2 shows the increase in pacing in the years 1972-1976, expressed in new implants per million of population per annum. The thicker line, rising from approximately 10 per million to 45 per million per annum, is the rise in implantation rate for the total population of 2,000,000. The top line represents the rise in that area of Wales (South Glamorgan) immediately adjacent to the University Hospital of Wales. This area includes the city of Cardiff. It represents a population of approximately half a million and the incidence of permanent pacing has now reached nearly 90 new implants per annum per million population. The other lines represent the rise in incidence of permanent pacing in the other counties of Wales. You will see that there has been a steady rise in all these areas over this period. While the total number of permanent implantations per annum is still considerably less than what one might take as an average Western European figure (approximately 100-115 new patients per million per annum), it seems likely that within two years we will have reached this level.

When you take this figure and use predictions for the survival of pacemaker patients, you arrive at some rather frightening figures for the predicted patient load for our clinic in the future. There is controversy about the expected survival of patients with permanent pacemakers, as we heard yesterday. However recent

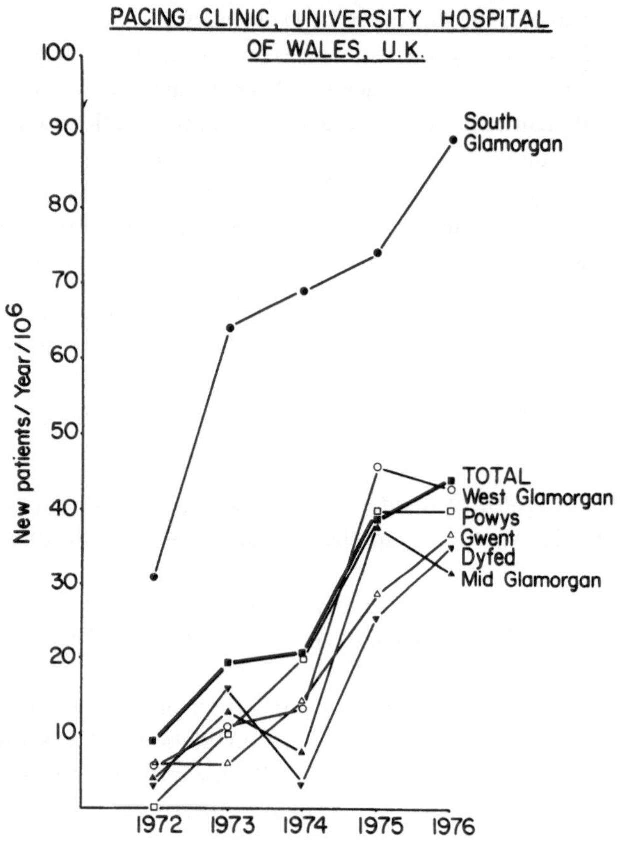

Figure 2.

data from St. George's Hospital and other centres in France have suggested that, if you exclude patients under the age of sixty, and only consider the older age group and those that present with Stokes-Adams attacks as opposed to congestive failure, the expected mortality of these patients is not very different from that of their peer-age group. In Wales the annual mortality per thousand population in the over-65's is 67 per annum. In fact the expected survival for people of the age of 80 is six years for males and seven years for females. At the age of 85 it is 3.6

for males and 5.6 for females. One can therefore make some predictions of the patient load for the pacemaker clinic in the future. In five years we expect to have – using relatively conservative figures – somewhere around 750 patients over the age of 60 attending our clinic. In ten years we will have 1,250. This of course only takes into account those patients who are over 60 at the time of the first implantation.

This load presents certain problems to us. However I suspect that these problems are not exclusive to our unit. One is the utilization of beds. Due to an administrative error some years ago in the planning of the University Hospital, there are only 48 beds for all cardiology and cardiac surgery. There is therefore a considerable limit on the number of implantations and changes of pacemaker units that can be performed without increasing the waiting list for other cardiac and cardiac surgical patients. In addition you will see (Figure 3) that the location

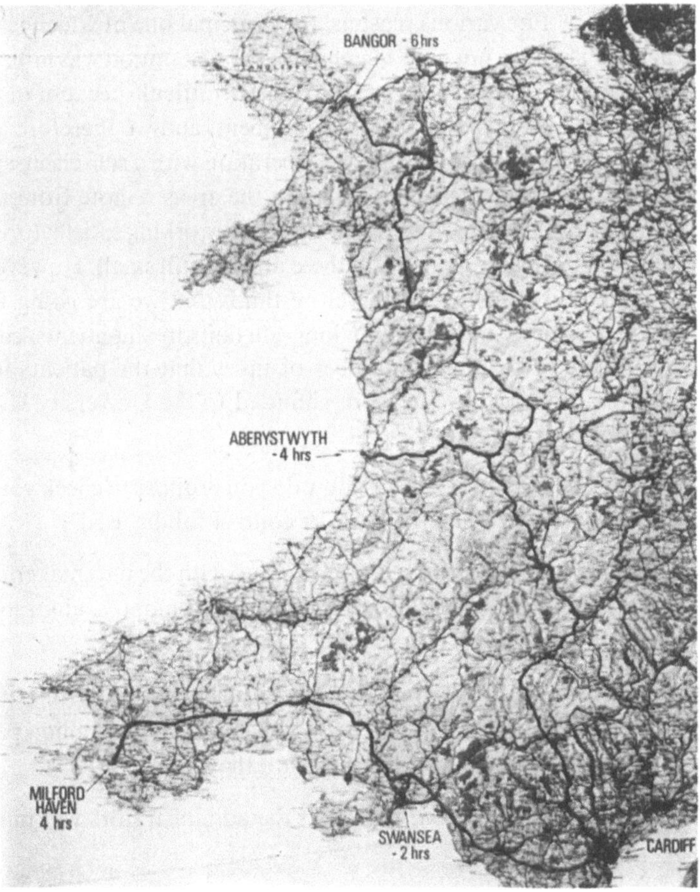

Figure 3.

of Cardiff, the capital of Wales, could hardly be worse for the planning of a regional pacemaker service. The dark lines represent the main roads which connect us with the District General Hospitals throughout Wales. A considerable proportion of our patients are referred from these hospitals. The figures attached to each District General Hospital represent a very optimistic estimate of the time it takes to move a patient in an ambulance to the University Hospital of Wales in Cardiff. While the distance from Bangor in North Wales to Cardiff is only 370 km., the journey takes no less than six hours. The road crosses several beautiful mountain ranges, and winds down some of the most lovely river valleys, but it is not the ideal route, particularly in the tourist season, for the rapid movement of patients. You clearly cannot move patients of the pacemaker age group this distance and back in one day. So we were faced in the planning of our service with a major problem. How were we going to cope with this? We had three options; telephone analysis of pacemakers, or patient self-check systems, or the setting up of satellite clinics. For various reasons, the principal one of which is that many people in these areas do not have telephones, the first option was not acceptable. The second option would have been extremely difficult because many of our elderly patients are frightened of new equipment, and we therefore considered that we would have, in practice, poor co-operation with a self-check system. We therefore had to establish satellite clinics in the areas remote from the central clinic in Cardiff. At the present time this system is working satisfactorily because the total number of paced patients in these areas is still small. However I do not see it remaining like this, and I therefore think that we are going to have to consider the possibility of implanting long-life units in all patients, certainly up to the age of 80, to reduce the number of times that the patients have to be checked in the clinic or have to be re-admitted to the University Hospital for replacement of their units.

CHAIRMAN: Thank you, Dr. Muir. How do you propose to check your patients in the clinic? What type of surveillance or control will be used?

J.R. MUIR *(Cardiff, England):* At the present, with the pacemakers with mercury cells they are seen, the first three months, then six months, nine months, nine months, six, three.

CHAIRMAN: I was not referring to the schedule, I was referring to the technique. Do you do photo analysis? What if you go to 300 per million per annum, like in the United States? Wales will sink into the sea.

J.R. MUIR *(Cardiff, England):* I think, the administrators will jump off the docks.

CHAIRMAN: We have not yet heard from Dr. Zoll and I do not think I have to introduce him to any of you. I always remember with great interest my contacts with him about modern pacing systems. He was very critical of transvenous pacing, early on, because of dislodgement problems. Here I find myself confessing to a 7% dislodgement last year. He was also very critical, I recall, of computer systems; I'll bet you have not changed your mind, Paul. I would very much appreciate hearing from you about your attitude concerning the surveillance problems.

P.M. ZOLL *(Boston, U.S.A.)*: I think our organization of the pacemaker clinic, which we do not call a clinic, is very much like that of Dr. Pinto. It comes down, basically, to the interchange of information between the patient and his physician. And that goes both ways. The patient wants to know what to expect and what he should do, in case of various eventualities. The physician wants to know how his treatment is proceeding. We primarily ask the patient about symptoms related to his pacemaker and particularly about his pulse rate. We still find that a daily check of the pulse rate by the patient – the only equipment required there being a timepiece with a second hand and somebody who can count to 100 more or less – is a very useful piece of information. In patients who have a fixed rate pacemaker and who are fully dependent on the pacemaker, the pulse rate is useful. In patients who have demand pacemakers, the pulse rate is useful: it tells us, if it is above the escape rate of the pacemaker, that the pacemaker is not being used; or, if it is irregular, that it is being used intermittently. If the pulse rate is well below the escape rate, we know there is a problem. So, it is useful even in patients with demand pacemakers.

We do the usual studies of pulse wave form analysis. We do this with rather simple equipment. It takes primarily an electrocardiograph machine, a small oscilloscope – I have a small, portable oscilloscope that I carry around with me – and maybe a magnet and a couple of other accessory pieces of equipment. We find that information of great value.

I would like to point out, however, an area that has really not been stressed very much; careful analysis of the various aspects of the pacemaker-electrode-patient system that lead to failure. We have heard a great deal about the pulse generator, but the connecting wire, the electrode, the myocardial tissue around the electrode are all sources of failure. I believe that in many clinics some of these aspects are not carefully examined. We take every opportunity to investigate each one of these, particularly when there is some suggestion of a failure in the system, a failure to sense or a failure to stimulate. We look carefully at the pulse generator, as I said and when it comes to surgery, to primary implantation, to replacement, to revision of the system, we examine every aspect of the system that we can. When we take a pulse generator out, we examine it carefully before we send it back to the manufacturer, because there seems to be an inordinate incidence of loss of defective pulse generators in manufacturers' hands. We often do not get a report, even though I know we should. We look carefully at the wire from the electrode to the external component. When we do not remove the wire, we measure the voltage and current simultaneously and thereby get an indication of the impedance, which gives us some indication about possible wire fracture. We look carefully for displacement and then we are left with the tissue reaction that may give a high threshold.

I think it is unfortunate that people still use the term "exit block," which primarily, I believe, means failure to stimulate. But it suggests that it is on a biological basis, like exit block around natural intrinsic pacemaker. If we do not know the reason why there is failure to stimulate, we should simply say "ineffective stimulation" or "intermittent ineffective stimulation." If we do know the reason, we should say so again, but we should not cover our ignorance with a technical term like "exit block," unless we do know that there is excessive tissue reaction around the electrode and, in that case, we should say so.

When the electrode is available we should take every opportunity we have to make all these measurements and, when the system has completely failed and a new one is inserted, to remove as much of the electrode as is possible. I have heard that this is, sometimes, extremely difficult, but it would be very valuable to do so. I have seen any number of instances in which electrodes were in the hands of the surgeon or a catheter cardiologist who successfully removed it and discarded it thereafter without any kind of an examination as to what went wrong. That is because they usually have fixed in their minds that the reason for the failure to stimulate was exit block.

CHAIRMAN: Do you follow your patients, or do the people of the Beth Israel follow their patients in an organized fashion, in a clinic?

P.M. ZOLL *(Boston, U.S.A.):* We have a rather disorganized system, because we have several men interested in pacemakers, each of whom thinks he knows best how to do things. And nobody will argue with the others about that. We do have a pacemaker clinic. Many of us follow our own patients individually. It really does not matter very much, so long as there is an interested and well trained cardiologist who takes the time to discuss the situation, to get as much information as he can from his patient. This is one of the reasons why I have a little hesitation, still, about computer systems. I would welcome very much the removal of paper work from my shoulders, but I am afraid with all those forms which, to my simple mind – in spite of Dr. Green's reassurances – are overwhelming, that I would spend my time looking at the forms and not at the patient; and that would be a loss.

CHAIRMAN: Any comments? Any questions? Dr. Green leaps to his feet!

G.D. GREEN *(Glasgow, Scotland):* I would like to comment on the exit block question. To me, exit block is perfectly explicit, as I have said in print and on many other occasions. I mean that pacing is not satisfactory, in spite of the fact that, from all your measurements, the pacemaker itself does not change, neither in its output, nor in its characteristics. That there is nothing wrong, technically, with the pacemaker itself, and that it has not moved in any way as far as one can judge from vector measurements, from X-ray measurements, ECG examination and so on. In other words, nothing has changed, except something at the interface between the electrodes and the patient and that is what we mean by exit block. We believe that it is due to the growth of tissue around the electrodes, which has therefore reduced the intensity of the current flowing through active muscle. That is exit block; perfectly explicit. I should hate to see "intermittent stimulation" used, because one can stimulate, in fact one often stimulates, but you do not get ventricular contractions. So, let us not talk about stimulation, let us not confuse those two issues.

CHAIRMAN: Thank you Dr. Green. There seems to be no comment from the panel here. I am just curious about Dr. Zoll's feeling that patients should be taking their pulse each day. I seem to spend my life trying to reassure patients to forget about the pacemaker, in the hope that they will not become pacer dependent in the emotional sense and every one of them is already extremely anxious, their families are extremely anxious. I am forever trying to reassure them that we will look after things through the clinic or through telephone monitoring. I wonder if other people tell patients to monitor their pulse. Most of the time it is pretty inaccurate and most of the time they are calling in some daughter-in-law or child to come and take their pulse for them. I respect your wisdom and years, Dr. Zoll, but I wonder if this really is the thing to do, in this follow-up era.

P.M. ZOLL *(Boston, U.S.A.):* We do not seem to have that problem, although we ask them to count the pulse once a day. After the first few months, many of them do not. But if we get a pulse count once a week, that is pretty good, too. Most patients seem to be reassured when they do indeed find the pulse at what I have explained to be an acceptable level.

CHAIRMAN: These are attitude differences that are rather important and I do not know if a person can ever be talked out of his attitudes. I more or less agree with you, Dr. Goldman, that it is the physician's responsibility to do the monitoring and I would let the patient rely on him. For that reason, I have always taken a stand against self-monitoring systems and against proprietary agencies doing the monitoring for me. But, there are lots of people who do not agree with that, as we have heard today.

Does anybody else wish to comment on this?

We have not heard yet from a few other people. Dr. Ector, would you like to comment about electrode problems?

H. Ector *(Leuven, Belgium):* Besides the specific problems of the pacemakers, you can also have some specific problems of late electrode malfunctions. We collected, in the last 60 months, twenty-seven cases of electrode malfunctions occurring one or more years after implantation.

A first important point is that, in our hospital, General Electric bipolar systems accounted for twenty cases of these twenty-seven cases of malfunction. Secondly, ten of these twenty F.E. failures are related to the demand function: eight cases of false inhibition and two cases with loss of R-wave detection. For this reason, we connect, whenever this is possible, a fixed-rate pacemaker to a G.E. lead. My feeling is that such bipolar leads are prone to some specific defects. These defects are probably due to corrosion, which preferably occurs in the anodal wire. If this is true, I would suggest as a conclusion and a point of discussion for the panel that, for long-term pacing, we have to prefer unipolar pacing systems.

Chairman: Does anyone else have experience with General Electric electrodes like that? I do not have more than a dozen, in my whole experience and they are mostly out. I do not know – and I hope I am not stepping on toes – if General Electric units are still in production in the United States. I think we cannot buy them anymore.

H. Ector *(Leuven, Belgium):* They have stopped production.

Chairman: Does anyone else have comments about the G.E. electrodes? How did you explain this phenomenon? What do you think happens?

H. Ector *(Leuven, Belgium):* Most cases of false inhibition are intermittent changes in the lead-patient circuit, in the same way as Dr. Barold explained it to us this morning: incomplete wire fracture.

Chairman: I would like to hear from some of the other people on the panel. Dr. Rodrigo, would you like to have a few words?

F.A. Rodrigo *(Leiden, The Netherlands):* Photo-analysis is mentioned this afternoon several times as a tool for determining pulse height, pulse width and pulse frequency. I want to draw your attention to the determination of pulse slope of the so-called voltage pulse generators; important for the knowledge of lead and electrode. For this determination some characteristics of the composition of the pulse must be known; viz.

a. the end of the pulse (pulse width more than 1.5 ms) has a logarithmic slope dependent on the capacity of the pulse generator and the ohmic resistance of the system.

b. the first part is not logarithmic and depends on polarization at the electrode.

c. the pulse, recorded via one of the Einthoven leads, is mostly rounded off (figure 4).

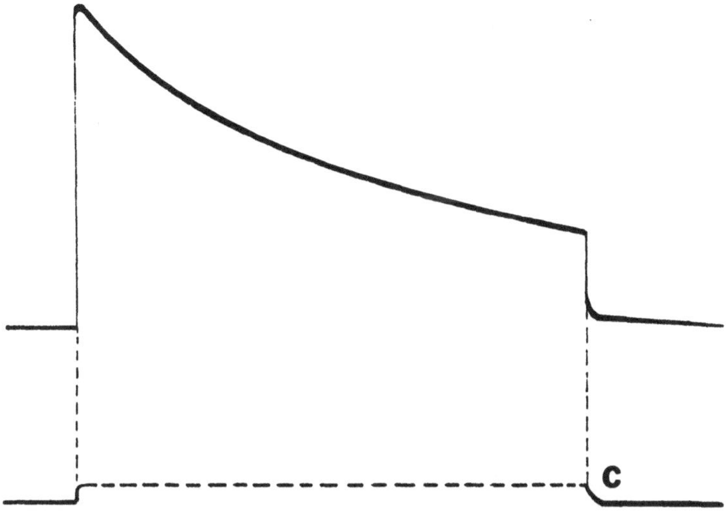

Figure 4. Upper curve: Reproduction of a pacemaker pulse, recorded via an Einthoven lead. Lower curve: Hypothetical base line shifting. C marks the beginning of the rounding at the trailing edge.

The phenomenon, mentioned under c, is a property of electrolyte solutions and depends on the distance between the pacemaker electrodes and their surface areas; the shorter the distance and the bigger the areas the bigger the roundings. This deformation may be looked upon as a base-line shifting, in figure 1 drawn under the pulse curve; the roundings are fully drawn and in between, as a first approximation, a straight line is dashed. To determine the slope of a pulse, one has to find first point C (the beginning of the roundings of the trailing edge) and then to draw the base line. An example, in which this correction only leads to the right conclusion, is shown in figure 5; two pulses of the same patient, the second one taken 6 months after the first one. Not until correction lines are drawn (the dashed lines in figure 5), a considerable difference in slope is clear, suggesting a big leakage. The shape of the pulse (the enormous rounding at the trailing edge) indicates a short distance between the electrodes. The conclusion from this photo-analysis was that there most probably should be an isolation leakage of the lead situated in the pocket near the pulse generator.

Actually the leakage is found in the pocket; the isolation was bursted open over a length of 2.5 cm.

CHAIRMAN: Thank you very much, Dr. Rodrigo for your interesting observations. I would like to call on Dr. Meibom who has a few comments to make about his explantation experience in 1976. I think it might be a fitting way to conclude this round table.

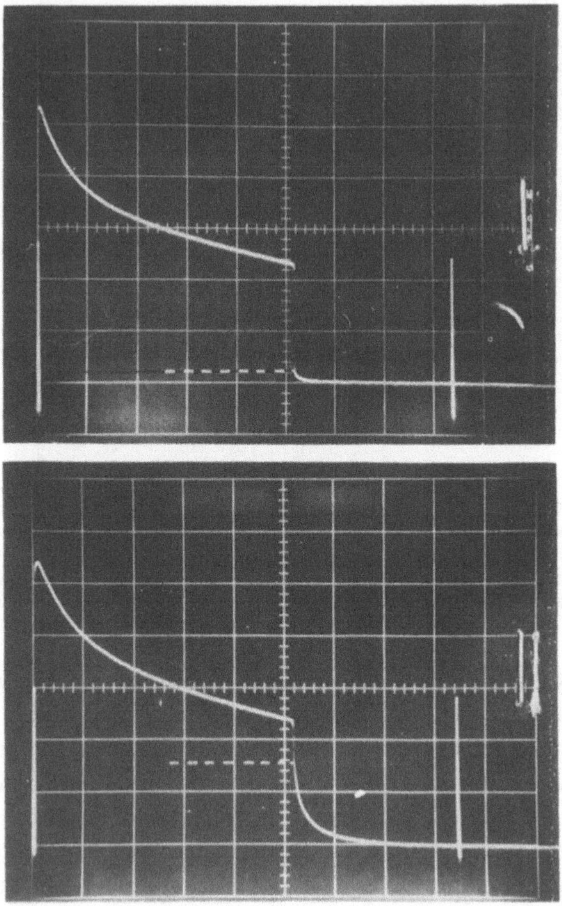

Figure 5. Pacemaker pulses of the same patient (Einthoven lead II), the lower picture is taken 6 months after the upper one. Correction for base line shifting is indicated (dashed lines) Calibration: Height 20 mV/div.; Time base 0.5 ms/div.

J. MEIBOM *(Copenhagen, Denmark):* Thank you, Mr. Chairman. At the outpatient clinic of the Rikshospital in Copenhagen, in 1976, we performed about 1500 examinations on about 350 patients with pacemaker systems of up to fourteen years of age. I will try to draw some additional conclusions which have not been mentioned at this meeting sofar.

I told you of 99 pacemakers which had to be explanted because of exhausted batteries. Out of these, 74 were explanted after an analysis in the outpatient clinic. The remaining 25 came by themselves or had been referred by the general practitioner.

It is remarkable that half of the pacemakers had a decrease in their rate which was greater than or equal to exhaustion of the cell as seen on slide 1. Follow-up showed that 18 out of 42 pacemakers, which were checked once a month, had a rate decrease of more than 10 b.p.m. and four had a rate decrease of more than 20 b.p.m.

The conclusions of pacemaker replacement because of exhausted batteries are:

1. the rate of the pacemakers, at the explantation time, was in about 50% of the cases disquietingly low.
2. 40% of the pacemakers checked every month had a rate decrease of more than ten per minute, within one month.

Altogether we had 41 other complications that needed surgical intervention. These are divided into complications found by the outpatient clinic, by the patient himself or by the general practitioner. The figures in brackets indicate the age of the system, in months. As shown here roughly, the outpatient clinic found equally as many complications as the patient himself or the general practitioner.

Some complications, we know, arise suddenly and give only very few possibilities of prediction, with the present technical means, like for example broken cable or displacement of endocardial electrodes. Other types of complications: threatening perforation, infection, exhausted batteries and insulation defects must and can be found before the pacemaker system has failed. We check our patients reasonably frequently in our opinion and, if the security has to be increased, the frequency of the checkups will rise further than the resources of the department will allow. If the security has to be better, we believe the solution lies in intensifying information of the patient and education of the general practitioner.

This data just mentioned may be discouraging from our patient-clinic point of view. But we must not forget that, until now, we have only dealt with technical problems. It is important to emphasize that the clinical evaluation of the pacemaker patient presumably is a most important point of the activity of the outpatient clinic. The survival of the patients is, primarily, dependent on their cardiac condition and it is essential to minimize the degree of congestive heart failure. A perfectly functioning and well-checked pacemaker system only fits a well-managed patient, not one disabled by heart insufficiency.

CHAIRMAN: I think we will conclude the panel with those remarks. I would like to thank the panel very much. Dr. Thalen has asked for the microphone for a few minutes.

H.J.TH. THALEN *(Groningen, The Netherlands)*: I usually do not ask for the microphone at the end of a session, but I have a special reason. All of us together here know that with us we have what you could call "the father of pacing," and that is Paul Zoll.

When we go back in history, it was in 1952 that, for the first time in the New England Journal of Medicine a publication appeared about pacing called: Resuscitation of the heart in ventricular standstill by external electric stimulation. It was written by Dr. P.M. Zoll.

We are now exactly 25 years later and in this panel still active and alert the same Dr. P.M. Zoll is giving us his wise advices. During this meeting – in a separate session – the contact persons for the World Symposia on Cardiac Pacing in Tokyo (1976) and Montreal (1979) have met and have signed the legal start of the International Society on Cardiac Pacing.

On behalf of all people involved in cardiac pacing and present at this meeting I would like to present some books to Dr. Paul Zoll to commemorate his 25 active years in cardiac pacing and to thank him for the fantastic work he started and that reached another milestone at this meeting with the establishment of the International Society on Cardiac Pacing.

OFFICIAL CLOSURE

IMPORTANCE OF COLLOQUIUM FOR THE CLINICIAN

J. Nieveen *(Groningen, The Netherlands)*

Ladies and Gentlemen, at the end of the Second European Pacemaker Colloquium, I have been asked to say a few words, as a clinician. As I already stated in my opening address at the First Colloquium, in Arnhem in '75, I think the scientific colloquium bringing together all kinds of people working on the subject of the colloquium is far more worthwhile than all those pounds of advertising material dumped every year in our mailboxes. In this pacemaker symposium, the new developments of the last few years are discussed in a short time, leaving the possibility to talk to many colleagues interested in the same field of cardiology.

The most salient things were stressed, and of importance for the clinician, are, to my feeling, the necessity to use more and more His Bundle Recordings in the diagnosis of unexplained fainting and the probability of using increasingly reliable atrial pacing equipment in the near future. Efforts to standardize pacemaking would be very worthwhile, and this as soon as possible, so that data from different centers could be more comparable than they are now. Further development of national data banks, automatization and telephone control of pacemaker patients are, in my opinion, desirable. It is a pity that our Dutch health authorities were not here during these days; if that had been the case, they could have heard that more personnel instead of less – as is their goal – is necessary to fulfill all the requirements I mentioned above.

Every time I am involved in a symposium like this Pacemaker Colloquium, I am increasingly convinced of the usefulness of these relatively small sessions. Most congresses are so large that one cannot see the woods for the numerous trees. Also, the number of papers and the literature are so augmented that it is difficult to read all of them in time. So I think – and I am convinced I speak for my fellow clinicians – that the initiative to organize this Second European Colloquium has been very important for us, clinicians and, as I believe, for the technicians who are here.

I would therefore like to thank the Vitatron people very much for organizing this symposium and hope this shall not be the last activity of theirs in this field. If they are planning another colloquium, it would, in my opinion, be better not to overload the program. As a clinician, I saw during these days many tired people.

Whether this was the result of the program and/or the activities of the evenings and late nights, I cannot say. Be it as it may, I do want to conclude by saying that this Colloquium was very succesful and would therefore like to thank all those who have organized it.

IMPORTANCE OF COLLOQUIUM FOR RESEARCH AND DEVELOPMENT

A.C.M. RENIRIE *(Dieren, The Netherlands)*

Ladies and Gentlemen. The ultimate success of this Colloquium will not be determined by the number of papers presented, or even by the number of persons attending the meetings, but it will be judged on the success in applying the knowledge acquired during these two days. The purpose was to bring together the many disciplines necessary to effectively serve the pacemaker field.

The benefit from such a colloquium, for our technical group, is to have the opportunity to exchange ideas with clinicians, technicians and other support groups who are sincerely interested in this exchange of ideas and advancing the art of pacing.

We feel the Colloquium has been an effective catalyst in initiating new ideas and concepts which may lead to the development of new and improved pacemaker devices. Two days is a very short time to exchange these ideas and therefore we are looking forward to a continuing dialogue with many of you, in the near future.

CLOSURE

J.N. HOMAN VAN DER HEIDE *(Groningen, The Netherlands)*

Ladies and Gentlemen, the official closure of the Second European Pacemaker Colloquium does not mean that we have reached an end, because the exchange of ideas and the results obtained today, inside this building, tomorrow, outside this room, will go on forever. The only thing we are really going to do is to withdraw and prepare for the opening of the next symposium. It is a great privilege for me to thank all speakers, the audience, the participants in the discussions and our hosts for their invaluable support in making this meeting a scientific and a social success. When I do not thank personally all those who have, with their work, made this symposium possible, it is not a sign of ingratitude, but a recognition of the fact that such a meeting cannot be organized by a few men and women. Through Mr. Wiersma, I compliment all the organizers of this meeting who have contributed to it.

The importance of the Second Colloquium for the clinic and for Research and Development has been explained to you by two experts. I have nothing to add to this. However, I have the exclusive privilege to explain what the participants of this Colloquium feel towards the management of Vitatron Medical, our host for the last two days. Gratitude alone does not express our feelings because it is mixed with admiration and respect for the magnificent achievements in pacemaker stimulation and technology by Vitatron Medical. Though every person engaged in health care has a certain brand loyalty, the fact remains that industry and the medical profession have separate responsibilities which may run parallel, but cannot be mixed.

We have, every time again, to choose the best possible pacemaker for our particular patients. This may or may not be a Vitatron. For this reason, we have highly appreciated the possibility afforded us by Vitatron to discuss freely our medical, surgical and technical problems with no strings attached. The management team of Vitatron is now due to recharge their batteries. As we are still here as the medical profession, we have, as a tribute to the whole team, made up a special prescription for two of the team, Mr. Blankestijn and Mr. Renirie. I have fetched up the bottles containing the secret tonic myself, because I was afraid somebody would steal the recipe. The engraved date on the collar makes it easy to get the exact refill when you want it. No harmful after-effects are known. The medicine is working when you get the feeling that everybody else can go to hell. At that moment, you are recharging. And when you have recharged, the bottle remains as a visible token of the respect and gratitude of the participants of this Colloquium. I now declare this Second Pacemaker Colloquium closed.

FAREWELL

A.J. BLANKESTIJN *(Dieren, The Netherlands)*

Ladies and Gentlemen. This is the end of this Colloquium. I hope you enjoyed it. From our side, we were impressed with the high attendance and high degree of interest on the part of the participants. As you all know, these two things do not have to go together. However, I have to say that the tiring programs of yesterday and today left a few victims along the wayside. I think the interest is the biggest compliment the contributors could get from the side of the participants. For us, it was nice to see at one session so many different people from different battery companies who all supply excellent power sources with either competitive or different interesting characteristics. Finally, the pacemaker industry can choose the power supply for their pacemaker out of alternative, competitive sources, just as you are able to do with the pacemakers you buy. Competition is the best way to progress. Therefore, I would especially thank Dr. Schneider, the inventor of the lithium-iodine battery, Dr. Greatbatch who recognized the importance of this power source for pacemaker application and brought this source to where it is today and Mr. Lehmann for their contribution. I would like to thank the speakers for their excellent contributions and the time and effort that they spent to make this Colloquium successful. I would also like to thank all those who made this symposium run smoothly. I can tell you from my experience that it is not easy; it is a lot of work. But I think they did it with pleasure.

I would like to give special thanks to Dr. Thalen, who organized the scientific program, and to Professor Homan van der Heide for the vital and wise way he oversaw the organization of this Colloquium.

Thank you all. Have a good trip home and we hope to meet you again at one of our next colloquiums.

INDEX